Introductory Food Toxicology

THE AUTHOR

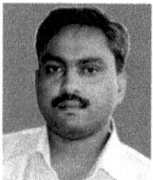

Dr. Lokesh Kumar Mishra obtained his Post-Graduate and Doctorate degree in Biochemistry from Narendra Deva University of Agriculture and Technology, Faizabad, Uttar Pradesh. The dissertation work of the author focused on the impact of fertilizers on the nutritional components of the cereal crops mainly wheat. He started his academic career as Assistant Professor in Biochemistry at ND University, Faizabad. He later on served as Assistant Professor at VBS Purvanchal University Jaunpur, UP. Presently he is working as Assistant Professor (Biochemistry) at Central Agricultural University, Imphal, Manipur. He is involved in teaching Biochemistry for the last eight years and allied disciplines like Food Toxicology, Food Analysis, Human Physiology and Clinical Nutrition for the last four years. The author is also handling Research projects funded by different agencies of the Government of India. He has authored several research papers and review articles in International and National Journals of repute and is associated with many national and international Societies in the field of Plant Biochemistry. Dr. Mishra has recently been selected for The DBT Overseas Visiting Associateship to work in the North Dakota State University, Fargo, United States.

Introductory Food Toxicology

Lokesh Kumar Mishra

2016

Daya Publishing House®

A Division of

Astral International Pvt. Ltd.

New Delhi-110002

Cataloging in Publication Data--DK

Courtesy: D.K. Agencies (P) Ltd. <docinfo@dkagencies.com>

Mishra, Lokesh Kumar, author.

Introductory food toxicology / Lokesh Kumar Mishra.

pages cm

Includes bibliographical references.

ISBN 978-93-5130-887-4 (International Edition)

1. Food--Toxicology. I. Title.

RA1258.M57 2015   DDC 615.954   23

Published by	:	**Daya Publishing House®**
		A Division of
		Astral International Pvt. Ltd.
		– ISO 9001:2008 Certified Company –
		4760-61/23, Ansari Road, Darya Ganj
		New Delhi-110 002
		Ph. 011-43549197, 23278134
		E-mail: info@astralint.com
		Website: www.astralint.com
Laser Typesetting	:	**SSMG Computer Graphics,** Delhi - 110 084
Printed at	:	**Replika Press Pvt Ltd**

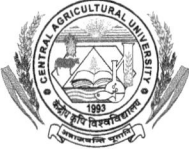

CENTRAL AGRICULTURAL UNIVERSITY

IROISEMBA, IMPHAL-795004, MANIPUR (INDIA)

Dr. S.N. Puri, FNAAS

Vice-Chancellor

Tel: (0385) 2415933(O)

2410450(R)

Gram: AGRIVARSITY

Fax : 2410450

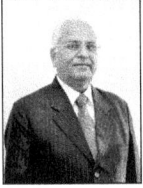

Foreword

Food has a pre-eminent position in the daily life of humankind and regarded as the most important need for human beings. In addition to provide primary energy and nutrient source, food has a great impact on our emotional and spiritual life. The quest for ensuring the availability of food to the exponentially growing world population has led to the development of diverse technologies, which not only focus on the extension of the shelf life of food, but also have the ability to develop novel foods. The benefits of these technologies have come to the mankind with associated risks. These technologies have inadvertently made food more susceptible to contamination with non nutrient components which may be toxic to consumers. The study of these hazardous elements in food has made the discipline of "Food Toxicology" a very important field. The need for research and sharing of information in this field has become even more important due to the increasing exposure of human life to pollutants and chemicals in almost every walk of life. Considering these facts "Food Toxicology" has been introduced in the undergraduate and post graduate curricula of the agricultural and general universities.

I congratulate Dr. Lokesh Kumar Mishra for preparing this comprehensive and informative compilation. The compilation is a dedicated effort to present the different aspects of the "Food Toxicology" in a very concise and relevant manner. I believe that the students and scientists working in the area of food sciences, nutrition and food biochemistry will find this book as a source of useful and authentic information.

I appreciate the efforts of Dr. Mishra in compiling this important document.

(Dr .S.N.Puri)

Preface

"Vasudhaiv Kutumbakam" is the underlying principle of Indian philosophy which stresses on the need for the world to work together for the common goal of peace prosperity and well being of human kind. The phenomena which closely seems to follow this principle at least in letter is the process of "Globalization". This is the prominent trend in every sphere of life. The Food industry which used to be local has now gone global and involves mega processing industries to meet the demand of the citizens of the "Global Village". Several efforts (GMP, HACCP, TFQM) are taken to ensure the production and distribution of hygienic and high standard food/food products. Despite the sincere efforts food gets contaminated when it reaches the consumer. This contamination many times is unintentional but one cannot rule out the role of deliberate acts of contamination in food. The science of Food Toxicology deals with the study of this contamination and also elaborates upon the numerous nutrients and non nutrients in food which may play an important role in determining the health of the consumers.

This book is an effort to give simple, concise and updated information about the aspects relevant to food toxicology. The book consists of 15 chapters. The Chapter 1-3 deal with the basic understanding of the science of toxicology, different sub-disciplines of toxicology and the different categories of toxic agents found in food. Chapter 4 deals with the current challenges confronting the food toxicologists and the solutions which have evolved by the application of emerging fields of genomics and information technology in food toxicology. Chapters 5-7 have been dedicated to update the information regarding the core topics of food allergy, compounds mimicking human hormones found in food and common toxicants in food. The field of Genetic Engineering and its impact on the food quality has been covered in Chapter 8 with effort to incorporate the latest developments in the field. Microbial damage to food can be directly attributed as the major cause of greatest threat in terms of mortality and morbidity in the world. Microbes due to their dramatic ability to evolve have managed to survive even the best and most hygienic manufacturing processes. They continue to remain the most potent threat to ensuring safe food to majority of population world over. Chapter 9 describes the important microbial toxins and gives an update of the developments in this important aspect. Food is more than a nutrient. In addition to providing energy and nursing our body certain components of food have been known to improve health and in many cases fight the most complex diseases known to mankind. Chapter 10 enumerates these fantastic components of food also called as chemopreventives in detail considering their importance and the immense focus they have received recently globally. Chapters 11-14 deals with the toxic components present in food due to environmental contamination, steps during food processing, and failure to follow SOP during manufacturing of food. Chapter 15 deals exclusively with the marine toxins that occur in food.

I hope the book serves a good source of information to food scientists and students studying food technology, biotechnology, biochemistry, food and nutrition and scholars interested in food safety.

I extend sincere appreciation to Dr. B B Singh and Mr. Surya Mittal for their continued help in preparation of this manuscript and encouraging me to take up this task. I gratefully acknowledge the guidance and motivation provided by Dr. K Sheela (Dean, College of Home Science, Central Agricultural University) in this task.

Words fail to describe the relentless support and encouragement provided by my wife Seema daughter Aishanee and son Ashwani during the arduous task of focusing to compile this book in spite of the tough challenges confronting us as a family.

I accept full responsibility for the unintentional errors, shortcomings in interpretation of facts and any omissions. I hope these are minimal and welcome the suggestions for improvement.

Lokesh Kumar Mishra

Contents

1

Toxicology: An Introduction

Toxicology is a branch of biology, chemistry, and medicine concerned with the study of the adverse effects of chemicals on living organisms. It is the study of symptoms, mechanisms, treatments and detection of poisoning, especially the poisoning of people. Dioscorides, a Greek physician in the court of the Roman emperor Nero, made the first attempt to classify plants according to their toxic and therapeutic effect. Ibn Wahshiya wrote the Book on Poisons in the 9th or 10th century.

Mathieu Orfila is considered to be the Modern Father of toxicology, having given the subject its first formal treatment in 1813 in his Traité des poisons, also called Toxicologie générale.

In 1850, Jean Stas gave the evidence that the Belgian Count Hippolyte Visart de Bocarmé killed his brother-in-law by poisoning him with nicotine.

Theophrastus Phillipus Auroleus Bombastus von Hohenheim (1493–1541) (also referred to as Paracelsus, from his belief that his studies were above or beyond the work of Celsus - a Roman physician from the first century) is also considered "the father" of toxicology. He is credited with the classic toxicology maxim, "Alle Dinge sind Gift und nichts ist ohne Gift; allein die Dosis macht, dass ein Ding kein Gift ist." which translates as, "All things are poison and nothing is without poison; only the dose makes a thing not a poison." This is often condensed to: "The dose makes the poison" or in Latin "Sola dosis facit venenum".

The relationship between dose and its effects on the exposed organism is of high significance in toxicology. The chief criterion regarding the toxicity of a chemical is the dose, i.e. the amount of exposure to the substance. All substances are toxic under the right conditions. The term LD refers to the dose of a toxic substance that kills 50 percent of a test population (typically rats or other surrogates when the test concerns human toxicity).

The conventional relationship (more exposure equals higher risk) has been challenged in the study of endocrine disruptors. Toxicity is species-specific, lending cross-species analysis problematic. Newer methods are available to bypass animal-testing.

What is Toxicology?

Toxicology is the study of how natural or man-made poisons cause undesirable effects in living organisms.

Harmful or adverse effects: Harmful or adverse effects are those that are damaging to either the survival or normal function of the individual.

Toxicity: The word "toxicity" describes the degree to which a substance is poisonous or can cause injury. The toxicity depends on a variety of factors: dose, duration and route of exposure, shape and structure of the chemical itself, and individual human factors.

Toxic: This term relates to poisonous or deadly effects on the body by inhalation (breathing), ingestion (eating), or absorption, or by direct contact with a chemical.

Toxicant: A toxicant is any chemical that can injure or kill humans, animals, or plants. The term "toxicant" is used when talking about toxic substances that are produced by or are a by-product of human-made activities. For example, dioxin (2,3-7,8-tetrachlorodibenzop-dioxin {TCDD}), produced as a by-product of certain chlorinated chemicals, is a toxicant. On the other hand, arsenic, a toxic metal, may occur as a natural contaminant of groundwater or may contaminate groundwater as a by-product of industrial activities. If the second case is true, such toxic substances are referred to as toxicants, rather than toxins.

Toxin: The term "toxin" usually is used when talking about toxic substances produced naturally. A toxin is any poisonous substance of microbial (bacteria or other tiny plants or animals), vegetable, or synthetic chemical origin that reacts with specific cellular components to kill cells, alter growth or development, or kill the organism.

Toxic Symptom: This term includes any feeling or sign indicating the presence of a poison in the system.

Toxic Effects: This term refers to the health effects that occur due to exposure to a toxic substance; also known as a poisonous effect on the body.

Selective Toxicity: "Selective toxicity" means that a chemical will produce injury to one kind of living matter without harming another form of life, even though the two may exist close together.

How Does Toxicity Develop? Before toxicity can develop, a substance must come into contact with a body surface such as skin, eye or mucosa of the digestive or respiratory tract. The dose of the chemical, or the amount that comes into contact with, is important when discussing how "toxic" an substance can be.

What is a dose? The dose is the actual amount of a chemical that enters the body. The dose received may be due to either acute (short) or chronic (long-term) exposure. An acute exposure occurs over a very short period of time, usually 24 hours. Chronic exposures occur over long periods of time such as weeks, months, or years. The amount of exposure and the type of toxin will determine the toxic effect.

Dose-response: Dose-response is a relationship between exposure and health effect, that can be established by measuring the response relative to an increasing dose. This relationship is important in determining the toxicity of a particular substance. It relies on the concept that a dose, or a time of exposure (to a chemical, drug, or toxic substance), will cause an effect (response) on the exposed organism. Usually, the larger or more intense the dose, the greater the response, or the effect. This is the meaning behind the statement "the dose makes the poison."

Threshold dose: Given the idea of a dose-response, there should be a dose or exposure level below which the harmful or adverse effects of a substance are not seen in a population. That dose is referred to as the 'threshold dose'. This dose is also referred to as the no observed adverse effect level (NOAEL), or the no effect level (NEL). These terms are often used by toxicologists when discussing the relationship between exposure and dose. However, for substances causing cancer (carcinogens), no safe level of exposure exists, since any exposure could result in cancer.

Individual susceptibility: This term describes the differences in types of responses to hazardous substances, between people. Each person is unique, and because of that, there may be great differences in the response to exposure. Exposure in one person may have no effect, while a second person may become seriously ill, and a third may develop cancer.

Sensitive sub-population: A sensitive sub-population describes those persons who are more at risk from illness due to exposure to hazardous substances than the average, healthy person. These persons usually include the very young, the chronically ill, and the very old. It may also include pregnant women and women of childbearing age. Depending on the type of contaminant, other factors (e.g., age, weight, lifestyle, sex) could be used to describe the population.

The Field of Toxicology

Toxicology addresses a variety of questions. For example, in agriculture, toxicology determines the possible health effects from exposure to pesticides or herbicides, or the effect of animal feed additives, such as growth factors, on people. Toxicology is also used in laboratory experiments on animals to establish dose-response relationships. Toxicology also deals with the way chemicals and waste products affect the health of an individual.

Sub-disciplines of Toxicology

The field of toxicology can be further divided into the following sub-disciplines or subspecialities:

\#	**Environmental Toxicology** is concerned with the study of chemicals that contaminate food, water, soil, or the atmosphere. It also deals with toxic substances that enter bodies of waters such as lakes, streams, rivers, and oceans. This sub-discipline addresses the question of how various plants, animals, and humans are affected by exposure to toxic substances.

Occupational (Industrial) Toxicology is concerned with health effects from exposure to chemicals in the workplace. This field grew out of a need to protect workers from toxic substances and to make their work environment safe. Occupational diseases caused by industrial chemicals account for an estimated 50,000 to 70,000 deaths, and 350,000 new cases of illness each year in the United States.

Regulatory Toxicology gathers and evaluates existing toxicological information to establish concentration-based standards of "safe" exposure. The standard is the level of a chemical that a person can be exposed to without any harmful health effects.

Food Toxicology is involved in delivering a safe and edible supply of food to the consumer. During processing, a number of substances may be added to food to make it look, taste, or smell better. Fats, oils, sugars, starches and other substances may be added to change the texture and taste of food. All of these additives are studied to determine if and at what amount, they may produce adverse effects. A second area of interest includes food allergies. Almost 30% of the American people have some food allergy. For example, many people have trouble digesting milk, and are lactose intolerant. In addition, toxic substances such as pesticides may be applied to a food crop in the field, while lead, arsenic, and cadmium are naturally present in soil and water, and may be absorbed by plants. Toxicologists must determine the acceptable daily intake level for those substances.

Clinical Toxicology is concerned with diseases and illnesses associated with short term or long term exposure to toxic chemicals. Clinical toxicologists include emergency room physicians who must be familiar with the symptoms associated with exposure to a wide variety of toxic substances in order to administer the appropriate treatment.

Descriptive Toxicology is concerned with gathering toxicological information from animal experimentation. These types of experiments are used to establish how much of a chemical would cause illness or death. The United States Environmental Protection Agency (EPA), the Occupational Safety and Health Administration (OSHA), and the Food and Drug Administration (FDA), use information from these studies to set regulatory exposure limits.

Forensic Toxicology is used to help establish cause and effect relationships between exposure to a drug or chemical and the toxic or lethal effects that result from that exposure.

Analytical Toxicology identifies the toxicant through analysis of body fluids, stomach content, excrement, or skin.

\#   **Mechanistic Toxicology** makes observations on how toxic substances cause their effects. The effects of exposure can depend on a number of factors, including the size of the molecule, the specific tissue type or cellular components affected, whether the substance is easily dissolved in water or fatty tissues, all of which are important when trying to determine the way a toxic substance causes harm, and whether effects seen in animals can be expected in humans.

2

Principles of Toxicology

While food is an essential source of energy, nutrients, building materials, and even pleasure, it also contains compounds that can potentially evoke greater or lesser health disorders. Toxins can originate from the raw materials or invade during processing, transportation, and storage. They can be intentionally added in the form of "harmless" food preservatives or health-promoting functional ingredients that can become toxic in combination or under environmental stressors. The continuous physical and biochemical processes that food undergoes indicate that there is always the chance for toxicity in even the most innocuous foods.

The intent of this chapter is to provide a concise description of the basic principles of toxicology and to illustrate how these principles are used to make reasonable judgments about the potential health hazards and the risks associated with chemical exposures.

Definitions and Terminology

The literal meaning of the term toxicology is "the study of poisons." The root word toxic entered the English language around 1655 from the Late Latin word toxicus (which meant poisonous), itself derived from toxikón, an ancient Greek term for poisons into which arrows were dipped. The early history of toxicology focused on the understanding and uses of different poisons, and even today most people tend to think of poisons as a deadly potion that when ingested causes almost immediate harm or death. As toxicology has evolved into a modern science, it has expanded to encompass all forms of adverse health effects that substances might produce, not just acutely harmful or lethal effects.

The following definitions reflect this expanded scope of the science of toxicology:

Toxic—having the characteristic of producing an undesirable or adverse health effect.

Toxicity—any toxic (adverse) effect that a chemical or physical agent might produce within a living organism.

Toxicology—the science that deals with the study of the adverse effects (toxicities) chemicals or physical agents may produce in living organisms under specific conditions of exposure. It is a science that attempts to qualitatively identify all the hazards (i.e., organ toxicities) associated with a substance, as well as to quantitatively determine the exposure conditions under which those hazards/toxicities are induced. Toxicology is the science that experimentally investigates the occurrence, nature, incidence, mechanism, and risk factors for the adverse effects of toxic substances.

As these definitions indicate, the toxic responses that form the study of toxicology span a broad biologic and physiologic spectrum. Effects of interest may range from something relatively minor such as irritation or tearing, to a more serious response like acute and reversible liver or kidney damage, to an even more serious and permanent disability such as cirrhosis of the liver or liver cancer. Given this broad range of potentially adverse effects to consider, it is perhaps useful for those unfamiliar with toxicology to define some additional terms:

Exposure—to cause an adverse effect, a toxicant must first come in contact with an organism. The means by which an organism comes in contact with the substance is the route of exposure (e.g., in the air, water, soil, food, medication) for that chemical.

Dose—the total amount of a toxicant administered to an organism at specific time intervals. The quantity can be further defined in terms of quantity per unit body weight or per body surface area.

Internal/absorbed dose—the actual quantity of a toxicant that is absorbed into the organism and distributed systemically throughout the body.

Delivered/effective/target organ dose—the amount of toxicant reaching the organ (known as the target organ) that is adversely affected by the toxicant.

Acute exposure—exposure over a brief period of time (generally less than 24 h). Often it is considered to be a single exposure (or dose) but may consist of repeated exposures within a short time period.

Subacute exposure—resembles acute exposure except that the exposure duration is greater, from several days to one month.

Subchronic exposure—exposures repeated or spread over an intermediate time range. For animal testing, this time range is generally considered to be 1–3 months.

Chronic exposure—exposures (either repeated or continuous) over a long (greater than 3 months) period of time. With animal testing this exposure often continues for the majority of the experimental animal's life, and within occupational settings it is generally considered to be for a number of years.

Acute toxicity—an adverse or undesirable effect that is manifested within a relatively short time interval ranging from almost immediately to within several days following exposure (or dosing). An example would be chemical asphyxiation from exposure to a high concentration of carbon monoxide (CO).

Chronic toxicity—a permanent or lasting adverse effect that is manifested after exposure to a toxicant. An example would be the development of silicosis following a long-term exposure to silica in workplaces such as foundries.

Local toxicity—an adverse or undesirable effect that is manifested at the toxicant's site of contact with the organism. Examples include an acid's ability to cause burning of the eyes, upper respiratory tract irritation, and skin burns.

Systemic toxicity—an adverse or undesirable effect that can be seen throughout the organism or in an organ with selective vulnerability distant from the point of entry of the toxicant (i.e., toxicant requires absorption and distribution within the organism to produce the toxic effect). Examples would be adverse effects on the kidney or central nervous system resulting from the chronic ingestion of mercury.

Reversible toxicity—an adverse or undesirable effect that can be reversed once exposure is stopped. Reversibility of toxicity depends on a number of factors, including the extent of exposure (time and amount of toxicant) and the ability of the affected tissue to repair or regenerate. An example includes hepatic toxicity from acute acetaminophen exposure and liver degeneration.

Delayed or latent toxicity—an adverse or undesirable effect appearing long after the initiation and/or cessation of exposure to the toxicant. An example is cervical cancer during adulthood resulting from in utero exposure to diethylstilbestrol (DES).

Allergic reaction—a reaction to a toxicant caused by an altered state of the normal immune response. The outcome of the exposure can be immediate (anaphylaxis) or delayed (cell-mediated).

Idiosyncratic reaction—a response to a toxicant occurring at exposure levels much lower than those generally required to cause the same effect in most individuals within the population. This response is genetically determined, and a good example would be sensitivity to nitrates due to deficiency of NADH (reduced-form nicotinamide adenine dinucleotide phosphate)–methemoglobin reductase.

Mechanism of toxicity—the necessary biologic interactions by which a toxicant exerts its toxic effect on an organism. An example is carbon monoxide (CO) asphyxiation due to the binding of CO to hemoglobin, thus preventing the transport of oxygen within the blood.

Toxicant—any substance that causes a harmful (or adverse) effect when in contact with a living organism at a sufficiently high concentration.

Toxin—any toxicant produced by an organism (floral or faunal, including bacteria); that is, naturally produced toxicants. An example would be the pyrethrins, which are natural pesticides produced by pyrethrum flowers (i.e., certain chrysanthemums) that serve as the model for the man made insecticide class pyrethroids.

Hazard—the qualitative nature of the adverse or undesirable effect (i.e., the type of adverse effect) resulting from exposure to a particular toxicant or physical agent. For example, asphyxiation is the hazard from acute exposures to carbon monoxide (CO).

Safety—the measure or mathematical probability that a specific exposure situation or dose will not produce a toxic effect.

Risk—the measure or probability that a specific exposure situation or dose will produce a toxic effect.

Risk assessment—the process by which the potential (or probability of) adverse health effects of exposure are characterized.

What Toxicologists Study

Toxicology has become a science that builds on and uses knowledge developed in other related disciplines of medical sciences, such as physiology, biochemistry, pathology, pharmacology, medicine, and epidemiology, to name only a few. Given its broad and diverse nature, toxicology is also a science where a number of areas of specialization have evolved as a result of the different applications of toxicological information that exist within society today. It might be argued, however, that the professional activities of all toxicologists fall into three main areas of endeavor: descriptive toxicology, research/mechanistic toxicology, and applied toxicology.

Descriptive toxicologists are scientists whose work focuses on the toxicity testing of chemicals. This work is done primarily at commercial and governmental toxicity testing laboratories, and the studies performed at these facilities are designed to generate basic toxicity information that can be used to identify the various organ toxicities (hazards) that the test agent is capable of inducing under a wide range of exposure conditions. A thorough "descriptive toxicological" analysis would identify all possible acute and chronic toxicities, including the genotoxic, reproductive, teratogenic (developmental), and carcinogenic potential of the test agent. It would also identify important metabolites of the chemical that are generated as the body attempts to break down and eliminate the chemical, as well as analyze the manner in which the chemical is absorbed into the body, distributed throughout the body and accumulated by various tissues and organs, and then ultimately excreted from the body. Hopefully appropriate dose–response test data are generated for those toxicities of greatest concern during the completion of the descriptive studies so that the relative safety of any given exposure or dose level that humans might typically encounter can be determined.

Basic research or mechanistic toxicologists are scientists who study the chemical or agent in depth for the purpose of gaining an understanding of how the chemical or agent initiates those biochemical or physiological changes within the cell or tissue that result in the toxicity (adverse effect). They identify the critical biological processes within the organism that must be affected by the chemical to produce the toxic properties that are ultimately observed. Or, to state it another way, the goal of mechanistic studies is to understand the specific biological reactions (i.e., the adverse chain of events) within the affected organism that ultimately result in the toxicity under investigation. These experiments may be performed at the molecular, biochemical, cellular, or tissue level of the affected organism, and thus incorporate and apply the knowledge of a number of many other related scientific disciplines within the biological and medical sciences (e.g., physiology, biochemistry, genetics, molecular biology). Mechanistic studies ultimately are the bridge of knowledge that connects functional observations made during descriptive toxicological studies to the extrapolations of dose–response information that is used as the basis of risk assessment and exposure guideline development (e.g., occupational health guidelines or governmental regulations) by applied toxicologists.

Applied toxicologists are scientists concerned with the use of chemicals in a "real world" or nonlaboratory setting. For example, one goal of applied toxicologists is to control the use of the chemical in a manner that limits the probable human exposure level to one in which the dose any individual might receive is a safe one. Toxicologists who work in this area of toxicology, whether they work for a state or federal agency, a company, or as consultants, use descriptive and mechanistic toxicity studies to develop some identifiable measure of the safe dose of the chemical. The process whereby this safe dose or level of exposure is derived is generally referred to as the area of risk assessment.

Within applied toxicology a number of subspecialties occur. These are: forensic toxicology, clinical toxicology, environmental toxicology, and occupational toxicology. Forensic toxicology is that unique combination of analytical chemistry, pharmacology, and toxicology concerned with the medical and legal aspects of drugs and poisons; it is concerned with the determination of which chemicals are present and responsible in exposure situations of abuse, overdose, poisoning, and death that become of interest to the police, medical examiners, and coroners. Clinical toxicology specializes in ways to treat poisoned individuals and focuses on determining and understanding the toxic effects of medicines and simple over-the-counter (nonprescription) drugs. Environmental toxicology is the subdiscipline concerned with those chemical exposure situations found in our general living environment. These exposures may stem from the agricultural application of chemicals (e.g., pesticides, growth regulators, fertilizers), the release of chemicals during modern-day living (e.g., chemicals released by household products), regulated and unintentional industrial discharges into air or waterways (e.g., spills, stack emissions, NPDES discharges, etc.), and various nonpoint emission sources (e.g., the combustion byproducts of cars). This specialty largely focuses on those chemical exposures referred to as environmental contamination or pollution. Within this area there may be even further subspecialization (e.g., ecotoxicology, aquatic toxicology, mammalian toxicology, avian toxicology). Occupational toxicology is the subdiscipline concerned with the chemical exposures and diseases found in the workplace.

Regardless of the specialization within toxicology, or the types of toxicities of major interest to the toxicologist, essentially every toxicologist performs one or both of the two basic functions of toxicology, which are to (1) examine the nature of the adverse effects produced by a chemical or physical agent (hazard identification function) and (2) assess the probability of these toxicities occurring under specific conditions of exposure (risk assessment function). Ultimately, the goal and basic purpose of toxicology is to understand the toxic properties of a chemical so that these adverse effects can be prevented by the development of appropriate handling or exposure guidelines.

The Importance of Dose and Dose-Response Relationship

It is probably safe to say that among lay individuals there exists considerable confusion between the terms poisonous and toxic. If asked, most lay individuals would probably define a toxic substance using the same definition that one would apply to highly poisonous chemicals, that is, chemicals capable of producing a serious injury or death quickly and at very low doses. However, this is not a particularly useful definition because all chemicals may induce some type of adverse effect at some dose, so all chemicals may be described as toxic. As we have defined toxicants (toxic chemicals) as agents capable of producing an adverse effect in a biological system, a reasonable question for one to ask becomes "Which group of chemicals do we consider to be toxic?" or "Which chemicals do we consider safe?" The short answer to both questions, of course, is all chemicals; for even relatively safe chemicals can become toxic if the dose is high enough, and even potent, highly toxic chemicals may be used safely if exposure is kept low enough. As toxicology evolved from the study of just those substances or practices that were poisonous, dangerous, or unsafe, and instead became a more general study of the adverse effects of all chemicals, the conditions under which chemicals express toxicity became as important as, if not more important than, the kind of adverse effect produced. The importance of understanding the dose at which a chemical becomes toxic (harmful) was recognized centuries ago by Paracelsus (1493–1541), who essentially stated this concept as "All substances are poisons; there is none which is not a poison. The right dose differentiates a poison and a remedy." In a sense this statement serves to emphasize the second function of toxicology, or risk assessment, as it indicates that concern for a substance's toxicity is a function of one's exposure to it. Thus, the evaluation of those circumstances and conditions under which an adverse effect can be produced is key to considering whether the exposure is safe or hazardous. All chemicals are toxic at some dose and may produce harm if the exposure is sufficient, but all chemicals produce their harm (toxicities) under prescribed conditions of dose or usage. Consequently, another way of viewing all chemicals is that provided by Emil Mrak, who said "There are no harmless substances, only harmless ways of using substances."

These two statements serve to remind us that describing a chemical exposure as being either harmless or hazardous is a function of the magnitude of the exposure (dose), not the types of toxicities that a chemical might be capable of producing at some dose. For example, vitamins, which we consciously take to improve our health and well-being, continue to rank as a major cause of accidental poisoning among children, and essentially all the types of toxicities that we associate with the term "hazardous chemicals" may be produced by many of the prescription medicines in use today.

Defining Dose and Response

Because all chemicals are toxic at some dose, what judgments determine their use? To answer this, one must first understand the use of the dose–response relationship because this provides the basis for estimating the safe exposure level for a chemical. A dose–response relationship is said to exist when changes in dose produce consistent, nonrandom changes in effect, either in the magnitude of effect or in the percent of individuals responding at a particular level of effect. For example, the number of animals dying increases as the dose of strychnine is increased, or with therapeutic agents the number of patients recovering from an infection increases as the dosage is increased. In other instances, the severity of the response seen in each animal increases with an increase in dose once the threshold for toxicity has been exceeded.

Components of Tests Generating Dose

The design of any toxicity test essentially incorporates the following five basic components:

1. The selection of a test organism

2. The selection of a response to measure (and the method for measuring that response)

3. An exposure period

4. The test duration (observation period)

5. A series of doses to test

Possible test organisms range from isolated cellular material or selected strains of bacteria through higher-order plants and animals. The response or biological endpoint can range from subtle changes in organism physiology or behavior to death of the organism, and exposure periods may vary from a few hours to several years. Clearly, tests are sought (1) for which the response is not subjective and can be consistently determined, (2) that are conclusive even when the exposure period is relatively short, and (3) (for predicting effects in humans) for which the test species responds in a manner that mimics or relates to the likely human response. However, some tests are selected because they yield indirect measurements or special kinds of responses that are useful because they correlate well with another response of interest; for example, the determination of mutagenic potential is often used as one measure of a chemical's carcinogenic potential.

Fortunately or unfortunately, each of the five basic components of a toxicity test protocol may contribute to the uniqueness of the dose–response curve that is generated. In other words, as one changes the species, dose, toxicity of interest, dosage rate, or duration of exposure, the dose-response relationship may change significantly. So, the less comparable the animal test conditions are to the exposure situation you wish to extrapolate to, the greater the potential uncertainty that will exist in the extrapolation you are attempting to make. For example, the organ toxicity observed in the mouse and the severity of that toxic response change with the air concentration of chloroform to which the animals are exposed. Both of these characteristics of the response—organ type and severity—also change as one changes the species being tested from the mouse to the rat.

In the mouse the liver is apparently the most sensitive organ to chloroform-induced systemic toxicity; therefore, selecting an air concentration of 3 ppm to prevent liver toxicity would also eliminate the possibility of kidney or respiratory toxicity. If the concentration of chloroform being tested is increased to 100 ppm, severe liver injury is observed, but still no injury occurs in the kidneys or respiratory tract of the mouse. If test data existed only for the renal and respiratory systems, an exposure level of 100 ppm might be selected as a no-effect level with the assumption that an exposure limit at this concentration would provide complete safety for the mouse. In this case the assumption would be incorrect, and this allowable exposure level would produce an adverse exposure condition for the mouse in the form of severe liver injury.

Note also that a safe exposure level for kidney toxicity in the mouse, 100 ppm, would not prevent kidney injury in a closely related species like the rat. This illustrates the problem in assuming that two similar rodent species like the mouse and rat have very similar dose–response curves and the same relative organ sensitivities to chloroform. For example, an investigator assuming both species have the same dose–response relationships might, after identifying liver toxicity as the most sensitive target organ in the mouse, use only clinical tests for liver toxicity as the biomarker for safe concentrations in the rat. Following this logic, the investigator might erroneously conclude that chloroform concentrations of 100 ppm were completely protective for this species (because no liver toxicity was apparent), although this level would be capable of producing nasal and kidney injury.

This simple illustration emphasizes two points. First, it emphasizes the fact that dose–response relationships are sensitive to, and dependent on, the conditions under which the toxicity test was performed. Second, given the variety of the test conditions that might be tested or considered and the variety of dose–response curves that might ultimately be generated with each new test system, the uncertainty inherent in any extrapolation of animal data for the purpose of setting safe exposure limits for humans is clearly dependent on the wideness of toxicity studies performed and the number of different species tested in those studies. This underscores the need for a toxicologist, when attempting to apply animal data for risk assessment purposes, to seek test data where the response is not subjective, has been consistently determined, and has been measured in a species that is known to, or can reasonably be expected to, respond qualitatively and quantitatively the way humans do.

Because the dose–response relationship may vary depending on the components of the test, it is, of course, best to rely on human data that have been generated for the same exposure conditions of interest. Unfortunately, such data are rarely available. The human data that are most typically available are generated from human populations in some occupational or clinical setting in which the exposure was believed at least initially, to be safe. The exceptions, of course, are those infrequent, unintended poisonings or environmental releases.

This means that the toxicologist usually must attempt to extrapolate data from as many as four or five different categories of toxicity testing (dose–response) information for the safety evaluation of a particular chemical. These categories are: occupational epidemiology (mortality and morbidity) studies, clinical exposure studies, accidental acute poisonings, chronic environmental epidemiology studies, basic animal toxicology tests, and the less traditional alternative testing data (e.g., invertebrates, in vitro data). Each type or category of toxicology study has its own advantages and disadvantages when used to assess the potential human hazard or safety of a particular chemical.

How Dose-Response Data Can Be Used

Dosages are often described as lethal doses (LD), where the response being measured is mortality; toxic doses (TD), where the response is a serious adverse effect other than lethality; and sentinel doses (SD), where the response being measured is a non- or minimally-adverse effect. Sentinel effects (e.g., minor irritation, headaches, drowsiness) serve as a warning that greater exposure may result in more serious effects. Construction of the cumulative dose–response curve enables one to identify doses that affect a specific percent of the exposed population. For example, the LD_{50} is the dosage lethal to 50 percent of the test organisms, or one may choose to identify a less hazardous dose, such as LD_{10} or LD_{01}.

Dose–response data allow the toxicologist to make several useful comparisons or calculations. Comparisons of the LD50 doses of toxicants A, B, and C indicate the potency (toxicity relative to the dose used) of each chemical. Knowing this difference in potency may allow comparisons among chemicals to determine which is the least toxic per unit of dose (least potent), and therefore the safest of the chemicals for a given dose. This type of comparison may be particularly informative when there is familiarity with at least one of the substances being compared. In this way, the relative human risk or safety of a specific exposure may be approximated by comparing the relative potency of the unknown chemical to the familiar one, and in this manner one may approximate a safe exposure level for humans to the new chemical. For toxic effects, it is typically assumed that humans are as sensitive to the toxicity as the test species. Given this assumption, the test dose producing the response of interest [in units of milligrams per kilogram of body weight (mg/kg)], when multiplied by the average human weight (about 70 kg for a man and 60 kg for a woman), will give an approximation of the toxic human dose.

A relative ranking system developed years ago uses this approach to categorize the acute toxicity of a chemical. Using this ranking system, an industrial hygienist might get some idea of the acute danger posed by a workplace exposure. Similarly, if chronic toxicity is of greatest concern, that is, if the toxicity occurring at the lowest average daily dose is chronic in nature, combining a measure of this toxic dose (e.g., TD50) and appropriate safety factors might generate an acceptable workplace air concentration for the chemical. Often the dose–response curve for a relatively minor acute toxicity such as odor, tearing, or irritation involves lower doses than more severe toxicities such as coma or liver injury, and much lower doses than fatal exposures.

The difference in dose between the toxicity curve and a sentinel effect represents the margin of safety. Typically, the margin of safety is calculated from data, by dividing TD50 by the SD50. The higher the margin of safety, the safer the chemical is to use (i.e., greater room for error). However, one may also want to use a more protective definition of the margin of safety (for example, TD10/SD50 or TD01/SD100) depending on the circumstances of the substance's use and the ease of identifying and monitoring either the sentinel response or the seriousness of the toxicity produced. Changing the definition to include a higher percentile of the sentinel dose–response curve (e.g., the SD100) and correspondingly lower percentile of the toxic dose–response curve (e.g., the TD10 or the TD01) forces the margin of safety to be protective for the vast majority of a population.

Margin of safety = TD50 SD50

Or redefine it as = TD01 SD100

Finally, the use of dose–response curves allows for the estimation of the threshold dose or exposure. The threshold is the lowest point on the dose–response curve, or that dose below which an effect by a given agent is not detectable. Thus, all doses, or exposures producing doses, less than the threshold dose should represent safe doses and exposures. As explained in more detail later in this chapter, the safety of extrapolating from the threshold dose is enhanced by dividing it by uncertainty factors, a procedure that is equivalent to selecting a lower dose from the no-effect region of the dose–response curve.

Avoiding Incorrect Conclusions from Dose–Response Data

While the dose–response relationship can be determined for each adverse health effect of a toxicant, one must be cognizant of certain limitations when using these data:

1. If only single values from the dose–response curves are available, it must be kept in mind that those values will not provide any information about the shape of the curve.

2. Acute toxicity, which is often generated in tests because of the savings in time and expense, may not accurately reflect chronic toxicity dose–response relationships. The type of adverse response generated by a substance may differ significantly as the exposure duration increases in time. Chronic toxicities are often not the same as acute adverse responses. For example, both toluene and benzene cause depression of the central nervous system, and for this acute effect toluene is the more potently toxic of the two compounds. However, benzene is of greater concern to those with chronic, long-term exposure, because it is carcinogenic while toluene is not.

3. There is usually little information for guidance in deciding what animal data will best mimic the human response. For example, a question that often arises initially in the study of a chemical is the following: Is the test species

less sensitive or more sensitive than humans? The dose of chloroform that is lethal to 50 percent of the test animals (i.e., the LD_{50}) varies depending on the species and strain of animal tested. Estimation of the fatal human dose based on the animal results would overstate the toxicity of chloroform when using the rabbit or CD-1 mouse data, and underestimate the toxicity of chloroform if projecting lethality using data from the two remaining mouse strains or the two rat strains tested.

Unfortunately, there are anatomical, physiological, and biochemical differences among animal species. These differences may confound the animal to human extrapolation by increasing the uncertainty and concern we have for the accuracy of the extrapolation being made. For example, some laboratory animals possess certain anatomical features that humans lack, such as the Zymbal gland and a forestomach. So, when a chemical produces organ toxicity or cancer within these structures, the relevance to humans is unknown. Similarly, male rats produce a protein known as α-2-microglobulin, which has been shown to interact with the metabolites of certain chemicals in a manner that results in repeated cellular injury within the kidney. This reaction is believed to be responsible for the kidney tumors seen in the male rat after chronic exposure to these chemicals. Because this unique protein from these animals does not occur to any appreciable extent in female rats or in mice, kidney tumors are not seen in female rats or male and female mice. From these important sex and species differences, regulatory agencies have concluded the male rat kidney tumors are of limited relevance to humans, a species which is also deficient in α-2-microglobulin. Finally, certain animal strains are uniquely sensitive to certain types of cancer. For example, a large proportion of B6C3F1 mice develop liver tumors before they die, and this sensitivity appears to be due in part to the fact that the H-ras oncogene in this mouse strain is hypomethylated, allowing this oncogene to be expressed more easily, especially during recurrent hepatocellular injury. Similarly, 100 percent of strain A mice typically develop lung tumors before these animals die, and so a chemical that promotes the early development of lung tumors in this strain of mice may not produce any lung tumors in other strains. To summarize, then, there are a number of important species differences that may cause changes in (1) basal metabolic rates; (2) anatomy and structure; (3) physiology and cellular biochemistry; (4) the distribution of chemicals to certain tissues and pharmacokinetics of the chemical in the animal; (5) the metabolism, bioactivation, and detoxification of the chemical; and (6) ultimately the cellular, tissue, or organ response to actions of the chemical at the biochemical, cellular, tissue, or organ level.

This problem of species-specific responses to chemicals creates somewhat of a paradox in toxicological research. We use animals as models to study the toxicities of many chemicals; yet, the proper selection of the animal to serve as the test system ideally requires prior knowledge of which animal species most closely resembles humans with respect to the chemical interaction of interest.

Thus, the toxicologist is almost always faced with a dilemma. The goal of the toxicologist's study is the prediction of chemical effects on humans by using animal studies. However, selection of the right animal for that study requires a prior knowledge of the fate and effects of the chemical in humans (the goal), as well as its fate and effects in various animals. Thus, once data are generated in a test species, there are always inherent limitations to extrapolating the observed effects to humans. This is especially problematic when, as sometimes happens, one of the species tested is susceptible to a very undesirable effect, such as cancer or birth defects, yet several other species show no such effects. In that situation, determining or choosing which species represents the human response most accurately has, of course, a great impact on the estimated risk.

Factors Influencing Dose–Response Curves

Organism-Related Factors

Characteristics of the test species or the human population may alter the dose–response curve or limit its usefulness. The following variables should be considered when extrapolating toxicity data:

Route of Exposure: The exposure pathway by which a substance comes in contact with the body determines how much of it enters (rate and extent of absorption) and which organs are initially exposed to the largest concentration of the substance. For example, the water and lipid solubility characteristics of a chemical affect its absorption across the lungs (after inhalation), the skin (after dermal application), or the gastrointestinal (GI) tract (after oral ingestion), and the effect differs for each organ. The rate and site of absorption (organ) also may in turn determine the rate of metabolism and excretion of the chemical. So, changing the route of exposure may alter the dose required to produce toxicity. It may also alter the organ toxicity that is observed. For example, the organ with generally the greatest capacity for the metabolism and breakdown of chemicals is the liver. Therefore, a chemical may be more or less toxic per unit of dosage when the chemical is given orally or peritoneally, routes of administration that ensure the chemical absorbed into the bloodstream passes through the liver before it perfuses other organs within the animal. If the capacity of the liver to metabolize the chemical within the bloodstream is great, this leads to what is referred to as a first-pass effect, in which the liver metabolizes a large proportion of the chemical as it is absorbed and before it can be distributed to other tissues. If the metabolism of this chemical is strictly a detoxification process, then the toxic potency of the chemical (i.e., toxicity observed per unit of dose administered) may be reduced relative to its potency when administered by other routes (e.g., intravenously). On the other hand, if the metabolism of that dose generates toxic, reactive metabolites, then a greater toxic potency may be observed when the chemical is given orally relative to inhalation, dermal, or intramuscular administrations of the chemical.

All of these chemicals were administered to the same test species so that differences relating to the route of exposure may be compared. The studies showed in some instances the potency changes very little with a change in the route of administration (e.g., potency is similar for the pesticide DFP for all routes except dermal), in other instances—DDT, for example—the potency decreases 10-fold when changing the route of administration from intravenous to oral, and another 10-fold when moving from oral to dermal.

Sex Gender characteristics may affect the toxicity of some substances. Women have a larger percent of fat in their total body weight than men, and women also have different susceptibilities to reproduction system disorders and teratogenic effects. Some cancers and disease states are sex-linked. Large sex-linked differences are also present in animal data. One well-known pathway for sex-related differences occurs in rodents where the male animals of many rodent strains have a significantly greater capacity for the liver metabolism and breakdown of chemicals. This greater capacity for oxidative metabolism can cause the male animals of certain rodent strains to be more or less susceptible to toxicity from a chemical depending on whether oxidative metabolism represents a bioactivation or detoxification pathway for the chemical at the dose it is administered. For example, in the rat, strychnine is less toxic to male rats when administered orally because their greater liver metabolism allows them to break down and clear more of this poison before it reaches the systemic circulation. This allows them to survive a dose that is lethal to their female counterparts. Alternatively, this greater capacity for oxidative metabolism renders male rodents more susceptible to the liver toxicity and carcinogenicity of a number of chemicals that are bioactivated to a toxic, reactive intermediate during oxidative metabolism.

Older age people have differences in their musculature and metabolism, which change the disposition of chemicals within the body and therefore the levels required to induce toxicity. At the other end of the spectrum, children have higher respiration rates and different organ susceptibilities [generally they are less sensitive to central nervous system (CNS) stimulants and more sensitive to CNS depressants], differences in the metabolism and elimination of chemicals, and many other biological characteristics that distinguish them from adults in the consideration of risks or chemical hazards. For example, the acute LD50 dose of chloroform is 446 mg/kg in 14-day-old Sprague–Dawley rats, but this dose increases to 1188 mg/kg in the adult animal.

Effects of Chemical Interaction (Synergism, Potentiation, and Antagonism): Mixtures represent a challenge because the response of one chemical might be altered by the presence of another chemical in the mixture. A synergistic reaction between two chemicals occurs when both chemicals produce the toxicity of interest, and when combined, the presence of both chemicals causes a greater-than-additive effect in the anticipated response. Potentiation describes that situation when a chemical that does not produce a specific toxicity nevertheless increases the toxicity caused by another chemical.

Modes of Chemical Interaction: Chemical interactions can be increased or decreased in one of four ways:

1. Functional—both chemicals affect the same physiologic function.

2. Chemical—a chemical interaction between the two compounds affects the toxicity of one of the chemicals.

3. Dispositional—the absorption, metabolism, distribution, or excretion of one of the chemicals is altered by the second chemical.

4. Receptor-mediated—when two chemicals bind to the same tissue receptor, the second chemical, which differs in activity, competes for the receptor and thereby alters the effect produced by the first chemical.

Like alcohol, smoking may also alter the effects of other chemicals, and the incidence of some minor drug-induced side effects have been reported to be lower in individuals who smoke. For example, smoking seems to diminish the effectiveness of propoxyphene (Darvon) to relieve pain, and it lowers the CNS depressant effects of sedatives from the benzodiazepine and barbiturate families. Smoking also increases certain metabolic pathways in the liver and so enhances the metabolism of a number of drugs. Examples of drugs whose metabolism is increased by smoking include antipyrine, imipramine, nicotine, pentazocine, and theophylline.

Genetic Makeup: We are not all born physiologically equal, and this provides both advantages and disadvantages. For example, people deficient in glucose-6-phosphate dehydrogenase (G6PD deficiency) are more susceptible than others to the hemolysis of blood by aspirin or certain antibiotics, and people who are genetically slow acetylators are more susceptible to neuropathy and hepatotoxicity from isoniazid.

Health Status: In addition to the genetic status, the general well-being of an individual, specifically, their immunologic status, nutritional status, hormonal status, and the absence or presence of concurrent diseases, are features that may alter the dose–response relationship.

Chemical-Specific Factors

We have seen that a number of factors inherent in the organism may affect the predicted response; certain chemical and physical factors associated with the form of the chemical or the exposure conditions also may influence toxic potency (i.e., toxicity per unit of dose) of a chemical.

Chemical Composition: The physical (particle size, liquid or solid, etc.) and chemical (volatility, solubility, etc.) properties of the toxic substance may affect its absorption or alter the probability of exposure. For example, the lead pigments that were used in paints decades ago were not an inhalation hazard when applied because they were encapsulated in the paints. However, as the paint aged, peeled, and chipped, the lead became a hazard when the paint chips were ingested by small children. Similarly, the hazards of certain dusts can be reduced in the workplace with the use of water to keep finely granulated solids clumped together.

Exposure Conditions: The conditions under which exposure occurs may affect the applied dose of the toxicant, and as a result, the amount of chemical that becomes absorbed. For example, chemicals bound to soils may be absorbed through the skin poorly compared to absorption when a neat solution is applied because the chemical may have affinity for, and be bound by, the organic materials in soil.

Concentration, type of exposure (dermal, oral, inhalation, etc.), exposure medium (soil, water, air, food, surfaces, etc.), and duration (acute or chronic) are all factors associated with the exposure conditions that might alter the applied or absorbed dose.

Descriptive Toxicology: Testing Adverse Effects of Chemicals and Generating Dose–Response Data

Since the dose–response relationship aids both basic tasks of toxicologists—namely, identifying the hazards associated with a toxicant and assessing the conditions of its usage—it is appropriate to summarize toxicity testing, or descriptive toxicology. While a number of tests may be used to assess toxic responses, each toxicity test rests on two assumptions:

1. The Hazard Is Qualitatively the Same. The effects produced by the toxicant in the laboratory test are assumed to be the same effects that the chemical will produce in humans. Therefore, the test species or organisms are useful surrogates for identifying the hazards (qualitative toxicities) in humans.

2. The Hazard Is Quantitatively the Same. The dose producing toxicity in animal tests is assumed to be the same as the dose required to produce toxicity in humans. Therefore, animal dose–response data provide a reliable surrogate for evaluating the risks associated with different doses or exposure levels in humans.

Which tests or testing scheme to follow depends on the use of the chemical and the likelihood of human exposure. In general, part or all of the following scheme might be required in a descriptive toxicology testing program.

Level 1: Testing for acute exposure

a. Plot dose–response curves for lethality and possible organ injuries.

b. Test eyes and skin for irritation.

c. Make a first screen for mutagenic activity.

Level 2: Testing for subchronic exposure

a. Plot dose–response curves (for 90-day exposure) in two species; the test should use the expected human route of exposure.

b. Test organ toxicity; note mortality, body weight changes, hematology, and clinical chemistry; make microscopic examinations for tissue injury.

c. Conduct a second screen for mutagenic activity.

d. Test for reproductive problems and birth defects (teratology).

e. Examine the pharmacokinetics of the test species: the absorption, distribution, metabolism, and elimination of chemicals from the body.

f. Conduct behavioural tests.

g. Test for synergism, potentiation, and antagonism.

Level 3: Test for chronic exposure

   a.   Conduct mammalian mutagenicity tests.

   b.   Conduct a 2-year carcinogenesis test in rodents.

   c.   Examine pharmacokinetics in humans.

   d.   Conduct human clinical trials.

   e.   Compile the epidemiologic data of acute and chronic exposure.

Establishing the safety and hazard of a chemical is a costly and time-consuming effort. For example, the rodent bioassay for carcinogenic potential requires 2–3 years to obtain results, at a cost of between $3,000,000–$7,000,000 and when completed the results, if positive, may in the end severely limit or prohibit the use of the chemical in question. Thus, this final test may entail additional costs if now a replacement chemical must be sought that does not have significant carcinogenic activity.

Extrapolation of Animal Test Data to Human Exposure

Several models can be used to extrapolate the human risks from chemical exposure on the basis of toxicity tests in animals. The model chosen is primarily determined by the health hazard of most concern. In the past, however, two basic methods for extrapolation were used. The first type consisted of extrapolating the human risk directly from either the threshold dose or some no-observable-effectlevel (NOEL) dose. This method was applied to most toxicities or health hazards (except cancer), since thresholds were assumed to be present for all of these health hazards. The second type of model was generally used to assess the risk associated with carcinogens. Since the regulatory approach to carcinogens has been to assume that no identifiable threshold exists for this type of toxicity, any exposure was assumed to involve some quantifiable amount of risk. This concept dictated that the mathematical models used to extrapolate to exposures far below the dosages that induce observable responses in the test animal population involve some form of linear extrapolation at low doses. For noncancer-causing toxicants (those with threshold toxicity), the models for extrapolating risk are relatively simple and similar to the methods that have been suggested or used by the National Academy of Sciences (NAS) and various governmental agencies such as the Food and Drug Administration (FDA) or the Environmental Protection Agency (USEPA). These models derive a safe dosage by dividing the threshold (or NOEL/LOEL) by uncertainty factors. The purpose of adding these uncertainty factors is to ensure that the allowable human dose is one that falls within the no-effect region of the human dose–response curve. Basically, this type of calculation assumes that humans are as sensitive as the test species used; so, the amount of a chemical ingested by the test animal that gives no toxic response is considered the safe upper limit of exposure for humans (especially after inclusion of appropriate safety factors).

Calculating Safety for Threshold Toxicities: The Safe Human Dose Approach The calculation of a safe human dose essentially makes an extrapolation on the basis of the size differential between humans and the test species. Usually this is a straightforward body-weight extrapolation, but a surface area scalar for dose could also be used. The calculation is similar to the following:

SHD =NOAEL = (mg/kg per day) 70 kg UF = N mg/day where NOAEL = threshold dose or some other no-observable-adverse-effect-level selected from the no-effect region of the dose–response curve SHD = safe human dose UF = the total uncertainty factor, which depends on the nature and reliability of the animal data used for the extrapolation N = number of milligrams consumed per day (Note: In this example we are extrapolating for an average adult male, and so we have assumed a 70kg body weight.)

Typically, the uncertainty factor used varies from 10 to 10,000 and is dependant on the confidence placed in the animal database as well as whether there are human data to substantiate the reliability of the animal no-effect levels that have been reported. Of course, the number calculated should use chronic exposure data if chronic exposures are expected. This type of model calculates one value, the expected safe human dosage, which regulatory agencies have referred to as either the acceptable daily intake (ADI) or the reference dose (RfD). Exposures which produce human doses that are at or below these safe human dosages (ADIs or RfDs) are considered safe.

3

Classification of Toxic Agents

Toxic substances are classified into the following:

Heavy Metals

Metals differ from other toxic substances in that they are neither created nor destroyed by humans. Their use by humans plays an important role in determining their potential for health effects. Their effect on health could occur through at least two mechanisms: first, by increasing the presence of heavy metals in air, water, soil, and food, and second, by changing the structure of the chemical. For example, chromium III can be converted to or from chromium VI, the more toxic form of the metal.

Solvents and Vapors

Nearly everyone is exposed to solvents. Occupational exposures can range from the use of "white-out" by administrative personnel, to the use of chemicals by technicians in a nail salon. When a solvent evaporates, the vapors may also pose a threat to the exposed population.

Radiation and Radioactive Materials

Radiation is the release and propagation of energy in space or through a material medium in the form of waves, the transfer of heat or light by waves of energy, or the stream of particles from a nuclear reactor.

Dioxin/Furans

Dioxin, (or TCDD) was originally discovered as a contaminant in the herbicide Agent Orange. Dioxin is also a by-product of chlorine processing in paper producing industries.

Pesticides

The EPA defines pesticide as any substance or mixture of substances intended to prevent, destroy, repel, or mitigate any pest. Pesticides may also be described as any physical, chemical, or biological agent that will kill an undesirable plant or animal pest.

Plant Toxins

Different portions of a plant may contain different concentrations of chemicals. Some chemicals made by plants can be lethal. For example, taxon, used in chemotherapy to kill cancer cells, is produced by a species of the yew plant.

Animal Toxins

These toxins can result from venomous or poisonous animal releases. Venomous animals are usually defined as those that are capable of producing a poison in a highly developed gland or group of cells, and can deliver that toxin through biting or stinging. Poisonous animals are generally regarded as those whose tissues, either in part or in their whole, are toxic.

Subcategories of Toxic Substance Classifications

All of these substances may also be further classified according to their:

- Effect on target organs (liver, kidney, hematopoietic system),
- Use (pesticide, solvent, food additive),
- Source of the agent (animal and plant toxins),
- Effects (cancer mutation, liver injury),
- Physical state (gas, dust, liquid),
- Labeling requirements (explosive, flammable, oxidizer),
- Chemistry (aromatic amine, halogenated hydrocarbon), or
- Poisoning potential (extremely toxic, very toxic, slightly toxic)

General Classifications of Interest to Communities

- Air pollutants
- Occupation-related
- Acute and chronic poisons

All chemicals (or any chemical) may be poisonous at a given dose and through a particular route. For example, breathing too much pure oxygen, drinking excessive amounts of water, or eating too much salt can cause poisoning or death.

4

Emerging Challenges in Food Toxicology

Rapid advances in science and technology have produced enormous benefits but have also created undesirable hazardous side-effects that impact human health and the environment. The toxicological sciences strive to understand and evaluate the health and environmental effects of chemical and physical agents. The impact of this expanding body of science on society has grown enormously in the last 100 years, and with that have arisen corresponding financial, legal, and individual implications. Despite the increased scientific data and understanding, decision making has become more difficult and complex. It is thus increasingly important to consider the ethical, legal, and social issues that confront toxicologists, public health professionals, and decision makers.

The fundamental principles that an ethical toxicologist should consider can be summarized as: 1) dignity, which includes respect for the autonomy of human and animal subjects; 2) veracity, an adherence to transparency and presentation of all the facts so all parties can discover the truth; 3) justice, which includes an equitable distribution of the costs, hazards, and gains; 4) integrity, an honest and forthright approach; 5) responsibility, an acknowledgment of accountability to all parties involved; and 6) sustainability, consideration that actions can be maintained over a long period of time.

Beyond these basic principles it is important to have a vision of environmental health that is grounded in ethical considerations.

Historical Perspective

Looking back, it is easy to see the beginnings of an ethical framework for decision making in the Greek physician Hippocrates (460-377 BC), who studied the effects of food, occupation, and climate on causation of disease and is credited with the basic medical tenet of "do no harm." Bernardo Ramazzini (1633 - 1714), an Italian physician, examined the health hazards of chemicals, dust, metals, and other agents encountered by workers in 52 occupations, which he documented in his book *De Morbis Artificum Diatriba* (Diseases of Workers).

Aldo Leopold, considered by many to be America's first bio-ethicist, summarized ethical responsibilities in a simple statement in 1949. "A thing is right when it tends to preserve the integrity, stability, and beauty of the biotic community. It is wrong when it tends otherwise." It can be extrapolated from this ethical statement that exposing people, particularly children, to harmful agents robs them of their "integrity, stability, and beauty," indeed their potential, and is therefore wrong. Health, ecological, and ethical concerns about chemical exposures were highlighted by Rachel Carson (photo, left) in *Silent Spring*, first published in 1962. Carson sounded one of the first alarms about the effects of environmental contaminants and catalyzed numerous regulatory changes related to chemical use. Her writings include the following statements: "It is the public that is being asked to assume the risks ... the public must decide whether it wishes to continue on the present road and it can only do so when in full possession of the facts..." "Only within the moment of time represented by the present century has one species - man - acquired significant power to alter the nature of his world."

The next major book to capture public attention on this subject was *Our Stolen Future* by Theo Colborn, Dianne Dumanoski, and John Peter Meyers, first published in 1996. This book focused on the reproductive and developmental effects of synthetic chemicals and raised awareness and concern about endocrine disruptors.

At the same time, there were ongoing efforts to define a more philosophical and ethical approach to managing the chemicals we have grown dependent upon. The idea for an Earth Charter was first proposed in 1987 as an approach to creating a broad ethical statement with the goal of establishing a global civil society. The Earth Charter took a step forward in 1992 at The Earth Summit in Rio de Janeiro, also known as the Rio Summit or Rio Conference, which produced the 27 Principles of the Rio Declaration. Principle 15 defined the precautionary principle as an approach to protect human health and the environment. In January 1998, the Wingspread Conference on the Precautionary Principle was held in Racine, Wisconsin to define the precautionary principle.

"When an activity raises threats of harm to the environment or human health, precautionary measures should be taken even if some cause and effect relationships are not fully established scientifically."

Legal Issues

There is a wide range of laws and regulations that shape the role of toxicology in society. One of the first laws dealing with toxicology, passed in 82 BCE by the Roman Emperor Sulla, was intended to deter intentional poisonings because women were poisoning men to acquire their wealth. In 1880, food poisonings spurred Peter

Collier, chief chemist, U.S. Department of Agriculture, to recommend passage of a national food and drug law. In 1938, the Federal Food, Drug, and Cosmetic Act was adopted following an incident in which Elixir Sulfanilamide, containing the poisonous solvent diethylene glycol, killed 107 people, many of whom were children. The need to control chemical contamination was recognized in the 1976 when the U.S. Congress passed the Toxic Substances Control Act (TSCA)to "prevent unreasonable risks of injury to health or the environment associated with the manufacture, processing, distribution in commerce, use, or disposal of chemical substances." TSCAbecame largely ineffective following court decisions and there is now an effort to pass chemical policy reform legislation. Mean while Europe has moved forward with REACH, Registration Evaluation and Authorization of Chemicals, a system that requires testing and evaluation of chemicals before their introduction into commerce.

Social Considerations

Toxicologists and public health professionals play an important role in society in protecting and promoting public health. There has been an extra focus on ethical and social issues related to children's health. The U.S. Society of Toxicology code of ethics indicates that toxicologists should be thoughtful public health advocates. While seldom explicitly stated, professional codes of ethics such as those for SOT are often based on the following social responsibilities: 1) to share and use knowledge, 2) to promote the health and well being of children, and 3) to maintain the right of all species to reach and maintain their full potential.

Additional Ethical Considerations

A toxicologist is also concerned with issues of integrity and honesty in the conduct and interpretation of toxicological studies. It is important to examine and acknowledge conflicts of interest. Toxicology associations as well state and federal agencies, nonprofits, and universities have statements and guidelines on conflict of interest and disclosure. In addition, toxicologists must adhere to rules and regulations regarding the use of animals and humans in scientific studies. The conduct of studies involving humans has a rich history that has become increasingly well defined and regulated to ensure adequate knowledge and consent of subjects involved.

The purest of ethical behavior and decision making requires the thoughtful development and articulation of fundamental principles upon which to base any action. The ethical toxicologist must consider and integrate basic ethical principles into the decision making process. This approach moves beyond what is legally required: an ethical approach requires ongoing discussion and considerations as the toxicological sciences and society evolve. Toxicologists must not only be familiar with the rules and regulations regarding the ethical conduct of research, but also with the underlying ethical principles. The challenge is to move beyond a purely legal adherence to the rules but toward an ethical approach grounded in carefully considered and articulated ethical principles that drive the responsible conduct and application of research in modern societies.

RESEARCH ISSUES

Research on or using toxicogenomics raises three categories of ethical issues. First, toxicogenomic research not involving human subjects may raise issues common to all biomedical research, including research integrity, conflicts of interest, and commercial relations and disclosures. Second, toxicogenomic research involving human subjects raises generally applicable human subject issues, such as the Common Rule and the Health Insurance Portability and Accountability Act of 1996 (HIPAA) Privacy Rule, equitable selection of subjects, informed consent, privacy and confidentiality, and special protections for vulnerable populations. Third, toxicogenomic research with human subjects involves distinct issues related to the collection and use of biorepositories in research, special issues of informed consent in genetics research, community consultation when doing genetics research in discrete subpopulations, and the duty to notify sample donors and their relatives of research findings.

Research Priorities

One myth about scientific research is that science is value neutral—that new scientific understandings await discovery, that these discoveries have no independent moral significance, and that they take on moral significance only when individuals and groups of individuals assign weight to scientific findings. One flaw in this argument is that there are seemingly limitless areas for scientific inquiry, yet there are finite numbers of scientists and limited resources to pursue research. Therefore, scientists and society must set priorities for research, and those priorities are a function of societal values. Even though scientists often make adventitious discoveries, they generally discover what they are looking for, and what they look for are the things that science and society value discovering.

Pharmacogenomics provides a good illustration. Pharmaceutical researchers may discover numerous polymorphisms in the gene for a particular drug target. Before spending tens or hundreds of millions of dollars on studying a particular polymorphism, any revenue-conscious biotech or pharmaceutical company will try to ascertain the population frequency of these drug targets. Consequently, initial drug development does not focus on genetic variations found most often among individuals in developing countries, where most people do not have the money to pay for basic medicines, let alone expensive new products that treat persons with particular genotypes. Even in developed countries, without some external support from government or private sources, developing drugs directed at rare genotypes is not cost-effective.

Another way to set research priorities is to focus on the nature of the harm to be prevented. It has been asserted that a disproportionate share of health resources (research and treatment) are directed at specific diseases simply because of the effectiveness of advocacy groups working on behalf of affected individuals Similarly, environmental policy may be influenced by considering certain environmental risks to be of greater societal concern than others. For example, it has been argued that U.S. environmental policy is flawed because we spend millions of dollars on a relatively few Superfund sites in need of remediation but insufficient sums on air and water pollution, which is a more widespread threat to public health. Undoubtedly, the targets of toxicogenomic research will be influenced by a myriad of social factors, and priority setting will be influenced by economic and political concerns.

Biorepositories

Biorepositories are repositories of human biologic materials collected for research. According to the most recent and widely cited estimate, more than 300 million specimens are stored in the United States, and the number grows by 20 million per year. Because the ability to access large numbers of well-characterized and annotated samples is an essential part of new genomic research strategies, biorepositories are increasingly important. Although biorepositories raise numerous issues involving research ethics and social policy, three issues are especially important to toxicogenomics, pharmacogenomics, and related research.

First, biorepositories collect samples and data for unspecified, unknown, future research and thereby differ from traditional biomedical research, which generally contemplates a single, discrete project for which a single process of informed consent is used. Thus, the question that arises is whether it is permissible under the Common Rule for researchers to obtain informed consent for future uses of specimens collected by a biorepository. Under the Common Rule, a research subject may consent to future, unspecified research. Nevertheless, IRBs generally do not approve "blanket consent" for all possible research on the grounds that consent about unknown future uses by definition is not "informed". Using "tiered" or "layered" consent, research subjects are presented with a menu of possible future research categories, such as cancer research, AIDS research, and genetic research. They can then indicate for which types of research it is permissible to use their sample. Because of the growth of biorepositories and new methods of informed consent, researchers need to monitor the understanding of research subjects and the effectiveness of the informed consent process to determine whether changes or improvements in the informed consent process are needed.

Under the HIPAA Privacy Rule, however, each new research project requires a new authorization. Thus, tiered consent does not satisfy the Privacy Rule. Although researchers can obtain a waiver of the authorization requirement (meaning that the researchers do not need to recontact each sample donor for each new research project) (45 C.F.R. §164.512[l][2][ii]), a separate waiver from an IRB or Privacy Board is needed for each proposed new use. Therefore, the inconsistency between the Common Rule and the Privacy Rule complicates compliance for researchers, especially when toxicogenomic research may involve large repositories of individually identifiable specimens that may be used for multiple research projects.

A second key ethical issue about biorepositories concerns if or when researchers have a duty to recontact sample donors to notify them that research using their samples has identified health risk information of clinical or social significance to them or their relatives. If the samples are deidentified, it will be impossible to notify any individual of sample-specific research findings, but there still may be a duty to notify all sample donors of the overall conclusions of the study and the potential desirability of consulting a physician. The greatest challenge, however, involves individually identifiable samples. Because it is too late to develop a recontact policy after a discovery has been made, the most prudent course is for researchers to ask sample donors at the time of sample collection if they want to be recontacted in certain circumstances (for example, when there is a predictive test or therapy) and, if so, whether the contact should be through their physician or personally.

A third set of issues on which there has been considerable debate in the bioethics literature, is who owns the property rights to tissue samples and whether researchers have a duty to undertake any type of "benefit sharing" with individual donors or groups of donors. For example, over and above informed consent, who ultimately controls the use, distribution, and disposal of donated tissue samples? In one of the first judicial decisions to address this issue, a federal district court recently held that the research institute, not the individual researcher or tissue donor, "owns" donated tissue samples (Washington University v. Catalona, 2006 U.S. Dist. LEXIS 22969 [E.D. Mo. 2006]). Some tissue donors, especially those who are members of identifiable groups such as Native Americans, are now insisting that they retain the property rights in their donated tissues as a precondition for providing samples for research.

A related question concerns those instances in which research on biorepository samples has led to commercially valuable discoveries: are sample donors entitled to some share of the proceeds (see Greenberg v. Miami Children's Hospital Research Institute, Inc., 264 F. Supp. 2d 1064 [S.D. Fla. 2003]; Moore v. Regents of Univ. of Cal., 793 p.2d 479 (Cal. 1990)? There have been a few documented cases in which one individual's sample has been extremely valuable in developing cell lines or other research products (Moore v. Regents of Univ. of Cal., 793 p.2d 479 [Cal. 1990]; Washington 1994). It is far more likely, however, for analyses of numerous samples to be needed for development of any commercially viable finding. Whether it is ethical for individual research subjects to waive all their interests in the products of discovery remains unclear, although it is common for informed consent documents to so provide. Regardless of the language in the informed consent document, the principle of benefit sharing would be satisfied if researchers declare in advance that they will set aside a small percentage of revenues derived from commercialization for dona tion to a charitable organization that, for example, provides health care to indigent individuals with the condition that is the target of the research.

Intellectual Property

The development, exploitation, and protection of intellectual property are important elements of contemporary research strategy. Many of the contentious intellectual property issues, such as publication, timing of filing, ownership, and licensing, arise "downstream," after the discovery of a patentable invention. These issues are not unique to toxicogenomic and pharmacogenomic research. Nevertheless, because many toxicogenomic applications involve assays that produce large amounts of data, often involving large numbers of genes or proteins, obtaining intellectual property rights to all the materials used in an assay could be particularly burdensome and problematic for researchers and platform manufacturers in the field of toxicogenomics.

An important, "upstream" issue, and one that needs to be addressed specifically in the context of toxicogenomic and pharmacogenomic research, is whether to have an "open access" policy to raw samples and data and, if so, how open it should be and how it would work. Traditionally, both toxicologic and pharmaceutical research have been undertaken with closed access, with private companies maintaining proprietary control over their research until a patent has been filed or a company has decided to disclose information for some other reason. Increasingly, however, there is pressure to make preliminary data from government-funded (and even some privately funded) research more widely available to researchers in general. For example, the Human Genome Project (public), the Pharmacogenetics Research Network (public), and the SNP Consortium (private) have adopted the policy of making research findings available online promptly for other researchers to use.

The Committee on Emerging Issues and Data on Environmental Contaminants of the National Research Council held a Workshop on Intellectual Property in June 2006 at the National Academies. Among other issues, the workshop discussed the position of the National Institutes of Health (NIH) in support of immediate (or prompt) release of and free access to human genome sequence data. These policies, embodied in the so-called Bermuda Principles, have been endorsed by the International Human Genome Organization and other organizations. They also have been applied more broadly, and they form the basis of the National Human Genome Research Institute's policies of prompt or immediate disclosure of genomic information generated by NIH-supported research or collected in NIH-supported repositories.

No standard policy for data release has been developed for toxicogenomic and pharmacogenomic research. In the absence of such a policy, the default position is nondisclosure. Consequently, affirmative steps should be undertaken to ensure that toxicogenomic and pharmacogenomic data are promptly and freely made available to all researchers whenever possible.

ETHICAL AND SOCIAL ISSUES

A number of ethical and social issues may apply to toxicogenomics. These issues include privacy and confidentiality, issues related to socially vulnerable populations, health insurance discrimination, employment discrimination, individual responsibility, issues related to race and ethnicity, and implementation.

Privacy and Confidentiality

Privacy has many dimensions. In the information sense, privacy is the right of an individual to prevent the disclosure of certain information to another individual or entity. Increasingly, the bioethics literature also has recognized a negative right of informational privacy—that is, the right "not to know" certain information about oneself. Toxicogenomics affects both of these aspects of privacy. Individuals may want to restrict the disclosure of their toxicogenomic or pharmacogenomic information that was obtained in a research, clinical, workplace, or other setting. They also may not want to know of certain risks, especially when nothing can be done to prevent the risk of harm (for example, where there was past occupational or environmental exposure).

Confidentiality refers to a situation in which information obtained or disclosed within a confidential relationship (for example, physician-patient) generally will not be redisclosed without the permission of the individual. With regard to toxicogenomics, the most important relationship is the physician-patient relationship. Restrictions on redisclosure are an important ethical precept of health care professionals, and maintaining the confidentiality of health information is important in preventing intrinsic and consequential harm to individuals. Although toxicogenomic and pharmacogenomic information would be covered under the "genetic privacy" laws several states have enacted, these laws afford limited and inconsistent protection.

It should also be noted that DHHS is taking the lead in promoting widespread adoption of electronic health records and creation of a national infrastructure to support a system of interoperable, longitudinal, comprehensive health records. In such an environment, privacy and confidentiality protections are even more important because detailed health information can be disclosed to numerous sources instantaneously.

Although it is important to safeguard the security of health records to prevent unauthorized disclosure of information, breaches of confidentiality through authorized disclosures may be an even greater problem. For example, in health care settings, not all employees (for example, billing clerks, meal service employees, maintenance employees) need the same degree of access to patient health records. Thus, the degree of access needs to comport with the need to know about protected health information. "Role-based access restrictions" help to limit the scope of disclosure.

In non-health care settings, individuals often are required to execute an authorization for disclosure of their medical records as a condition of employment or insurance. Development and application of "contextual access criteria" will help to limit these disclosures to the health information relevant to the purpose of the disclosure (for example, ability to perform a job).

Socially Vulnerable Populations

Many genetic loci of actual or potential significance to toxicogenomics and pharmacogenomics have a differential allelic frequency in discrete subpopulations. Due to ancestral patterns of endogamy (marrying within a social group), migration, geographic isolation, and other elements of ancestral origins, some genetic traits have a higher frequency among subpopulations socially defined by race or ethnicity. Thus, there is great potential for stigma when an increased risk of a particular undesirable health condition is associated with a particular population group, especially when the group is a racial or ethnic minority in a society. These population groups are then said to be "vulnerable" with respect to a particular health condition.

A socially vulnerable population also can be based on shared somatic mutations. For example, workers with an acquired mutation or biomarker based on a particular occupational exposure or residents of a certain area with toxic exposures who demonstrated the subclinical effects of a particular exposure may also be said to be socially vulnerable populations. These polymorphisms may not be phenotypically obvious and often do not correlate with race, ethnicity, and other traditional social categories.

The notion of vulnerable populations based on toxicogenomics and pharmacogenomics raises numerous ethical concerns, including the ethical principles of justice, respect for persons, and beneficence. Because of the social risks to vulnerable populations from research, special efforts are needed to obtain infor mation about community interests and concerns. Community engagement and consultation are essential elements of ethical research. In addition, if environmental or pharmaceutical exposures have already adversely affected a subpopulation or a subpopulation has been identified to be at greater risk, ethical considerations might require that vulnerable populations have fair access to health care for diagnostic and treatment measures; that steps be taken to prevent unfair discrimination in employment, insurance, and other opportunities; that there is adequate compensation for harms; that feasible remediation be undertaken; and that effective protections are in place for protecting privacy and confidentiality (Weijer and Miller 2004).

Health Insurance Discrimination

The leading concern among individuals at a genetically increased risk of illness is that they will be unable to obtain or retain their health insurance (Rothstein and Hornung 2004). In the United States, individuals obtain health care coverage mostly through government-funded programs (for example, Medicare, Medicaid) or employer-sponsored group health insurance. A relatively small percentage (about 10%) of those with health coverage have individual health insurance policies. Although this group is the only one in which individual medical underwriting takes place, individuals who currently have group coverage might be legitimately concerned that if they lost their job and their group health insurance, they would need to obtain individual health insurance.

To address the concern about discrimination in health insurance, nearly every state has enacted a law prohibiting genetic discrimination in health insurance. These laws have a fatal flaw: they prohibit discrimination only against individuals who are asymptomatic. If an individual later becomes affected by a condition, he or she is no longer protected by the law and is at risk of rate increases or even cancellation in accordance with general provisions of state insurance law.

Health insurance discrimination is very difficult to resolve. As long as a key element of our system of health care finance is individually underwritten, optional, health insurance, then it will contain less favorable access for individuals at an increased risk of future illness. Meaningful reform would require major changes in health care financing.

Employment Discrimination

Employers have two concerns about employing individuals who are at a genetic risk of future illness. First, employee illness and disability of any etiology represents significant costs in terms of lost productivity, lost work time, high turnover, and increased health care costs. Genetic testing makes it possible to predict future risks and would make it more attractive for employers to exclude at-risk individuals from their workforces. To combat such discrimination, about two-thirds of the states have enacted laws prohibiting genetic discrimination in employment. These laws are seriously deficient because, although they make discrimination based on genetic information illegal, they do not prohibit employers from lawfully obtaining genetic information contained within the comprehensive health records that employers may require individuals to disclose as a condition of employment. Consequently, at-risk individuals, who might benefit from genetic testing, are often reluctant to do so because a future employer can lawfully obtain the results.

Second, employers may be reluctant to hire or assign individuals to work where they are at an increased risk of occupational illness because of their genetics. In addition to the employers' illness concerns listed above, occupational illness could result in additional costs based on workers' compensation, compliance with the Occupational Safety and Health Act of 1970, personal injury litigation, and reduced employee morale. With regard to toxicogenomics in the workplace, is it lawful or ethical for employers to request or require workers to undergo genetic testing?

There are two ethical cross-currents in the laws regulating the workplace: paternalism and autonomy. Much workplace health and safety regulation may be characterized as paternalistic, including child labor laws, minimum wage laws, and the Occupational Safety and Health Act. A greater appreciation for worker autonomy in the workplace is reflected in the Supreme Court's leading decision in International Union, UAW v. Johnson Controls, Inc. (1991). The Court held that the employer discriminated on the basis of sex, in violation of Title VII of the Civil Rights Act of 1964 (42 U.S.C. § 2000e), by excluding all fertile women from jobs with exposure to inorganic lead because of concerns that a woman could become pregnant and give birth to a child with deformities caused by maternal workplace exposures. According to the Court: "Congress made clear that the decision to become pregnant or to work while being either pregnant or capable of becoming pregnant was reserved for each individual woman to make for herself" (499 U.S. at 206).

A middle position between permitting employers to mandate genetic testing and prohibiting all employee genetic testing is that a worker who is currently capable of performing the job should have the option of learning whether he or she is at increased risk of occupational disease based on genetic factors. Optional genetic testing would be conducted by a physician or laboratory of the individual's choice; the testing would be paid for by the employer; and the results would be available only to the individual. The individual would then have the option of deciding whether to assume any increased risk of exposure. Only if employment of the individual created a direct and immediate threat of harm to the individual or the public would the employer be justified in excluding the individual based on future risk (Chevron U.S.A. Inc v. Echazabal 2002).

Individual Responsibility

To what extent should individuals have a responsibility to learn if they are at increased risk from certain exposures, to avoid those exposures, and to deal with the consequences of illness caused by those exposures? To what extent does society have a duty to respect the autonomy of individuals to decline to learn of possible increased risks or to accept those risks? To what extent is society obligated to provide special protections for such individuals and health care if they become sick?

Several of these policy choices have been settled in the workplace setting for some time. Under workers' compensation law, an employer "takes the employee as is," and therefore it is no defense that the individual was at an increased risk of illness (Perry v. Workers' Comp. App. Bd. 1997). Under the Occupational Safety and Health Act, health standards, at least in theory, are designed to protect all workers (29 U.S.C. § 655 [c][5]). Under HIPAA, employer-sponsored group health plans may not charge employees different rates or have different levels of coverage based on their health status, including genetic predisposition (42 U.S.C. § 300gg-1[a] and [b]). Nevertheless, even with regard to employment, many issues remain to be resolved, including the role of individual variation in setting permissible exposure levels.

It may be even more difficult to develop rules of general applicability beyond the workplace setting. Both scientific evidence (for example, absolute risk, relative risk, severity, latency, treatability) and context-specific social conceptions of reasonable conduct in the face of increased risk are likely to affect the development of public policy. For example, if members of a low-income family with a genetic predisposition to illness and with few options of places to live "voluntarily" agree to accept the increased risk of living in the vicinity of toxic emissions, it is doubtful that society would shift the moral blame from the polluter to the individuals harmed by the pollutants. On the other hand, if toxicogenomic testing indicated that a particular individual would be much more likely to suffer serious harm from exposure to tobacco smoke and the individual started smoking or made no effort to stop, it is likely that at least some of the moral blame would shift to the cigarette smoker.

Race and Ethnicity

Concerns about race and ethnicity are subsumed under the heading of "socially vulnerable populations," discussed above, but they are raised in distinctive ways by pharmacogenomics. All humans are genetically 99.9% alike. There is more genetic diversity within certain socially defined groups (for example, race, ethnicity) than between groups. The individual and group differences, however, are measurable and may be significant. Among the traits for which subpopulation variance has been observed are those dealing with pharmacokinetics and pharmacodynamics.

Although pharmacogenomics holds great promise for increasing drug efficacy and decreasing adverse drug events, there is a risk of "racializing" medicine. It is facile to rely on race as a surrogate for genotype, but the social cost of doing so may be high. "By heedlessly equating race with genetic variation and genetic variation with genotype-based medications, we risk developing an oversimplified view of race-specific medications and a misleading view of the scientific significance of race". The controversy surrounding the FDA's approval of the drug BiDil in 2005 for self-identified African Americans demonstrates the currency of the issue.

Implementation Issues

Traditionally, pharmaceutical companies have searched for new blockbuster drugs to provide effective treatments for common conditions, such as hypertension, hypercholesterolemia, and musculoskeletal pain. A single product is designed to be safe and effective for substantially all members of the adult population. With pharmacogenomics, however, the potential market is segmented by genotype and many different companies may develop products for each affected population. Although virtually every biotech and pharmaceutical company is using genomic technologies in researching new products, whether "personalized medicine" will prove to be a viable business model remains to be seen.

Once medications that target people with particular genotypes are developed, it is not clear how widely they will be adopted. Targeted medications may eliminate the costly trial and error of current prescribing and dosing, but the substantial research and development costs almost certainly will result in more expensive medications. Whether private and public payers will include these therapies on their formularies will depend on several factors, including the condition being treated, the relative improvement in safety and efficacy over standard therapies, and cost. Patient demand produced by direct-to-consumer advertising and provider concerns about potential liability undoubtedly will increase adoption of the new products.

New technologies will also expand the responsibilities of physicians, nurses, pharmacists, and other health care providers to use genetic information in prescribing, dispensing, and administering medications. Professionals not only will need to integrate genetic information into their practices, they also will need to become competent in genetic counseling. In addition, even though genetic testing for medication purposes is more limited in scope than genetic tests for assessment or prediction of health status, the test results will still contain sensitive genetic information. For example, identifying someone as being more difficult or expensive to treat could lead to discrimination in employment or insurance. Consequently, pharmacogenomics could increase the demand for new protections for the confidentiality of health information.

Protection of Genetically Susceptible Individuals

Many regulatory programs specifically require protection of susceptible individuals. For example, the Clean Air Act requires that national ambient air-quality standards be set at a level that protects the most susceptible subgroups within the population. Under this program, the EPA focuses its standard-setting activities on susceptible subgroups such as children with asthma. Recent studies indicate a significant genetic role in susceptibility to air pollution, which may lead to air-quality standards being based on the risks to genetically susceptible individuals. Regulations under other environmental statutes, such as pesticide regulations under the Food Quality Protection Act and drinking water standards under the Safe Drinking Water Act, may likewise focus on genetically susceptible individuals in the future, as might occupational exposure standards promulgated by the Occupational Safety and Health Administration. Likewise, pharmaceutical approvals may require considering and protecting individuals with genetic susceptibilities to a particular drug.

The identification of genetic susceptibilities to chemicals, consumer products, pharmaceuticals, and other materials raises a number of regulatory issues. One issue is the question of the feasibility of protecting genetically susceptible individuals. On the one hand, protecting the most susceptible individuals in society may be extremely costly, and perhaps even infeasible without major, formidable changes in our industrial society. On the other hand, the concept of government regulators leaving the health of some individuals unprotected, who through no fault of their own are born with a susceptibility to a particular product or chemical, also seems politically and ethically infeasible. As more information on individual genetic susceptibility becomes available, regulators and society generally will confront difficult challenges in deciding whether and how to protect the most genetically vulnerable citizens in our midst.

A related set of issues will involve the extent to which we rely on societal regulation versus individual self-help in protecting genetically susceptible individuals. All regulatory programs confront choices between societal regulation and targeting high-risk individuals (Rose 1994), but these choices will be heightened by the identification of genetic susceptibilities to specific products or substances. For example, should products be labeled to warn people with particular genotypes to avoid using the product, just as diet sodas are labeled to warn people with the genetic disease phenylketonuria that the product contains phenylalanine? Should regulators approve for sale pharmaceuticals that are effective only for individuals with compatible genotypes and are ineffective or even hazardous for other people? Under what conditions and with what types of warnings? Will workers with genetic susceptibilities to specific workplace hazards be precluded from working in those jobs, or will they be required to accept personal responsibility for any harms that result? In all these scenarios relying on self-help, how will susceptible individuals discover they carry a particular genetic susceptibility? How will the privacy and confidentiality issues associated with such genetic knowledge be addressed? How well will people understand and adapt their behavior appropriately to information on their genetic susceptibilities? Policymakers, scientists, regulators, and other interested parties will need to address these and other questions raised by new knowledge about genetic susceptibilities.

Generic Regulatory Challenges

Several generic issues will confront all regulatory programs that use toxicogenomic data. One issue will be ensuring that toxicogenomic data are adequately validated. Each agency has its own procedures and criteria for ensuring data quality. In deciding whether and when toxicogenomic data are ready for "prime time" application in formulating federal regulations, agencies must balance the risk of premature use of inadequately validated data versus the harm from unduly delaying the use of relevant data by overly cautious policies. Agencies such as the EPA have been criticized for being too conservative in accepting new types of toxicologic data.

Another trade-off that agencies must face involves whether and when to standardize toxicogenomic platforms and assays (Gallagher et al. 2006). On the one hand, standardization is important in that it facilitates comparison between datasets on different substances and ensures consistent treatment of different substances. On the other hand, standardization runs the risks of prematurely freezing technology before it has fully matured.

A related issue is how regulatory agencies can encourage or require private parties to generate and submit toxicogenomic data. Many product manufacturers are likely to be concerned that toxicogenomic markers may detect biologic effects from their products or emissions at lower doses that may lead to increased regulatory scrutiny. To address such disincentives, agencies have adopted different approaches to encourage data submission. The FDA has adopted an approach under which the voluntary submission of certain types of toxicogenomic data will be for informational purposes only to help regulators and regulated parties better understand toxicogenomic responses, with an assurance that the data will not be used for regulatory purposes. The EPA has adopted an interim policy that it will not base regulatory decisions solely on genomic data, alleviating concerns that a new regulatory requirement may be imposed based solely on a toxicogenomic finding when no other indication of toxicity is present.

LITIGATION

Toxic tort litigation involves lawsuits in which one or more individuals (the plaintiffs) who have been allegedly injured by exposure to a toxic agent sue the entity responsible for that exposure (the defendant) for compensation. Both plaintiffs and defendants are likely to seek to use toxicogenomic data for various purposes in future toxic tort litigation.

Proving Exposure

Many toxic tort claims involving exposures to environmental pollutants fail because the plaintiffs are unable to adequately demonstrate and quantify their exposure to a toxic agent. Individuals exposed to contaminated drinking water, hazardous chemicals in the workplace, or toxic releases from an environmental accident often lack access to objective environmental monitoring data that can be used to quantify their exposures. In such cases, courts often dismiss claims because the plaintiffs are unable to prove sufficient exposure with objective data (Wright

v. Willamette Indus 1996). Some courts have endorsed, in principle, the possibility of using genetic biomarkers (for example, chromosomal aberrations) rather than environmental monitoring data to demonstrate and even quantify exposure (in re TMI litigation, 193 F. 3d 613, 622-623 [3d Cir. 1999] cert. denied, 530 U.S. 1225 [2000]).

Toxicogenomic data may be able to help prove or disprove exposure in appropriate cases. If a particular toxic agent creates a chemical-specific fingerprint of DNA transcripts, protein changes, or metabolic alterations, those biomarkers potentially could be used to demonstrate and perhaps even quantify exposure. Alternatively, a defendant could argue that the lack of a chemical-specific toxicogenomic marker in an individual proves that there was not sufficient exposure. However, a number of technical obstacles and data requirements need to be addressed before toxicogenomic data can be used reliably in this manner. The chemical-specific attribution of the toxicogenomic change would need to be validated, as would the platform used to quantify the changes. The potential variability in expression between cell types and individuals would also need to be addressed. Perhaps most significantly, the time course of toxicogenomic changes during and after exposure would need to be understood to correctly extrapolate an individual's exposure history from after-the-fact measurements of toxicogenomic changes.

Causation

The other major evidentiary challenge that plaintiffs in toxic exposure cases must overcome is to prove causation. Plaintiffs bear the burden of proof to demonstrate both general causation and specific causation. General causation involves whether the hazardous agent to which the plaintiff was exposed is capable of causing the adverse health effect the plaintiff has incurred. Specific causation concerns whether the exposure did in fact cause the health effect in that particular plaintiff. Courts generally consider these questions separately, and both inquiries frequently suffer from a lack of direct evidence, resulting in outcomes that are highly uncertain, speculative, and often unfair. Toxicogenomic data have potential applications for both general causation and specific causation.

General causation determinations are impaired by "toxic ignorance" in which valid scientific studies do not exist for many combinations of toxic substances and specific health end points. The lack of a valid published study evaluating whether the agent to which the plaintiff was exposed can cause the plaintiff's health condition will generally bar tort recovery for failure to demonstrate general causation. Toxicogenomic assays that can reliably be used for hazard identification may provide a relatively inexpensive and quick test result that could be used to fill the gaps in general causation. For example, a gene expression assay that can identify a particular type of carcinogen might be used to classify a chemical as a carcinogen (and hence establish general causation) in the absence of a traditional chronic rodent bioassay for carcinogenicity.

Toxicogenomic data can also play a role in proving or disproving specific causation. Current toxicologic methods are generally incapable of determining whether a toxic agent caused an adverse health effect in a specific individual for all but so-called "signature diseases" that usually have a single cause (for example, mesothelioma and asbestos; diethylstilbestrol and adenocarcinoma). Lacking any direct evidence of specific causation, courts generally adjudicate specific causation based on a differential diagnosis by an expert or based on epidemiologic evidence showing a relative risk greater than 2.0, which suggests that any individual plaintiff's disease was more likely than not caused by the exposure under study. Such methods are very imprecise and prone to under- and overcompensation depending on the facts of the case. A toxicogenomic marker could provide direct evidence of specific causation if an individual who develops a disease is shown to have the specific molecular signature of toxicity attributable to a specific agent.

Duty of Care

Toxic tort litigation involves judgments about the duty of care by an actor who creates risks to those who may be injured by those risks. Toxicogenomic data could affect or shift those judgments about duty of care in a number of con texts. For example, the finding that some members of the population may have a genetic susceptibility that makes them particularly sensitive to a product may impose new duties on the product manufacturer with regard to testing, labeling, and selling that product. Some individuals who alleged they had been harmed by the Lyme disease vaccine Lymerix brought lawsuits claiming that the vaccine manufacturer had a legal duty to warn vaccine users to obtain a genetic test for a polymorphism that allegedly affected the user's propensity to develop serious side effects from the vaccine. The litigation settled before a judgment was issued but likely contributed at least indirectly to the vaccine being removed from the market and was the first of what will likely be a new trend of plaintiffs claiming that a product manufacturer has additional duties to protect individuals genetically susceptible to their products. Alternatively, under the "idiosyncratic defense doctrine," defendants may be able to argue in some cases that they have no duty to protect individuals with a rare genetic susceptibility to a product. Under this line of cases, courts have held that a product manufacturer can be reasonably expected to ensure the safety of "normal" members of the population and not individuals with an unusual susceptibility to the agent in question.

The detection of toxicogenomic changes in exposed individuals using toxicogenomic technologies may also result in lawsuits seeking damages for an increased risk of disease or for medical monitoring. Historically, courts have been reluctant to award damages for an increased risk of disease that has not yet manifested in clinical symptoms, but courts in some states have recognized such a claim if the at-risk individual can sufficiently quantify a substantial increased risk of disease. It is possible that toxicogenomic data could support such a claim. A related type of claim is for medical monitoring, now recognized by more than 20 states, which requires a defendant responsible for a risk-creating activity to pay for periodic medical testing of exposed, at-risk individuals. Toxicogenomic assays could be used to identify at-risk individuals who would be entitled to ongoing medical evaluations, or the assays could serve as a periodic medical test for people who incurred a hazardous exposure.

Damages

Toxicogenomic data may also be relevant in the damages stage of toxic tort litigation. A defendant who is liable for a plaintiff's injuries may seek to undertake genetic testing of the plaintiff to identify potential predispositions to disease that might have contributed to his or her disease or that might otherwise reduce the plaintiff's life expectancy. Either of these findings could reduce the damages the defendant would be ordered to pay to the plaintiff. Although the plaintiff's genetic predispositions to disease may sometimes be pertinent (and may be used to benefit the plaintiff in some situations), there is a danger that defendants will undertake "fishing expeditions" in the plaintiff's genome that may reveal sensitive and private personal information and potentially violate the plaintiff's right not to know.

Legal, Policy, and Ethical Aspects of Toxic Tort Applications

The many potential applications of toxicogenomic data in toxic tort litigation raise a number of scientific, legal, policy, and ethical issues. One central concern is the potential for premature use of toxicogenomic data. Unlike regulatory agencies, which generally consider new types of data cautiously and deliberately, toxic tort litigants are unlikely to show similar restraint. A toxic tort case is a one-time event often involving large stakes that, once filed, tends to move forward expeditiously toward a decision under a court-ordered schedule. Therefore, toxic tort litigants have every incentive to use any available data that may help them prevail, regardless of how well those data have been considered and validated by the scientific community. Premature use of toxicogenomic data should obviously be discouraged, but it is important to note that current scientific evidence on issues in litigation such as causation are often inadequate, and toxicogenomic data have enormous potential to make the resolution of toxic tort litigation more scientifically informed, consistent, and fair.

The reliability of toxicogenomic data introduced in a court proceeding will be evaluated under the standards for admissibility of scientific evidence. In federal courts and many state courts, the evidence will be evaluated under the criteria for scientific evidence announced by the U.S. Supreme Court in the 1993 Daubert decision (Daubert v. Merrell Dow 1993). Under that standard, the trial judge is to serve as a gatekeeper for scientific evidence to ensure that any such evidence presented to a jury is both relevant and reliable. The Supreme Court identified the following four nonexclusive criteria that courts can use to evaluate the reliability of scientific evidence: (1) whether the evidence can and has been empirically tested, (2) whether it has a known rate of error, (3) whether it has been peer reviewed and published, and (4) whether it is generally accepted within the relevant scientific field. These criteria are consistent with general criteria used to validate toxicologic tests and, if applied rigorously, should help ensure against the premature or inappropriate use of toxicogenomic data in toxic tort litigation.

Specifically, a court might want to consider the following factors in deciding whether to admit toxicogenomic data in a toxic tort lawsuit.

a. Has the toxicogenomic response been shown to be associated with or predictive of a traditional toxicologic end point (for example, cancer, toxicity)?

b. Are there data showing that the observed toxicogenomic response is characteristic of exposure to the specific toxic agent at issue, with a similar time course of exposure as experienced by the plaintiff?

c. Have the data used or relied on for making the above determinations been published in peer-reviewed scientific journals?

d. Have one or more other laboratories replicated the same or similar results under similar conditions?

e. Has the toxicogenomic platform used been shown to provide consistent results to the platform used in any other studies relied on?

Ideally, all these questions would be answered affirmatively before toxicogenomic data were introduced into evidence. Given that it is not reasonable to impose greater barriers to the introduction of toxicogenomic data than other types of toxicologic evidence used in toxic tort litigation, data satisfying most of the above criteria would likely be sufficiently reliable to be admitted.

The use of toxicogenomic data in toxic tort litigation raises a series of other issues. For instance, the capability of lay jurors to adequately understand and apply toxicogenomic data in their decision making will present challenges. The potential privacy and confidentiality issues raised by genetic testing of plaintiffs create another set of concerns. Protective orders that protect sensitive information used at trials from being publicly disclosed will be needed to help protect the confidentiality of personal genetic information.

Product manufacturers may have concerns about future liabilities associated with toxicogenomic biomarkers. For example, a manufacturer may sponsor a study that detects a biomarker of unknown toxicologic significance today but that years later may become established as a validated biomarker of toxicity. The use of such data to impose liability retroactively could raise fairness concerns and may deter manufacturers from conducting toxicogenomic studies. At the same time, shielding manufacturers from such liability could create the wrong incentives by deterring them from investigating the risks of their products and taking appropriate mitigation measures and may deprive injured product users from being compensated for their injuries. These countervailing factors demonstrate the complex and sensitive role that potential liability can exert on scientific research and applications of toxicogenomics.

Communication and Education

The increasing scientific capability of making individualized predictions of risk from toxic substances raises the important question of how this information will be communicated to individuals and the public. Such predictions, tailored for the individual, may be years away. But it is still important to communicate with the public in advance about relevant scientific advancements to maintain public support for the science and to help educate members of the public for the day when many of them may have to make personal decisions based on their capacity to understand the customized predictions of the risk they face from one or more toxic hazards. A great deal of research is needed in this field. Among other things, we do not know how much information people want, in what form, their likely comprehension, their likely response, and the degree of variability in different socioeconomic and cultural groups. Nevertheless, some basic risk-communication principles are instructive.

Risk communication has been defined as "an interactive process of exchange of information and opinion among individuals, groups, and institutions" . Thus, the prescription for agencies, media, and others involved in risk communication is to abandon the traditional top-down, sender-based, "public education" model of risk communication (for example, launching a flurry of messages in an attempt to get the public to see things the way experts do). Instead, they should favor an approach that emphasizes greater understanding of the emotional reactions, concerns, and motivations of a segmented public who can seek (or even avoid), process, and evaluate critically the risk information they encounter and who have varying desires and capacities to do so. Indeed, "the degree to which individuals have the capacity to obtain, process, and understand basic health information and services needed to make appropriate health decisions" has become the prime definition of "health literacy" and has been proposed as an essential component of health and risk communication programs.

Thus, there are at least four key issues in risk communication: (1) sufficiency of information; (2) capacity of the individual or society to access, assess, and understand information; (3) emotional responses to risks; and (4) trust in scientific and mass media organizations that oversee communication channels.

It is important to understand that effective risk communication requires multiple messages tailored to a particular audience. People interpret health risks in light of their everyday events and experiences, and the messages must be framed within a familiar context. Health disparities and environmental justice issues are of heightened concern in some communities. In all communities, a person's emotional response to risk, such as worry, fear, anger, and hope, can determine risk perception as well as response to risk. The emotional response to risk is also a key factor in risk acceptability. Better understood and familiar risks may be more acceptable than dreaded, poorly understood risks of a lower magnitude.

Complicating any discussion of risk communication is the public's low level of scientific comprehension, low level of understanding probabilistic information, and low level of understanding basic numerical concepts. Thus, risk communication, especially about predictions of individualized risk from toxic substances, must include upfront efforts designed to help the public improve their health and risk literacy.

There are many dimensions to the translation of toxicogenomic and pharmacogenetic knowledge into health benefits. Research needs to focus on both individual-level and population-level educational and risk communication aspects of translation into medical and public health practice. For example, critical research issues on an individualized level are exemplified by research on genetic risk communication, in formed consent processes, the decision-making process and provider knowledge and awareness of genetics. These research arenas have direct practice implications for genetic education and genetic counseling, interventions incorporating genetic information, patient adherence to screening recommendations, effectiveness of decision supports and aids, and health care provider training.

Researchers and practitioners in the field of health behavior and health education can play a pivotal role in integrating toxicogenomics into practice to improve the public's health. Priority areas that are ripe for further exploration, understanding, and application include the following: (1) public and provider education about genetic information, (2) risk communication and interventions for behavior change, (3) sociologic sequelae of genetic testing, and (4) public health assurance and advocacy. An ecologic perspective should be considered when addressing the educational and communication issues involved in applying toxicogenomics to decrease health risks. Many different types of stakeholders and practitioners should be considered, and, consequently, many levels of intervention and analysis should be pursued.

Conclusions and Recommendations

Because this chapter presents a number of complex issues, the conclusion text precedes the corresponding, numbered recommendations.

It is critical to ensure adequate protections on the privacy, confidentiality, and security of toxicogenomic information in health records. Safeguarding this information will further important individual and societal interests. It will also prevent individuals from being dissuaded from participating in research or undergoing the genetic testing that is the first step in individualized risk assessment and risk reduction. The potential consequences of disclosure of toxicogenomic information are greater with the growth of electronic health records.

There is a lack of comprehensive legislation protecting the privacy, confidentiality, and security of health information, including genetic information. These protections are needed at all entities that generate, compile, store, transmit, or use health information, not just those affected by HIPAA.

1. Address the privacy, confidentiality, and security issues that affect the use of toxicogenomic data and the collection of data and samples needed for toxicogenomic research.

2. Role-based access restrictions should be used for the disclosure of health information in health care settings. Contextual access criteria should be developed and used for the disclosure of health information, pursuant to an authorization, beyond health care settings. Toxicogenomic research

often uses large biorepositories and databases in anonymous, deidentified, linked, or identifiable forms as well as phenotypic data in health records. Inconsistencies between the Common Rule informed consent requirement and the HIPAA Privacy Rule authorization requirement burden and interfere with toxicogenomic research.

3. Consider approaches to harmonize standards for deidentification and informed consent and authorization under the Federal Rule for the Protection of Research Subjects (Common Rule) and the HIPAA Privacy Rule, to minimize unnecessary barriers to research while continuing to protect the privacy and welfare of human subjects.

4. DHHS should explore new approaches to facilitate large-scale biorepository and database research while protecting the welfare and privacy of human subjects.

   Subpopulation groups considered socially vulnerable based on race or ethnicity, income, age, or other factors are at increased risk for discrimination, stigma, and other adverse treatment as a result of individualized toxicogenomic information.

5. In toxicogenomic research, especially involving or affecting socially vulnerable populations, special efforts should be made at community engagement and consultation about the nature, methods, and consequences of the research.

6. To minimize the risk of adverse impacts on socially vulnerable populations from toxicogenomic research and implementation, access to adequate health care for diagnostic and treatment purposes will be critical and should be a priority for funding agencies and legislators.

   The decision to use toxicogenomic testing to learn about one's individual risk should rest with the individual, including risk posed by the workplace setting. Employers have the primary responsibility, under the Occupational Safety and Health Act, to provide a safe and healthful workplace and, under the Americans with Disabilities Act, to provide nondiscriminatory employment opportunities and reasonable accommodations for individuals with disabilities.

7. When toxicogenomic tests to provide individualized risk information have been validated, individuals should be able to learn of their particular risk from workplace exposures without the information being disclosed to their current or potential employer. Upon learning of their individualized risk information they should be able to decide for themselves whether to accept the risk of such employment.

8. Only in extraordinary circumstances, when employing an individual with a risk would create a direct and immediate threat to the individual, cowork ers, or the public, would the employer be justified in excluding an individual from a particular employment based on increased risk.

Toxicogenomic data have many promising applications in regulation and litigation. These data have the potential to help fill many of the scientific uncertainties and gaps regarding exposure, causation, dose response, and extrapolation that currently limit the toxicologic knowledge critical for making sound regulatory and liability decisions.

9. Although caution, scrutiny, and validation are required to protect against premature, inappropriate, and unethical use of toxicogenomic data in regulatory and litigation contexts, care should also be taken to ensure that a higher standard of proof is not imposed for toxicogenomic data relative to other types of toxicologic data used in regulation and litigation.

10. A regulatory agency or court should give appropriate weight to the following factors in deciding whether to rely on toxicogenomic data:

    a. Has the toxicogenomic response been shown to be associated with or predictive of an adverse health outcome (for example, cancer, toxicity)?

    b. Has the specificity and sensitivity of the test been established to be within reasonable bounds?

    c. Are there data showing that the observed toxicogenomic response is characteristic of exposure to the specific toxic agent at issue, with a similar time course and level of exposure as experienced by the plaintiff?

    d. Have the data used or relied on for making the above determinations been published in peer-reviewed scientific journals?

    e. Have one or more other laboratories replicated the same or similar results under similar conditions?

    f. Has the toxicogenomic platform used been shown to provide results consistent with the platforms used in any other studies that were relied on?

Risk communication is an essential component of translating toxicogenomic information into reduced health risks for the public. Currently, the general public, as well as health care practitioners, are ill-equipped to understand and use toxicogenomic information to alter adverse health outcomes.

11. Research is needed on how to communicate toxicogenomic risk information to the public using culturally and psychologically appropriate methods.

12. Educational initiatives are needed for vulnerable subgroups and the general public to raise awareness about toxicogenomic findings that can affect their health.

13. Educational initiatives need to be developed and implemented to prepare the medical and public health workforce to use toxicogenomic information.

Finally, several areas of future research would address some of the issues raised in this chapter. These include the following:

14. Federal agencies should increase their support for research on the issues of ethical, legal, and social implications in applying toxicogenomic technologies, including public attitudes toward individualized risk, social effects of personalized information on increased risks, and regulatory criteria for toxicogenomics.

15. The National Institute of Environmental Health Sciences (or other federal agencies) should develop "points-to-consider" documents that identify and discuss the issues of ethical, legal, and social implications relevant to individual researchers, institutional review boards, research institutes, companies, and funding agencies participating in toxicogenomic research and applications.

5

Food Intolerance and Allergy

Food intolerance or non-allergic food hypersensitivity is a term used widely for varied physiological responses associated with a particular food, or compound found in a range of foods.

Food intolerance is a detrimental reaction, often delayed, to a food, beverage, food additive, or compound found in foods that produces symptoms in one or more body organs and systems, but it is not a true food allergy. A true food allergy requires the presence of Immunoglobin E (IgE) antibodies against the food, and a food intolerance does not.

Food intolerances can be classified according to their mechanism. Intolerance can result from the absence of specific chemicals or enzymes needed to digest a food substance, as in hereditary fructose intolerance. It may be a result of an abnormality in the body's ability to absorb nutrients, as occurs in fructose malabsorption. Food intolerance reactions can occur to naturally occurring chemicals in foods, as in salicylate sensitivity. Drugs sourced from plants, such as aspirin, can also cause these kinds of reactions. Finally, it may be the result of non-IgE-mediated immune responses.

Definitions

Non-allergic food hypersensitivity is the medical name for food intolerance, loosely referred to as food hypersensitivity, or previously as pseudo-allergic reactions. Non-allergic food hypersensitivity should not be confused with true food allergies. Food intolerance reactions can include pharmacologic, metabolic, and gastro-intestinal responses to foods or food compounds. Food intolerance does not include either psychological responses or foodborne illness.

A non-allergic food hypersensitivity is an abnormal physiological response. It can be difficult to determine the poorly tolerated substance as reactions can be delayed, dose-dependant, and a particular reaction-causing compound may be found in many foods.

- Metabolic food reactions are due to inborn or acquired errors of metabolism of nutrients, such as in diabetes mellitus, lactase deficiency, phenylketonuria and favism.

- Pharmacological reactions are generally due to low-molecular-weight chemicals which occur either as natural compounds, such as salicylates and amines, or to food additives, such as preservatives, colouring, emulsifiers and taste enhancers. These chemicals are capable of causing drug-like (biochemical) side effects in susceptible individuals.

- Gastro-intestinal reactions can be due to malabsorption or other GI Tract abnormalities.

- Immunological responses are mediated by non-IgE immunoglobulins, where the immune system recognises a particular food as a foreign body.

- Toxins may either be present naturally in food, be released by bacteria, or be due to contamination of food products. Toxic food reactions are caused by the direct action of a food or substance without immune involvement.

- Psychological reactions involve manifestation of clinical symptoms caused not by food but by emotions associated with food. These symptoms do not occur when the food is given in an unrecognisable form.

Elimination diets are useful to assist in the diagnosis of food intolerance. There are specific diagnostic tests for certain food intolerances.

Signs and Symptoms

Non-IgE-mediated food hypersensitivity (food intolerance) is more chronic, less acute, less obvious in its presentation, and often more difficult to diagnose than a food allergy. Symptoms of food intolerance vary greatly, and can be mistaken for the symptoms of a food allergy. While true allergies are associated with fast-acting immunoglobulin IgE responses, it can be difficult to determine the offending food causing a food intolerance because the response generally takes place over a prolonged period of time. Thus the causative agent and the response are separated in time, and may not be obviously related. Food intolerance symptoms usually begin about half an hour after eating or drinking the food in question, but sometimes symptoms may be delayed up to 48 hours.

Food intolerance can present with symptoms affecting the skin, respiratory tract, gastrointestinal tract (GIT) either individually or in combination. On the skin may include skin rashes, urticaria(hives), angioedema, dermatitis, and eczema. Respiratory tract symptoms can include nasal congestion, sinusitis, pharyngeal irritations, asthma and an unproductive cough. GIT symptoms include mouth ulcers, abdominal cramp, nausea, gas, intermittent diarrhea, constipation, irritable bowel syndrome, and may include anaphylaxis.

Food intolerance has been found to be associated with; irritable bowel syndrome and inflammatory bowel disease, chronic constipation, chronic hepatitis C infection, eczema, NSAID intolerance, respiratory complaints, including asthma, rhinitis and headache, functional dyspepsia, eosinophilic esophagitis and ENT illnesses.

Causes

Reactions to chemical components of the diet are more common than true food allergies They are caused by various organic chemicals occurring naturally in a wide variety of foods, both of animal and vegetable origin more often than to food additives, preservatives, colourings and flavourings, such as sulfites or dyes. Both natural and artificial ingredients may cause adverse reactions in sensitive people if consumed in sufficient amount, the degree of sensitivity varying between individuals.

Pharmacological responses to naturally occurring compounds in food, or chemical intolerance, can occur in individuals from both allergic and non-allergic family backgrounds. Symptoms may begin at any age, and may develop quickly or slowly. Triggers may range from a viral infection or illness to environmental chemical exposure. It occurs more commonly in women, which may be because of hormone differences, as many food chemicals mimic hormones.

A deficiency in digestive enzymes can also cause some types of food intolerances. Lactose intolerance is a result of the body not producing sufficient lactase to digest the lactose in milk; dairy foods which are lower in lactose, such as cheese, are less likely to trigger a reaction in this case. Another carbohydrate intolerance caused by enzyme deficiency is hereditary fructose intolerance.

Celiac disease, an autoimmune disorder caused by an immune response to the protein gluten, results in gluten intolerance and can lead to temporary lactose intolerance.

The most widely distributed naturally occurring food chemical capable of provoking reactions is salicylate, although tartrazine and benzoic acid are well recognised in susceptible individuals. Benzoates and salicylates occur naturally in many different foods, including fruits, juices, vegetables, spices, herbs, nuts, tea, wines, and coffee. Salicylate sensitivity causes reactions to not only aspirin and NSAIDs but also foods in which salicylates naturally occur, such as cherries.

Other natural chemicals which commonly cause reactions and cross reactivity include amines, nitrates, sulphites and some antioxidants. Chemicals involved in aroma and flavour are often suspect.

The classification or avoidance of foods based on botanical families bears no relationship to their chemical content and is not relevant in the management of food intolerance.

Salicylate-containing foods include apples, citrus fruits, strawberries, tomatoes, and wine, while reactions to chocolate, cheese, bananas, avocado, tomato or wine point to amines as the likely food chemical. Thus exclusion of single foods does not necessarily identify the chemical responsible as several chemicals can be present in a food, the patient may be sensitive to multiple food chemicals and reaction more likely to occur when foods containing the triggering substance are eaten in a combined quantity that exceeds the patient's sensitivity thresholds. People with food sensitivities have different sensitivity thresholds, and so more sensitive people will react to much smaller amounts of the substance.

Pathogenesis

The term food allergy is widely misused for all adverse reactions to food. Food allergy (FA) is a food hypersensitivity occurring in susceptible individuals, which is mediated by a classical immune mechanism specific for the food itself. The best established mechanism in FA is due to the presence of IgE antibodies against the offending food. Food intolerance (FI) are all other adverse reactions to food. Subgroups of FI are enzymatic (e.g. lactose intolerance due to lactase deficiency), pharmacological (e.g. reactions against biogenic amines, histamine intolerance), and undefined food intolerance (e.g. against some food additives). As knowledge of mechanisms and causes of food intolerance improve, nomenclature will be updated.[41] There is no worldwide scientific consensus on the pathogenesis of food intolerance.

Food intolerances can be caused by enzymatic defects in the digestive system, can also result from pharmacological effects of vasoactive amines present in foods (e.g. Histamine), among other metabolic, pharmacological and digestive abnormalities. (Pastar & Lipozenice, 2006)

A frequent misconception among the general public is confusion between cow's milk allergy (CMA) and cow's milk intolerance, which is usually intolerance to lactose. There are at least two, and possibly more, distinct pathologies. Hypersensitivity to milk is often broadly classified into immunoglobulin E (IgE)-mediated allergy and non-IgE-mediated intolerance. The immunopathological mechanisms of non-IgE-mediated intolerance in particular remain poorly understood, and this has hindered the development of simple and reliable diagnostics. Adults with non-IgE-mediated intolerance to milk tend to suffer ongoing reactions without the development of tolerance. The precise immunopathological mechanisms of non-IgE-mediated intolerance remain unclear. A number of mechanisms have been implicated, including type-1 T helper cell (Th1) mediated reactions, the formation of immune complexes leading to the activation of Complement, or T-cell/mast cell/neuron interactions inducing functional changes in smooth muscle action and intestinal motility. Food antigens contact the immune system throughout the intestinal tract via the gut associated lymphoid system (GALT), where interactions between antigen presenting cells and T cells direct the type of immune response mounted. Unresponsiveness of the immune system to dietary antigens is termed "oral tolerance" and is believed to involve the deletion or switching off of reactive antigen-specific T cells and the production of regulatory T cells (T reg) that quell inflammatory responses to benign antigens. In the case of IgE-mediated allergies, a deficiency in regulation and a polarisation of specific effector T cells towards type-2 T helper cells (Th2) lead to signalling of B-cells to produce milk protein-specific IgE. Whereas non-IgE-mediated reactions (intolerances) may be due to Th1 mediated inflammation. Dysfunctional T reg cell activity has been identified as a factor in both allergy/ intolerance mechanisms.

Diagnosis

Diagnosis of food intolerance can include hydrogen breath testing for lactose intolerance and fructose malabsorption, professionally supervised elimination diets, and ELISA testing for IgG-mediated immune responses to specific foods. It is important to be able to distinguish between food allergy, food intolerance, and autoimmune disease in the management of these disorders. Non-IgE-mediated intolerance is more chronic, less acute, less obvious in its clinical presentation, and often more difficult to diagnose than allergy, as skin tests and standard immunological studies are not helpful. Elimination diets must remove all poorly tolerated foods, or all foods containing offending compounds. Clinical investigation is generally undertaken only for more serious cases, as for minor complaints which do not significantly limit the person's lifestyle the cure may be more inconvenient than the problem.

The Hemocode Food Intolerance System and Rocky Mountain Analytical Food Allergy Test are unvalidated yet heavily marketed examples of ELISA testing of IgG4 to foods. IgG4 against foods indicates that the person has been repeatedly exposed to food proteins recognized as foreign by the immune system. However, its presence should not be considered a factor which induces intolerance. Food-specific IgG4 does not indicate food allergy or intolerance, but rather a normal physiological response of the immune system after exposure to food components. Although elimination of foods based on IgG-4 testing in IBS patients resulted in an improvement in symptoms, the positive effects of food elimination were more likely due to wheat and milk elimination than IgG-4 test-determined factors. The IgG-4 test specificity is questionable as healthy individuals with no symptoms of food intolerance also test positive for IgG-4 to several foods.

Diagnosis is made using medical history and cutaneous and serological tests to exclude other causes, but to obtain final confirmation a Double Blind Controlled Food Challenge must be performed. Treatment can involve long-term avoidance, or if possible re-establishing a level of tolerance.

The antigen leukocyte cellular antibody test (ALCAT) has been commercially promoted as an alternative, but has not been reliably shown to be of clinical value.

Prevention

There is emerging evidence from studies of cord bloods that both sensitization and the acquisition of tolerance can begin in pregnancy, however the window of main danger for sensitization to foods extends prenatally, remaining most critical during early infancy when the immune system and intestinal tract are still maturing. There is no conclusive evidence to support the restriction of dairy intake in the maternal diet during pregnancy in order to prevent. This is generally not recommended since the drawbacks in terms of loss of nutrition can out-weigh the benefits. However, further randomised, controlled trials are required to examine if dietary exclusion by lactating mothers can truly minimize risk to a significant degree and if any reduction in risk is out-weighed by deleterious impacts on maternal nutrition.

A Cochrane review has concluded feeding with a soy formula cannot be recommended for prevention of allergy or food intolerance in infants. Further research may be warranted to determine the role of soy formulas for prevention of allergy or food intolerance in infants unable to be breast fed with a strong family history of allergy or cow's milk protein intolerance. In the case of allergy and celiac disease others recommend a dietary regimen is effective in the prevention of allergic diseases in high-risk infants, particularly in early infancy regarding food allergy and eczema. The most effective dietary regimen is exclusively breastfeeding for at least 4–6 months or, in absence of breast milk, formulas with documented reduced allergenicity for at least the first 4 months, combined with avoidance of solid food and cow's milk for the first 4 months.

Management

Individuals can try minor changes of diet to exclude foods causing obvious reactions, and for many this may be adequate without the need for professional assistance. For reasons mentioned above foods causing problems may not be so obvious since food sensitivities may not be noticed for hours or even days after one has digested food. Persons unable to isolate foods and those more sensitive or with disabling symptoms should seek expert medical and dietitian help. The dietetic department of a teaching hospital is a good start.

Guidance can also be given to your general practitioner to assist in diagnosis and management. Food elimination diets have been designed to exclude food chemicals likely to cause reactions and foods commonly causing true allergies and those foods where enzyme deficiency cause symptoms. These elimination diets are not everyday diets but intended to isolate problem foods and chemicals. Avoidance of foods with additives is also essential in this process.

Individuals and practitioners need to be aware that during the elimination process patients can display aspects of food addiction, masking, withdrawals, and further sensitization and intolerance. Those foods that an individual considers as 'must have every day' are suspect addictions, this includes tea, coffee, chocolate and health foods and drinks, as they all contain food chemicals. Individuals are also unlikely to associate foods causing problems because of masking or where separation of time between eating and symptoms occur. The elimination process can overcome addiction and unmask problem foods so that the patients can associate cause and effect.

It takes around five days of total abstinence to unmask a food or chemical, during the first week on an elimination diet withdrawal symptoms can occur but it takes at least two weeks to remove residual traces. If symptoms have not subsided after six weeks, food intolerance is unlikely to be involved and a normal diet should be restarted. Withdrawals are often associated with a lowering of the threshold for sensitivity which assists in challenge testing, but in this period individuals can be ultra-sensitive even to food smells so care must be taken to avoid all exposures.

After two or more weeks if the symptoms have reduced considerably or gone for at least five days then challenge testing can begin. This can be carried out with selected foods containing only one food chemical, so as to isolate it if reactions occur. In Australia, purified food chemicals in capsule form are available to doctors for patient testing. These are often combined with placebocapsules for control purposes. This type of challenge is more definitive. New challenges should only be given after 48 hours if no reactions occur or after five days of no symptoms if reactions occur.

Once all food chemical sensitivities are identified a dietitian can prescribe an appropriate diet for the individual to avoid foods with those chemicals. Lists of suitable foods are available from various hospitals and patient support groups can give local food brand advice. A dietitian will ensure adequate nutrition is achieved with safe foods and supplements if need be.

Over a period of time it is possible for individuals avoiding food chemicals to build up a level of resistance by regular exposure to small amounts in a controlled way, but care must be taken, the aim being to build up a varied diet with adequate composition.

Prognosis

The prognosis of children diagnosed with intolerance to milk is good: patients respond to diet which excludes cow's milk protein and the majority of patients succeed in forming tolerance. Children with non-IgE-mediated cows milk intolerance have a good prognosis, whereas children with IgE-mediated cows milk allergy in early childhood have a significantly increased risk for persistent allergy, development of other food allergies, asthma and rhinoconjunctivitis.

A study has demonstrated that identifying and appropriately addressing food sensitivity in IBS patients not previously responding to standard therapy results in a sustained clinical improvement and increased overall well being and quality of life.

Epidemiology

Estimates of the prevalence of food intolerance vary widely from 2% to over 20% of the population. So far only three prevalence studies in Dutch and English adults have been based on double-blind, placebo-controlled food challenges. The reported prevalences of food allergy/intolerance (by questionnaires) were 12% to 19%, whereas the confirmed prevalences varied from 0.8% to 2.4%. For intolerance to food additives the prevalence varied between 0.01 to 0.23%.

Food intolerance rates were found to be similar in the population in Norway. Out of 4,622 subjects with adequately filled-in questionnaires, 84 were included in the study (1.8%) Perceived food intolerance is a common problem with significant nutritional consequences in a population with IBS. Of these 59 (70%) had symptoms related to intake of food, 62% limited or excluded food items from the diet. Tests were performed for food allergy and malabsorption, but not for intolerance. There were no associations between the tests for food allergy and malabsorption and perceived food intolerance, among those with IBS. Perceived food intolerance was unrelated to musculoskeletal pain and mood disorders.

According to the RACP working group, "Though not considered a "cause" of CFS, some patients with chronic fatigue report food intolerances that can exacerbate symptoms."

In 1978 Australian researchers published details of an 'exclusion diet' to exclude specific food chemicals from the diet of patients. This provided a basis for challenge with these additives and natural chemicals. Using this approach the role played by dietary chemical factors in the pathogenesis of chronic idiopathic urticaria (CIU) was first established and set the stage for futute DBPCT trials of such substances in food intolerance studies.

In 1995 the European Academy of Allergology and Clinical Immunology suggested a classification on the basis of the responsible pathogenetic mechanism; according to this classification, non-toxic reactions can be divided into 'food allergies' when they recognize immunological mechanisms, and 'food intolerances' when there are no immunological implications. Reactions secondary to food ingestion are defined generally as 'adverse reactions to food'.

In 2003 the Nomenclature Review Committee of the World Allergy Organization issued a report of revised nomenclature for global use on food allergy and food intolerance, that has had general acceptance. Food intolerance is described as a 'non allergic hypersensitivity' to food.

Uncovering Hidden Food Allergies and Sensitivities

Up to 4 percent of adults and 8 percent of children under the age of 5 suffer from food allergies, which can range in severity from mildly annoying to life threatening. They occur when your immune system mistakenly believes a food, such as peanuts, or a food component, such as lactose or gluten, is dangerous, and produces specific immunoglobulin E (IgE) antibodies to neutralize that substance.

As part of the neutralization process, your body will release histamine as well as other chemicals into your bloodstream anytime you eat the offending food, and it's these chemicals that cause the entire range of allergic symptoms, from a runny nose and rashes to anaphylactic shock.

Reactions to foods can be tricky, however, because it's possible to experience uncomfortable symptoms -- including symptoms you may not associate with the food you eat -- even when a true food allergy is not present.

Food Allergy vs. Food Sensitivity: What's the Difference?

A food allergy is an immune reaction to a specific food. It will occur each and every time you eat that food, even if only a tiny trace passes by your lips. With a food sensitivity, or intolerance, your immune system is not involved. Rather, typically the food will irritate your digestive system because you are unable to properly digest or break down the food.

Unlike with a true food allergy, if you have a food sensitivity you may be able to tolerate small amounts of a food without symptoms, but experience a reaction if larger quantities are consumed.

Food intolerance is incredibly common, impacting a far greater percentage of the population than true food allergies do. While a skin prick test or a blood test designed to detect IgE antibodies can determine if you have a food allergy, linking your symptoms with a specific food in the case of a sensitivity can require some detective work on your part.

Signs and Symptoms of a Food Allergy or Sensitivity

Many of the symptoms of food allergy and sensitivity overlap, including:

- Nausea
- Stomach pain
- Diarrhea

However, a food allergy may also produce rash or hives, itchy skin, wheezing, nasal congestion, swelling of face or throat, dizziness, shortness of breath and trouble breathing, and only true food allergies can produce life-threatening anaphylaxis. With a food intolerance, you're more likely to experience more digestive-type trouble such as gas, cramps, bloating, vomiting and heartburn, as well as headache and even emotional changes, such as irritability or nervousness.

Food sensitivities may also trigger chronic inflammation and changes to your immune system that can cause not only digestive upset but also possibly weight gain, asthma, joint pain, fatigue and even rheumatoid arthritis.

Food sensitivity has also been implicated as a potential cause of leaky gut syndrome, a condition in which damage to the intestinal lining allows bacteria, toxins, undigested food particles and more to "leak" into your bloodstream. This triggers an autoimmune reaction that can lead to bloating, gas, fatigue, joint pain, rashes and even more food sensitivities.

Common Food Allergens and Intolerances

The vast majority (90 percent) of all food allergies are caused by just eight foods:

- Milk
- Egg
- Peanut
- Tree nuts
- Fish
- Shellfish
- Wheat
- Soy

Food intolerances tend to be much more broad, but commonly include lactose, gluten (a protein found in wheat and certain other grains), preservatives and food additives. You can even be sensitive to incredibly common substances like sugar and caffeine.

People with lactose intolerance have a deficiency in lactase, an enzyme that breaks down lactose, or milk sugar, resulting in bloating, stomach pain and often diarrhea when dairy products are eaten. With gluten intolerance, the consumption of gluten in wheat, barley or rye leads to an autoimmune reaction that attacks the lining of the small intestine, resulting in diarrhea, nausea, abdominal pain and, over time, improper nutrient absorption, anemia, osteoporosis and more.

In other cases, the causes of food intolerances are largely unknown and reactions to foods may even fluctuate depending on your levels of physical and emotional stress.

How to Uncover Food Allergy or Sensitivity

Traditional allergy tests such as the IgE RAST blood test or skin prick test can uncover a true food allergy. However, if you're suffering from unexplained symptoms that you think may be related to a food allergy or sensitivity, an elimination diet may be in order.

The first step is to narrow down the foods you think may be causing a reaction. Keeping a precise journal of the foods you eat, along with any symptoms that appear soon after, can help you narrow this down.

Interestingly, often the foods you are sensitive to are those you tend to crave the most. It's not entirely clear why this is, but one theory suggests you can become addicted to histamine or other chemicals that are released by your body's allergic response to a food, causing you to crave more of it.

Another theory suggests that when only a small amount of antigen is present in your body it leads to the creation of large complexes of antibodies that increase symptoms. Food cravings could therefore be your body's way of introducing more antigens into your body to reduce the formation of large antibody complexes, as well as lessen symptoms (in the short-term at least, as ultimately giving in to the food craving will lead to continued symptoms).

Once you've determined which foods may be problematic, eliminate them from your diet and take note of your symptoms. Some people initially feel a worsening of symptoms when removing a sensitive food from their diet, but generally within a week or two your symptoms should improve.

Keep in mind that processed foods often contain hidden derivatives from sensitive foods under names you may not recognize, so you may need to avoid processed foods entirely until you determine which foods (or food additives) are problematic for you.

After two or three weeks, you can then slowly re-introduce the problematic foods, one at a time, into your diet while keeping a journal of symptoms. Foods that trigger a return of your symptoms are those you should avoid. In some cases, by avoiding a food for long enough – a few months to a year or two – the antibodies can actually disappear and you'll be able to go back to eating the food without problems. This is true only with food sensitivities, however. In the case of a true food allergy, the food will need to be avoided for life to avoid a potentially life-threatening reaction.

Food Allergy or Something Else?

It's pretty common to have a reaction to a certain food, but in most cases it's an intolerance rather than a true allergy. Why does it matter? Although they may have similar symptoms, a food allergy can be more serious.

These clues can help you figure out if it is an allergy or intolerance. A doctor can help you know for sure.

Food Allergy

- Usually comes on suddenly
- Small amount of food can trigger
- Happens every time you eat the food
- Can be life-threatening

Food Intolerance

- Usually comes on gradually
- May only happen when you eat a lot of the food
- May only happen if you eat the food often
- Is not life-threatening

Gluten-Free Diet for People with Gluten Allergies or Celiac Disease

Shared Symptoms

A food allergy and an intolerance both can cause:

- Nausea
- Stomach pain
- Diarrhea
- Vomiting

Different Symptoms

When a food irritates your stomach or your body can't properly digest it, that's an intolerance. You may have these symptoms:

- Gas, cramps, or bloating
- Heartburn
- Headaches
- Irritability or nervousness

A food allergy happens when your immune system mistakes something in food as harmful and attacks it. It can affect your whole body, not just your stomach. Symptoms may include:

- Rash, hives, or itchy skin
- Shortness of breath
- Chest pain
- Sudden drop in blood pressure, trouble swallowing or breathing – this is life-threatening.

Common Food Allergies and Intolerances

These triggers cause about 90% of food allergies.

- Peanuts
- Tree nuts (such as walnuts, pecans and almonds)
- Fish
- Shellfish
- Milk
- Eggs
- Soy
- Wheat

The most common food intolerance is lactose intolerance. It happens when people can't digest lactose, a sugar found in milk and dairy. Another kind of intolerance is being sensitive to sulfites or other food additives. Sulfites can trigger asthma attacks in some people.

What about a gluten allergy? While celiac disease -- a long-lasting digestive condition that's triggered by eating gluten -- does involve the immune system, it doesn't cause life-threatening symptoms.

Treatment for Food Allergy

Your doctor can find out if you have an allergy or intolerance. These things may help:

- Keep a diary of the foods you eat and the symptoms you have
- Stop eating some foods to help figure out which one is causing symptoms
- Have allergy tests

If you have a food allergy, you'll need to stop eating the food altogether. If you have a food intolerance, you'll need to avoid or cut back on that food in your diet. For lactose intolerance, you can look for lactose-free milk or take a lactase enzyme supplement.

With a food allergy, you could be at risk for anaphylaxis, a life-threatening reaction. Ask your doctor if you need to carry an Auvi-Q or Epi-Pen (epinephrine shot) that you could give yourself in an emergency.

How to Prevent Symptoms

- Learn which foods – and how much – cause you to have symptoms. Either avoid the food or only have as much as you can without triggering symptoms.

- When you eat out, ask your server about how your meal will be prepared. It may not always be clear from the menu whether some dishes contain problem foods.

- Learn to read food labels and check the ingredients for trigger foods. Don't forget to check condiments and seasonings. They may have MSG or another additive that can cause symptoms.

Difference between a Food Intolerance and Food Allergy?

Food reactions are common, but most are caused by a food intolerance rather than a food allergy. A food intolerance can cause some of the same signs and symptoms as a food allergy, so people often confuse the two.

A true food allergy causes an immune system reaction that affects numerous organs in the body. It can cause a range of symptoms. In some cases, an allergic food reaction can be severe or life-threatening. In contrast, food intolerance symptoms are generally less serious and are limited to digestive problems.

If you have a food allergy, even a tiny amount of the offending food can cause an immediate, severe reaction. Digestive signs and symptoms may include nausea, vomiting, cramping and diarrhea. Other signs and symptoms can include a tingling mouth, hives, and swelling of the lips, face, tongue and throat. A life-threatening allergic reaction known as anaphylaxis can cause breathing trouble and dangerously low blood pressure. If you have a food allergy, you'll need to avoid the offending food entirely.

Food intolerance symptoms generally come on gradually and don't involve an immune system reaction. If you have a food intolerance, you may be able to eat small amounts of the offending food without trouble. You may also be able to take steps that help prevent a reaction. For example, if you have lactose intolerance, you may be able to drink lactose-free milk or take lactase enzyme pills that aid digestion (such as Lactaid).

Causes of food intolerance include:

- **Absence of an enzyme needed to fully digest a food.** Lactose intolerance is a common example.

- **Irritable bowel syndrome.** This chronic condition can cause cramping, constipation and diarrhea.

- **Food poisoning.** Toxins such as bacteria in spoiled food can cause severe digestive symptoms.

- **Sensitivity to food additives.** For example, sulfites used to preserve dried fruit, canned goods and wine can trigger asthma attacks in sensitive people.

- **Recurring stress or psychological factors.** Sometimes the mere thought of a food may make you sick. The reason is not fully understood.

- **Celiac disease.** Celiac disease has some features of a true food allergy because it does involve the immune system. However, symptoms are mostly gastrointestinal, and people with celiac disease are not at risk of anaphylaxis. This chronic digestive condition is triggered by eating gluten, a protein found in wheat and other grains.

If you have a reaction after eating a particular food, see your doctor to determine whether you have a food intolerance or a food allergy.

If you have a food allergy, you may be at risk of a life-threatening allergic reaction (anaphylaxis) — even if past reactions have been mild. Learn how to recognize a severe allergic reaction and know what to do if one occurs. You may need to carry an emergency epinephrine shot (EpiPen, Twinject) for emergency self-treatment.

If you have a food intolerance, your doctor may recommend steps to aid digestion of certain foods or to treat the underlying condition causing your reaction.

Food Allergies

Food allergy is the body's response to a perceived invader. Culprits are certain food proteins like fish, seafood, nuts or eggs: the immune system misreads these proteins as 'foreign'. The response is to release antibodies intended to disable the foreign invaders - and the usual consequence is inflammation: tissue swelling, itching and fluid accumulation.

With true food allergy - second and subsequent occurrences are progressively more severe leading to the possibility of Anaphylaxis - a life-threatening condition where throat tissues become swollen, blocking breathing.

Prevalence of Food Allergy

Food Allergy: Sudden Onset Responses: 1% of people

- Is rare ~ 1% of people
- Is an immediate abnormal reaction to a food protein
- It is triggered by the immune system
- Severe cases are called Anaphylaxis and can be life-threatening

For the traditionally accepted view of food allergy (sudden onset and severe) it is estimated that around 3% of children and about 1% of adults are affected. These responses are generally brought on by the allergens (proteins) in eggs, milk, nuts, soy, corn, fish and shellfish. They can also be found in food additives like colours and preservatives.

Because of their sudden onset and the severity of symptoms, this type of food allergy is usually detected in very young babies, when they are first introduced to the food. Subsequent encounters with the allergen cause greater and greater reactions and severity - leading to the extreme **Anaphylactic shock**.

Prevalence of Food Intolerance

Food Intolerance: Delayed onset responses - up to 75%

- Is very common - up to 75% of people
- Is a slow-onset abnormal reaction to a protein or other food
- It may involve the immune system - as with Gluten intolerance
- Long-term cases progress to diseases like arthritis, depression or dia*betes*

Confusion arises - because many cases of **Food Intolerance** involve the immune system - so must be classified as 'allergic' responses. These are suffered by a much greater percentage of people - up to 75% (three in four people).

Many doctors like to classify conditions like dairy intolerance and gluten intolerance as non-allergic reactions. However the sufferers' blood tests always indicate immune response activity to the food proteins in question.

Food Allergies: Sudden Onset Responses

Food Allergy symptoms are sudden onset (within a few moments of eating the food) and severe. These can be:

- Sudden onset respiratory symptoms: wheezing, gasping, coughing and asthma
- Sudden onset skin problems: hives, rashes
- Sudden onset gastro-intestinal symptoms: nausea, vomiting, babies' projectile vomiting

The extreme reaction is **Anaphylactic shock** a life-threatening event: the tissues of the mouth and throat swell up obstructing breathing. Of course if you suffer this level of reaction to a food you would have known about it from a very young age - and will be managing it properly.

Food Intolerance: Delayed Reactions

However there are other allergic reactions which take much longer to appear - because the reaction is to a partially digested food molecule (e.g. a food protein like gluten or casein). **Food intolerance is the inability to fully digest a food.**

Of course this partly digested food only occurs well down in the gut - many hours after eating, typically in the small intestine where absorption happens. So *that is where the immune reaction takes place* - disrupting the digestive process.

In the case of Gluten - actual damage can be suffered by the small intestine - holes are torn in the lining - giving rise to a condition known as Leaky Gut. Once the gut is "leaky" the troublesome protein fragments spill into the bloodstream - where they should never be. They then are free to travel anywhere in the body and cause immune responses like autoimmune disease: rheumatoid arthritis, thyroiditis, diabetes type 1 and others.

Allergic Symptoms Masking Other Diseases

If you have a Food Allergy, chances are you were diagnosed in early childhood and have avoided the offending food ever since. However, allergy symptoms can mask other disease which have similar symptoms. It's important to relieve the symptoms of allergies so other disorders can be recognised.

Imagine if measles were confused with an allergic rash, or breathlessness caused by blood clot in the lung (pulmonary embolism) was misread as an allergic symptom in an allergic patient?

By correctly identifying allergens and keeping the symptoms under control the person is much more likely to be diagnosed quickly and correctly when other ailments arise. In addition, keeping symptoms under control allows children to participate in playtime and sports – an important activity for early childhood learning and development of social skills.

Test for Food Allergies

Food allergies are usually identified in babies when they are first introduced to a particular food. A food allergy is an immediate immune response caused by the body "misreading" a food protein as an enemy or toxic substance. Because they are fairly dramatic, sudden onset allergic responses are usually easily identified very early in life.

Doctors may use Blood tests, "patch testing" or other types of Clinical Testing to get actual proof. But the most reliable method is the Elimination Diet.

Food Intolerance: Delayed Onset Responses

Many adverse reactions caused by foods are delayed for hours or even days, making it difficult to connect the food with the response. This is *classic food intolerance* - because the reaction is happening much lower down in the gut - in the small intestine. And even when absorbed - the subsequent inflammatory reaction can take a day or more to show.

How to Treat Food Allergies

Treatment is generally one of three approaches:

- Avoidance of the allergen
- Symptom management with medication
- Auto-immune therapy – a series of vaccinations: extracts of the allergen are injected across many months in an attempt to de-sensitise the individual
- Anaphylactic shock requires emergency treatment – usually an injection of adrenaline to maintain breathing

Lactose Intolerance

Lactose intolerance is defined as "the inability to digest the milk sugar lactose" - due to a deficiency of the enzyme lactase. Prevalence of Lactose Intolerance is

75% - or three in four people. In certain ethnic groups it's even higher: up to 90% of African Americans and 80% in some Europeans. Most sufferers are unaware - leaving them vulnerable to illnesses like malabsorption and depression.

Prevalence of Lactose Intolerance

The US National Institute of Diabetes and Digestive and Kidney Diseases (NIDDK) states that 75% of the world's population has Lactose Intolerance. That is, three quarters of all people have difficulty digesting lactose. In certain ethnic groups it is even higher:

- Lactose intolerance affects 3 in 4 of all people
- Lactose intolerance affects more than 90% of African Americans
- In addition - Lactose intolerance affects ~ 80 - 90% of people of Chinese descent

Common symptoms like **Stomach Bloating** and **Flatulence** and **Diarrhea** and **Irritable Bowel Syndrome** are caused by lactose intolerance. Therefore milk and milk products are not suitable foods for the majority of people.

Symptoms of Lactose Intolerance

There can be many symptoms of Lactose Intolerance. They include:

Gastrointestinal symptoms:

- Nausea and vomiting
- Bloated stomach
- Diarrhea
- Gurgling stomach, flatulence
- Irritable Bowel Syndrome - regular bouts of diarrhea then constipation

Malabsorption symptoms- lack of nutrients:

- Low iron levels - or Anaemia
- Low calcium and other mineral levels
- Loss of bone density - brittle bonesm
- Osteoporosis
- Mood swings, the 'blues' and depression

Causes of Lactose Intolerance

Lactos intolerance occurs due to lactose deficiency, which may be generic or environmentally induced. The symptoms appear due to low levels of the enzyme lactose in devodenuar living. Lactose (diasaccharide found in milk and dairy products) cannot be directly absorbed through the wall of the small intestine into the blood. In the absence of the enzyme lactose (which can break it down to harmless glucose and galactose) it passes intail into the colon. Bailesia in the colon metabolise lactose and the resulting fermentation produces copious amount of gas (a mixure of hydrogen, CO_2 and methane) that causes diverse abdominal symptoms. The unabsorbed sugars and fermentation products also raise the osmotin pressure of the colon, causing an increased flow of water into bowels leading to diarrhoea.

How to Treat Lactose Intolerance

The simple **strategy** for Lactose Intolerance is to *remove Lactose from your diet.* The simplest solution is to switch to a Dairy-free diet (which is also Lactose-Free). Track your symptoms as you switch foods. The symptoms for Lactose intolerance can be the same as those for **Fructose intolerance** and **Wheat Sensitivity** and **Gluten Sensitivity** - so they often get mixed up.

Lactase enzyme additives: Some people take an enzyme preparation before eating dairy products. These products provide the enzyme your body does not have for digesting Lactose. So to eat dairy products you must take the lactase before every meal. However because lactose intolerance often goes together with casein allergy (milk protein sensitivity) - the ingestion of milk in any form causes adverse reactions.

Lactose Intolerance is not a 'disease' - so it does not need to be 'cured'. It is people eating foods they cannot fully digest. Like other food intolerances - it is genetic- like having curly hair, blue eyes or freckles. We cannot change our genes. But we can choose to eat appropriate foods which we can easily digest.

People with Lactose Intolerance get sick because the human body is simply *not equipped to process milk* after weaning. Even the cow's calf - which does have the right biological equipment to process cow's milk loses the ability to do so upon weaning.

Other mammalian milk: Lactose intolerance also applies to other mammalian milks like goat milk, sheep's milk, buffalo milk etc.

Dairy Sensitivity

The inability to fully digest milk products (dairy sensitivity) affects more than 70% of all people. Both lactose and casein (milk protein) can be troublesome. Dairy sensitivity is increasing due to strong marketing of milk products - and the mass production of foods containing low-cost dairy derivatives.

A. **Lactose:** Recent evidence indicates that up to **75%** of the world's population is Lactose Intolerant to some extent*. That is, three quarters ( ) of all people have difficulty digesting lactose. (Pribila et al, 2000)

B. **Casein:** Other people (~ 3%) are allergic to Casein (the protein found in milk). This is usually detected in babies by projectile vomiting, colic or other troublesome conditions but can be undiagnosed till later.

Dairy sensitivity is responsible for symptoms like bloating, flatulence, diarrhea and Irritable Bowel Syndrome in millions of people and appears more frequently now that thousands of processed foods contain dairy derivatives. Heavily subsidised dairy farming now produces millions of tons of milk derivitives - delivering low cost ingredients for manufacturers.

Symptoms of Dairy Sensitivity

A. **Lactose sensitivity**:

- Nausea, diarrhea, bloating, flatulence, Irritable Bowel Syndrome
- Malabsorption - nutrient deficiency like anaemia, bone density loss
- Mood swings, depression

B. **Casein allergy:**

- Common allergy symptoms like itchy skin, eczema
- Leaky Gut - malabsorption: bone density loss, anaemia
- Respiratory problems like coughing, asthma, sinusitis.

The symptoms of Dairy sensitivity can be confused with those of Fructose sensitivity and Gluten sensitivity, they all overlap. All food sensitivity symptoms - if left untreated - become worse with age.

How to Identify Dairy Sensitivity

A. **Lactose:** Some people get clinical tests including the Hydrogen breath test and stool acidity tests. Unfortunately most *clinical* testing for food sensitivity is not reliable. Breath tests are amongst the least trusted methods. However it easily identifies Lactose Sensitivity.

B. **Casein** allergy is often apparent with very young babies when they are first given cow's milk formula. But the sensitivity can remain undiagnosed until adulthood. Symptoms including hives, eczema, projectile vomiting, asthma, diarrhea and frequent infections like coughs and colds.

How One Gets Dairy Sensitivity?

A. **Lactose:** It's all in the genes. If your ancestry is Northern European (e.g. Dutch or Scandinavian), the chance of Lactose Sensitivity is only 25%. If not then generally you have a 75% chance of being Lactose Intolerant.

B. **Casein:** Milk protein allergy is also an inherited gene.

Comments: If you are Dairy sensitive and have children - then you have already passed on the gentic material to them. Make sure you alert them to the possibility so they can make well-informed health choices.

Dairy sensitive people improve dramatically on a Dairy-free diet. But it's best to get accurate answers before changing your diet.

How to Treat Dairy Sensitivity?

A. **Lactose:** The obvious and simple strategy for managing Dairy Sensitivity is to go Dairy-free. However because Dairy sensitivity has many of the same symptoms as Fructose sensitivity, you need to keep some notes. Track how your symptoms improve (or not) on a changed diet.

B. **Casein:** Obviously a dairy-free diet is the answer. However for Casein there needs to be more vigilance as Casein is now included in thousands of processed foods. Get into the habit of reading labels for dairy and milk derivatives.

Wheat Sensitivity and Wheat Allergy

Wheat Sensitivity

Wheat Sensitivity (or Wheat Intolerance) is a *delayed onset reaction* caused by gluten, contained in wheat, rye, barley, oats and other grains. It affects around 15% of people - or 1 in 7 people. (Pietzak, 2012)

Wheat Allergy

Wheat allergy is the very *rare severe sudden onset* allergic reaction to a certain protein component of wheat. It affects less than 0.5% of the population. However when most people speak of wheat allergy they may be referring to wheat (gluten) intolerance.

Difference between Wheat Allergy and Wheat Sensitivity

The main difference is *the response time - the time lapse between eating the food and the reaction.*

Wheat Allergy is a very rare sudden-onset response to a protein found in wheat. Most food allergies are discovered very early in life - e.g. when babies are first given solid foods. However - when people speak of wheat allergy - they are likely referring to the *inability to digest Gluten* - or Gluten intolerance. Gluten is a very complex protein found in wheat and other grains.

Wheat Sensitivity (including Gluten Sensitivity) is a common type of Food Intolerance. Despite claims that food intolerances do not involve the immune system - Gluten Sensitivity certainly does - because Gluten's breakdown proteins are seen as 'foreign' by the immune system.

This sets up inflammation and disrupts processes - and leads to a medical condition known as Leaky Gut Syndrome. Consequences are Chronic inflammatory disorders like Rheumatoid Arthritis, gastro-intestinal problems, heart disease, Depression, Eczema, low blood iron levels and others. Sometimes the first indication of Wheat or Gluten Sensitivity is diagnosis of low iron or anaemia.

Symptoms of Wheat Allergy and Wheat Sensitivity

Wheat Allergy: **Sudden onset** symptoms - vomiting, asthma, nausea, coughing, hives etc.

Wheat Sensitivity: frequently delayed reactions - hours later - up to 2 or 3 days later:

- Bloated stomach and Flatulence and Diarrhea, constipation etc.
- Constant infections like colds, 'flu, mouth ulcers, thrush
- Asthma, coughing, bronchitis

- Headaches, sinus pain and migraines
- Arthritis, back ache, "Restless legs syndrome"
- Skin rashes, Eczema, Psoriasis, itching flaky skin
- Chronic fatigue, lethargy
- Mood swings, cravings or Depression

How One Gets Wheat Sensitivity?

Wheat Sensitivity like **any Food Sensitivity - is genetic**. It's in your genes! Just like having brown eyes or freckles - you got it from your parents and grandparents. Also - if you have children – you have already passed on those genes to your sons and daughters. So make sure you **learn all about food intolerance** - so you can share the information with the family.

Agriculture - including the growing of grain crops (like wheat and barley) has only been practised for around ten thousand (10,000) years. Compared to how long humans have been eating other foods (e.g. digestion-friendly meat, fish, vegetables and fruits) - two and a half million years (2,500,000) - that's a very short time.

Our bodies have not evolved as fast as our ability to produce Modern Foods. In fact our capacity to grow grain crops like Wheat, Corn and rye has far outstripped our digestive system's development. That is, we do not yet have all the necessary *biological equipment* to process these proteins: the Glutens and other proteins. And that is why we experience food sensitivity!

Gluten is one of the largest and most complicated molecules we eat. Unfortunately it damages the small intestine - leading to Leaky Gut Syndrome - and from there to dozens of chronic inflammatory diseases.

How to Test for Wheat Allergy or Wheat Sensitivity?

Temporary treatment: Some people choose to *treat the symptoms* of Wheat sensitivity (or other food sensitivity) with medications like anti-histamines or supplements. But this gives only a few hours relief - and it means you have to keep buying and taking medications your whole life - and keep getting their side effects.

Permanent treatment: Choose the natural no-drug solution. The most preferable option is to *go to the source of the problem* - and simply remove it. That is - *identify your food intolerance* and then substitute that food for another delicious food.

Fructose Sensitivity

- Fructose Malabsorption may now be more common due to increased consumption of sugars
- Hereditary Fructose Intolerance (HFI) is rare - but can be serious if left undiagnosed

- Both lead to malabsorption illnesses - and both are easily treated by avoiding Fructose.

Hereditary Fructose Intolerance (HFI) is quite rare (less than one in 10,000). It is inherited (genetic) so you have it for life. HFI is an inborn error of fructose metabolism caused by deficiency of the enzyme aldolase B. The individuals suffering from HFI do not show any symptoms untill they ingest fructose, sucrose or sorbitol. Once fructose is ingested lack of aldolase B leads to accumulation of frutose-1-phosphate. This has undesirable impact on gluconeogenesis and regeneration of adenosiac triphsphate (ATP). HFI may include the symptoms such as vomitting, jaundice hypoglycemia, hemorrhage, hepatomegaly, hyperuricemia and kidney failure in extreme cases. HFI is an autosomal recessive condition caused by mutations in the ALDOB gene. The metabolic consequences of HFI may lead to death in infants and children. HFI in itself is not a clinically threatening condition but improper diagnosis often aggravates the condition. A positive diagnosis requires a stool test (DNA test) from your doctor.

Fructose Malabsorption is very common. Up to one in three people or 33% has some level of sugar sensitivity - most commonly to Fructose. However around half of these people may show no symptoms at all - until later in life. Fructose is found in some fruits and vegetables, and thousands of processed foods like soft drinks and confectionery.

Most sensitivity to sugars like lactose, fructose and sorbitol is undiagnosed, but can be responsible for unexplained stomach bloating, diarrhea and intestinal distress in millions. These sugars are used extensively in manufactured foods due to their sweetening power and low cost.

Difference between Two Types of Fructose Sensitivity

Hereditary Fructose Intolerance (HFI) is a rare genetic condition where the enzyme for breaking down Fructose is not produced. If you discover you have fructose sensitivity - you need to rule out HFI by seeing your doctor for a DNA test. With HFI it is vital to observe a very strict Fructose-free diet. Otherwise there is risk of serious disease including liver failure.

Fructose malabsorption on the other hand is much more common and affects about 30% of people. It especially affects young people who have many soft drinks per week including soda and mixers. With Fructose Malabsorption special cells (epithelial cells) on the surface of the intestine are not available to break down the fructose sugars.

Symptoms of Fructose Sensitivity

- Gastro-intestinal distress: flatulence, bloating, diarrhea
- Tiredness, Chronic fatigue
- Malabsorption issues: low iron (anaemia), osteoporosis or other nutrient deficiency

- Sugar cravings
- Poor skin, nails and hair
- Irritable Bowel Syndrome

How One Gets Fructose Sensitivity?

Blame the parents! Food Intolerance is genetic – so you got it from your parents and grandparents. A very small percentage of people have the hereditary Fructose Sensitivity (less than 1 in 10,000 people.)

Most Fructose sensitivity is the Malabsorption type. It may be somewhat self-imposed by our modern sugar-heavy diets. Humans have not yet evolved the biological equipment to cope with such high sugar consumption.

How to Test for Fructose Intolerance?

The hydrogen or H_2 breath test is often used. However many doctors now regard this test as unreliable. The doctor may also use stool analysis to check for HFI. If you find you are Fructose-sensitive it is vital to rule out HFI as there may be serious health issues.

However the simplest, most reliable and accurate test is the Elimination Diet.

How to Treat Fructose Sensitivity

A Fructose-free or low-sugar diet is the best treatment - and the best management - forlife. This is easy if you know which foods contain fructose - but many processed foods contain added Fructose under aliases like 'corn syrup'. You need a guide.

Fructose is present in many fruits and vegetables and thousands of processed foods, supplements and medications.

The uncommon HFI (Hereditary Fructose Intolerance) cannot be cured. For this a strict Fructose-free Diet must be maintained in the long term.

The much more common Fructose Malabsorption cannot be cured either. But it is much easier to manage. Using a journal and monitoring yourself, you will find a threshold level that is easy to live with. That is - you will be able to eat some Fructose without suffering symptoms.

It is important to keep a journal of food eaten and symptoms on a daily basis, until you come to know your body's limits. A Journal lets you discover your threshold of sensitivity - so you can eat some sweet foods without suffering symptoms.

Yeast Sensitivity (e.g. candida)

Up to one in three people suffers from Yeast Sensitivity - recurring yeast or fungal infections including thrush or tinea. Studies show that the cause of Yeast Sensitivity is a depressed immune system - often due to another underlying food intolerance - like Gluten or Dairy. Solving the underlying food intolerance cures the Yeast Sensitivity.

Yeast infection is extremely common. Up to one in three or 35% of people have yeast infections at any time. It is usually a strong indication that you have *another food intolerance* - one of the main intolerances.

Yeast (candida or other fungal) infections can appear as thrush (in babies and adults), as rashes and as tinea, jock itch and ringworm. Yeasts and other fungals are everywhere in the air we breathe and the foods we eat.

When you are not eating right for your body - Yeast and other fungal infections come back again and again. But with a little careful attention to the foods you eat - you can stop the recurrences and be free of them permanently. A temporary Yeast-free diet is an essential part of the healing - but it is just the first step in a two step process.

Many people misunderstand what a Yeast-free diet means and simply cut out bread and other yeast-raised foods. However a Yeast-free diet needs a little more attention and gives great results.

Symptoms of Yeast Sensitivity

Yeast infection carries the widest spectrum of symptoms of any food sensitivity:

- Skin problems like rashes and ringworm
- Genital fungal infections like thrush (candida albicans)
- Gastro-intestinal problems: Flatulence, Stomach Bloating, Constipation and Diarrhea
- Lethargy (extreme tiredness and lack of energy)
- Halitosis - bad breath
- Headaches - and bad taste in the mouth
- Breathing difficulties - Coughing, asthma
- Mood swings, memory loss, Depression

Many of these are the same as symptoms of other intolerances like Dairy, Gluten and Fructose. So be careful not to jump to conclusions. To differentiate among intolerances use the Journal Method.

How to Identify Yeast Sensitivity?

Although clinical testing is available it is generally inconclusive. Types of testing include blood tests and tissue swabs among others. However - the most useful indicator that you have Yeast sensitivity is *your history of yeast infections*: vaginal, ear or throat infections, jock itch, tinea, ringworm or other fungal infection.

Yeast (fungal) infections flourish when your immune system is under stress. This can be caused by a course of anti-biotics, or an illness. However - one source of immune system stress that is frequently overlooked is *some other underlying food intolerance*.

How One Gets Recurring Yeast?

The repeated appearances of *candida*, *tinea* or other fungal infection usually indicate a compromised immune system. Anything that weakens the immune system can trigger a yeast infection: repeated courses of antibiotics or hormonal changes. . . but read on:

Food intolerance stresses your immune system

However the most likely cause of recurring yeast infections is another *underlying food* intolerance like Gluten intolerance, or Fructose Malabsorption or Dairy intolerance. While your body battles one or more of these intolerances - your immune defences are impaired. So you have lower resistance to all kinds of infections: bacterial, viral and fungal (yeast).

If you suffer from regular infections of any type - you probably have untreated food intolerance. The way to get well permanently is to find out your food intolerance using the Journal Method.

How to Treat Candida?

The most effective way to be free of recurring Yeast infections *permanently* is:

STEP ONE :   Get rid of the Yeast infection:

      a. A prescription anti-fungal medication from your doctor - along with

      b. A Yeast-free diet for 2 - 3 weeks (no longer)

STEP TWO :   Find out your *other underlying food intolerance* (Journal Method) so you will never get candida again!

This two-pronged approach works well to rid your body of the yeast overgrowth.

Using a Yeast-Free Diet and a prescription anti-fungal from your doctor - you should be free of the yeast overgrowth within a week or two. That is STEP ONE achieved.

STEP TWO is to find out your *other underlying food intolerance* - the one that causes the repeat performances of *candida!*

Remember - a Yeast-free diet is always *a temporary measure* until your body recovers. Once the *candida* overgrowth is under control you can start the investigation of your other food intolerance. The trickiest thing about a yeast-free diet is knowing about 'hidden' yeast in foods and drinks. You need to 'starve' the yeast organism so it can no longer flourish in your body.

Yeast Infections and Your Immune System

The Candida yeast organism is normally kept in check by the human immune system. But sometimes, particularly when the immune system is compromised - yeasts will multiply rapidly and overwhelm our systems leading to a variety of unpleasant symptoms – collectively known as *candidiasis* or yeast infection.

Candida is opportunistic. That is, it jumps in and takes over when your immune defences are down - as with food intolerance like Dairy intolerance or Gluten intolerance. It can also strike following hormonal changes: as with hormone therapy, pregnancy or the contraceptive pill. Repeated courses of antibiotics can also be a trigger.

Nightshade Vegetable Sensitivity

Some people react badly to Nightshade Vegetables - meaning they are unable to digest them fully. These foods are only recently introduced to the Western diet from South America - so they fall into the category of "Modern Foods". . . those which cause the symptoms of food intolerance.

Nightshades are a diverse group of foods, herbs, shrubs and trees. It is actually the common name used to describe over 2,800 species of plants, many with very different properties and constitutions. The most famous food members of the nightshade vegetables group include potatoes, tomatoes, many species of sweet and hot peppers, eggplant, tomatillos (*Physallis ixocapra*) tomarillos (*Cyphomandra betacea*), pepimos (*Solanum muricatum*). These vegetables contain saporins, alkaloids and lectins which are not harmful to most of the people. But some persons are very sensitive to these components and they should avoid the nightshades in their regular diet.

There can be many symptoms of Nightshade Sensitivity. They overlap with the symptoms of other food intolerances like Gluten intolerance and Dairy intolerance - especially when these latter sensitivities have already caused Leaky Gut.

Gastrointestinal symptoms

- Nausea and indigestion
- Bloated stomach
- Diarrhea
- Gurgling stomach, flatulence
- Irritable Bowel Syndrome - regular bouts of diarrhea then constipation

Malabsorption symptoms- lack of nutrients

- Low iron levels - or Anaemia
- Low calcium and other mineral levels
- Loss of bone density - brittle bones
- Osteoporosis
- Arthritic Stiff or painful joints or back ache
- Headaches
- Mood swings, the 'blues' and depression

How do Nightshade Vegetables Cause Leaky Gut?

Nightshades contain alkaloids which are poisonous in large amounts. But they also contain saponins. Depending on the quantity eaten, the effect of saponins in these foods can damage the gut - tearing tiny holes in the tissue lining. This leads to a condition called Leaky Gut - and from there to inflammatory disease. Saponins in these foods have evolved to protect the plant from being decimated by insects. Their action is to dissolve the cell membranes of predatory insects so they die.

Unfortunately this same effect - damage to cell membranes - can also be suffered by mammals (like us!) frequently in the small intestine. The result is a gut lining that develops holes and allows the passage of foreign - often toxic - substances into our bloodstream - making us ill and condition is referred to as Leaky Gut. In addition some of this group of vegetables (e.g. potatoes) also contain lectins which cause additional gut damage in large amounts in some people. Remember - the effects of nightshade vegetables depend on the quantity eaten. Overindulgence - as with any 'modern food' may lead to problems.

How One Gets Nightshade Sensitivity?

Nightshade Vegetable Sensitivity - like all food intolerance - is genetic. You got it from your parents, grandparents and other ancestors - it's in your genes! If your cultural heritage is South American your chance of being Nightshade sensitive is low - because Nightshades are native to this continent. However they were only recently added to the Western diet (around 400 years ago - very recently in anthropological terms). That's why many of us do not have the biological equipment to fully digest these plants.

Nightshade Sensitivity is genetic - so if you have children - you may have already passed on those genes to your sons and daughters. So make sure you alert your children possibility. Being well informed allows them to make good choices for their health.

If you have Nightshade Sensitivity - you will improve dramatically by identifying which vegetable is the problem. You will not be sensitive to all Nightshades.

Gluten Sensitivity and Celiac (Coeliac) Disease

Difference between Celiac Disease and Gluten Sensitivity

Celiac Disease is defined as a positive result to a biopsy of the small intestine - damaged villi (structures which assist absorption).

Gluten sensitivity is defined as any sensitivity to Gluten - and includes Celiac Disease. Gluten sensitivity is a broad term which includes all kinds of sensitivity to Gluten. A very small proportion of Gluten intolerant people will test positive for Celiac Disease, and so are called Celiacs (less than 0.5% of the population).

But most Gluten sensitive people return negative or inconclusive results upon Celiac testing. The correct term for these people is Non-Celiac Gluten Sensitive (NCGS) and may be as many as ~15% of all people or 1 in 7.

The most accurate and effective way to identify NCGS is to use a Journal - an Elimination Diet.

Celiac Disease (CD) was the first type of Gluten sensitivity ever recognised. A special test was designed in the 1940s to observe whether the small intestine was damaged. it is called a biopsy and uses a tiny section of intestinal tissue.

Although Celiac testing is still used in many clinics as a first test for Gluten sensitivity, it only picks up the small percentage of Gluten-sensitive people who are Celiac. It misses the NCGS patients. Consequently this latter group is poorly diagnosed and misses out on discovering the simple and drug-free cure of a **Gluten-free Diet** for a dramatic recovery.

What is Gluten and which foods have it?

Gluten is a highly complex protein that occurs in four main grains: Wheat, rye, barley and oats. It is present in all types of Wheat grain like whole grain wheat, wheat bran, spelt, triticale and others.

This means Gluten is also present in all baked foods that are made from these grains: bread, pies, cake, breakfast cereals, porridge, cookies, pizza and pasta. There are thousands of processed foods which contain Gluten.

Gluten is one of the most complex proteins consumed by man. It is a very large molecule relative to other food molecules and for that reason is difficult for the human digestive system to break down. Problems begin when it reaches the small intestine. In sensitive individuals Gluten actually tears holes in the lining of the gut, creating Leaky Gut Syndrome. This allows foreign particles (and whatever else is in the gut, including bacteria) into the bloodstream. Of course that sets the body's immune system on 'high alert' - resulting in your symptoms.

Prevalence of Celiac Disease and Gluten Sensitivity

Around 0.5% of the world's population is Celiac. This means ~1 in 200 people. However new evidence shows *Non-Celiac Gluten Sensitivity (NCGS) is around 30 times more prevalent*. Up to 15% of people or 1 in 7 are Gluten Sensitive and suffer the same symptoms. These are people who test negative or inconclusive for Coeliac Disease. The most accurate and clinically effective way to identify NCGS is the Elimination Diet – or Journal Method.

All Gluten sensitive people improve dramatically on a Gluten-Free diet. Diagnosis of Gluten sensitivity in elderly patients is disproportionately high - because it is misdiagnosed and under-diagnosed by doctors. The symptoms of both Non-Coeliac Gluten Sensitivity (NCGS) and Coeliac Disease (CD) become worse with age if left undiagnosed.

Symptoms of Celiac disease and Gluten Sensitivity?

The symptoms for Gluten sensitivity are varied and usually have a delayed onset - up to 2 or 3 days later. This is why they are traditionally difficult for doctors to diagnose. They can be any combination of these:

- Gastro-intestinal: stomach bloating & pain, diarrhea, flatulence, constipation etc.
- Neurological: headache, memory loss, behavioural difficulties, depression
- Immune: poor resistance to infection, mouth ulcers
- Inflammatory disease: arthritis, colitis, thyroiditis etc.
- Skin rashes, eczema, psoriasis, itching flaky skin
- General: food cravings, tiredness, chronic fatigue, unwell feeling
- Infertility, miscarriage or difficulty conceiving
- 'Failure to thrive' in children - from poor absorption of nutrients

How to Test for Gluten Sensitivity?

Temporary treatment: Some people choose to *treat the symptoms* of Gluten sensitivity with medications like anti-histamines, pain relief or supplements. But this gives only a few hours relief - and it means you have to keep buying and taking medications your whole life - plus keep getting their side effects.

Permanent treatment: Choose the natural no-drug solution. We believe it's much better to *go to the source of the problem* - and simply remove it. That is - *identify your food intolerance* and then substitute that food for another delicious food.

All Gluten sensitivity is easily and accurately identified by an Elimination Diet (Journal Method).

However many people turn to blood tests as a first resort, expecting it will be quicker and more accurate. Unfortunately most testing for Gluten sensitivity is not reliable. DNA (stool) testing brings accurate results. Most of these tests are looking for markers of Celiac disease (blood tests and intestinal biopsy).

The prevalence of Celiac Disease is just a tiny fraction of Gluten sensitivity. Celiac Disease (CD) was the first type of Gluten sensitivity for which a diagnostic testing procedure was devised - way back in the 1940s. Although that same type of Celiac testing is still used in many clinics as a first test for Gluten sensitivity, it only picks up the small percentage of Gluten-sensitive people who are Celiac.

This old-fashioned test misses the Non-Celiac Gluten Sensitive patients. Therefore this latter group is poorly diagnosed and never gets to take advantage of the brilliant and free-of-drugs remedy - the Gluten-Free diet. Once on the right diet these people would begin getting well within days.

How One Gets Celiac Disease or Gluten Sensitivity?

Gluten sensitivity - both NCGS and Coeliac Disease is 'in the family', or genetically inherited. Indicators are European or Anglo-Celtic ancestry. If you are Gluten intolerant, then up to 10% of the immediate family will also be affected, even if they don't yet have any symptoms. Could this be you?

Some Gluten sensitivity is identified in children. But for others, it is not until much later in life that Gluten sensitivity is actually suspected. Frequently it is triggered by some 'life event' - like divorce, a death in the family, job loss or serious illness. One indicator can be persistently low iron levels or anaemia.

How to Treat Celiac Disease and Gluten Sensitivity?

No drugs or therapies are needed to treat Gluten sensitivity. The best treatment is to substitute all Gluten bearing foods in your diet for life . . . a Gluten-free diet. However it is not wise to jump to conclusions about your food intolerance. The best way to investigate your symptoms and get the right answer is by using a Journal - like the Detection Diet Journal.

While a Gluten-free Diet does mean avoiding things which contain Gluten - fortunately thousands of new and delicious Gluten-free products become available with every passing month. To eat Gluten-free with confidence - read all food labels and understand the traps and pitfalls.

We don't view Celiac - or Gluten sensitivity as a 'disease'. It is when people eat foods they cannot fully digest - foods which are inappropriate for them. So you don't need a cure, just a different diet. Gluten sensitivity is genetic – it's the way we are. Like having blue eyes, brown skin or freckles.

For your freckles you stay out of the sun. For your Gluten sensitivity, you avoid Gluten. After just a few weeks on a gluten-free diet symptoms diminish or disappear completely. Many Gluten sensitive people report feeling better than they have for years - once on the right diet. There is also a great deal of research evidence that they will be avoiding chronic disease later in life.

6

Estrogens and Antiestrogens in Food

Phytoestrogens are plant-derived xenoestrogens functioning as the primary female sex hormone (see estrogen) not generated within the endocrine system but consumed by eating phytoestrogenic plants. Also called "dietary estrogens", they are a diverse group of naturally occurring nonsteroidal plant compounds that, because of their structural similarity with estradiol (17-β-estradiol), have the ability to cause estrogenic or/and antiestrogenic effects.

Their name comes from the Greek phyto = plant and estrogen, the hormone which gives fertility to the female mammals. The word "estrus" -Greek οίστρος- means sexual desire and "gene" -Greek γόνο- is "to generate"). It has been proposed that plants use the phytoestrogens as part of their natural defence against the overpopulation of the herbivore animals by controlling the male fertility.

The similarities, at molecular level, of estrogens and phytoestrogens allow them to mildly mimic and sometimes act as antagonists of estrogen. Phytoestrogens were first observed in 1926, but it was unknown if they could have any effect in human or animal metabolism. In the 1940s, it was noticed for the first time that red clover (a phytoestrogens-rich plant) pastures had effects on the fecundity of grazing sheep. Researchers are exploring the nutritional role of these substances in the regulation of cholesterol, and the maintenance of proper bone density post-menopause. Evidence is accruing that phytoestrogens may have protective action against diverse health disorders, such as prostate, breast,bowel, and other cancers, cardiovascular disease, brain function disorders and osteoporosis, though there is no evidence to support their use in alleviating the symptoms of menopause.

Phytoestrogens cannot be considered as nutrients, given that the lack of these in diet does not produce any characteristic deficiency syndrome, nor do they participate in any essential biological function.

Analytical methods are available to determine phytoestrogen content in plants and food.

Structure

Phytoestrogens mainly belong to a large group of substituted natural phenolic compounds: the coumestans, prenylflavonoids and isoflavones are three of the most active in estrogenic effects in this class. The best-researched are isoflavones, which are commonly found in soy and red clover. Lignans have also been identified as phytoestrogens, although they are not flavonoids. Mycoestrogens have similar structures and effects, but are not components of plants; these are mold metabolites of Fusarium, a fungus that is frequently found in pastures as well as in alfalfa and clover. Although mycoestrogens are rarely taken into account in discussions about phytoestrogens, these are the compounds that initially generated the interest on the topic.

Mechanism of Action

Phytoestrogens exert their effects primarily through binding to estrogen receptors (ER). There are two variants of the estrogen receptor, alpha (ER-α) and beta (ER-β) and many phytoestrogens display somewhat higher affinity for ER-β) compared to ER-α.

The key structural elements that enable phytoestrogens to bind with high affinity to estrogen receptors and display estradiol-like effects are:

- The phenolic ring that is indispensable for binding to estrogen receptor
- The ring of isoflavones mimicking a ring of estrogens at the receptors binding site
- Low molecular weight similar to estrogens (MW=272)
- Distance between two hydroxyl groups at the isoflavones nucleus similar to that occurring in estradiol
- Optimal hydroxylation pattern

In addition to interaction with ERs, phytoestrogens may also modulate the concentration of endogenous estrogens by binding or inactivating some enzymes, and may affect the bioavailability of sex hormones by depressing or stimulating the synthesis of sex hormone-binding globulin (SHBG).

Emerging evidence shows that some phytoestrogens bind to and transactivate peroxisome proliferator-activated receptors (PPARs). *In vitro* studies show an activation of PPARs at concentrations above 1 µM, which is higher than the activation level of ERs. At the concentration below 1 µM, activation of ERs may play a dominant role. At higher concentrations (>1 µM), both ERs and PPARs are activated. Studies have shown that both ERs and PPARs influence each other and therefore induce differential effects in a dose-dependent way. The final biological effects of genistein are determined by the balance among these pleiotrophic actions.

Ecology

These compounds in plants are an important part of their defense system, mainly against fungi.

Phytoestrogens are ancient naturally occurring substances, and as dietary phytochemicals they are considered as co-evolutive with mammals. In the human diet, phytoestrogens are not the only source of exogenous estrogens. Xenoestrogens (novel, man-made), are found as food additives and ingredients, and also in cosmetics, plastics, and insecticides. Environmentally, they have similar effects as phytoestrogens, making it difficult to clearly separate the action of these two kind of agents in studies done on populations.

Food Sources of Phytoestrogens

According to a study by Canadian researchers about the content of nine common phytoestrogens in a Western diet, foods with the highest relative phytoestrogen content were nuts and oilseeds, followed by soy products, cereals and breads, legumes, meat products, and other processed foods that may contain soy, vegetables, fruits, alcoholic, and nonalcoholic beverages. Flax seed and other oilseeds contained the highest total phytoestrogen content, followed by soybeans and tofu. The highest concentrations of isoflavones are found in soybeans and soybean products followed by legumes, whereas lignans are the primary source of phytoestrogens found in nuts and oilseeds (e.g. flax) and also found in cereals, legumes, fruits and vegetables.

Phytoestrogen content varies in different foods, and may vary significantly within the same group of foods (e.g. soy beverages, tofu) depending on processing mechanisms and type of soybean used. Legumes (in particular soybeans), whole grain cereals, and some seeds are high in phytoestrogens. A more comprehensive list of foods known to contain phytoestrogens includes: soybeans and soy products, tempeh linseed (flax), sesame seeds, wheatberries, fenugreek, oats, barley, beans, lentils, yams, rice, alfalfa, mung beans, apples, carrots, pomegranates, wheat germ, rice bran, lupin, kudzu, coffee, licorice root, mint, ginseng, hops, bourbon, beer, fennel and anise.

An epidemiological study of women in the United States found that the dietary intake of phytoestrogens in healthy post-menopausal Caucasian women is less than one milligram daily.

Health Risks and Benefits

In human beings, phytoestrogens are readily absorbed, circulate in plasma and are excreted in the urine. Metabolic influence is different from that of grazing animals due to the differences between ruminant versus monogastric digestive systems.

In the last few years, there has been a great deal of research into the possible beneficial effects of phytoestrogens in both diabetes and coronary heart disease.

Males

A 2010 meta-analysis of fifteen placebo-controlled studies said that "neither soy foods nor isoflavone supplements alter measures of bioavailable testosterone concentrations in men." Furthermore, isoflavone supplementation has no effect on sperm concentration, count or motility, and leads to no observable changes in testicular or ejaculate volume.

A soy phytoestrogen-rich diet can substantially reduce testosterone levels in male rats in laboratory studies, while possibly having protective benefits against prostate cancer.

Females

There are conflicting studies, and it is unclear if phytoestrogens have any effect on the cause or prevention of cancer in females. Epidemiological studies showed a protective effect against breast cancer. In vitro studies concluded that females with current or past breast cancer should be aware of the risks of potential tumor growth when taking soy products, as they can stimulate the growth of estrogen receptor-positive cells in vitro. The potential for tumor growth was found related only with small concentration of genistein, and protective effects were found with larger concentrations of the same phytoestrogen. A 2006 review article stated the opinion that not enough information is available, and that even if isoflavones have mechanisms to inhibit tumor growth, in vitro results justify the need to evaluate, at cellular level, the impact of isoflavones on breast tissue in females at high risk for breast cancer. Recent epidemiologic studies suggest that consumption of soy estrogens is safe for patients with breast cancer, and may decrease mortality and recurrence rates. A Cochrane Review of the use of phytoestrogens to relieve the vasomotor symptoms of menopause (hot flashes) demonstrated that there was no evidence to suggest any benefit to their use. It has been reported that phytoestrogens such as genistein may help prevent photoaging in human skin, and also promote formation of hyaluronic acid.

Infant Formula

Some studies have found that some concentrations of isoflavones may have effects on intestinal cells. At low doses, genistein acted as a weak estrogen and stimulated cell growth; at high doses, it inhibited proliferation and altered cell cycle dynamics. This biphasic response correlates with how genistein is thought to exert its effects.

Some reviews express the opinion that more research is needed to answer the question of what effect phytoestrogens may have on infants, but their authors did not find any adverse effects. Multiple studies conclude that there are no adverse effects in human growth, development, or reproduction as a result of the consumption of soy-based infant formula compared to conventional cow-milk formula. While it should be noted that all infant formulas are inferior to human milk, soy formula presents no more risk than cow-milk formula. One of these studies, published at the *Journal of Nutrition*, concludes that:

"Comprehensive literature reviews and clinical studies of infants fed SBIFs [soy-based infant formulas] have resolved questions or raise no clinical concerns with respect to nutritional adequacy, sexual development, neurobehavioral development, immune development, or thyroid disease. SBIFs provide complete nutrition that adequately supports normal infant growth and development. FDA has accepted SBIFs as safe for use as the sole source of nutrition"

Clinical guidelines from the American Academy of Pediatrics state: "although isolated soy protein-based formulas may be used to provide nutrition for normal growth and development, there are few indications for their use in place of cow milk-based formula. These indications include (a) for infants with galactosemia and hereditary lactase deficiency (rare) and (b) in situations in which a vegetarian diet is preferred."

Ethnopharmacology

In some countries, phytoestrogenic plants have been used for centuries in the treatment of menstrual and menopausal problems, as well as for fertility problems. Plants used that have been shown to contain phytoestrogens include Pueraria mirifica, and its close relative, kudzu, Angelica, fennel and anise. In a rigorous study, the use of one such source of phytoestrogen, red clover, has been shown to be safe, but ineffective in relieving menopausal symptoms (black cohosh is also used for menopausal symptoms, but does not contain phytoestrogens. Panax Ginseng contains phytoestrogens and has been used for menopausal symptoms.

Estrogen: Functions and Synthesis

Estrogens (alternate spellings: oestrogens or œstrogens) are a group of steroid compounds, named for their importance in the estrous cycle, and functioning as the primary female sex hormone.

Estrogens are used as part of some oral contraceptives, in estrogen replacement therapy of postmenopausal women, and in hormone therapy for transsexual women.

Like all steroid hormones, estrogens readily diffuse across the cell membrane; inside the cell, they interact with estrogen receptors.

Table 6.1: Foods high in phytoestrogens content

Phytoestrogen food sources	Phytoestrogens content (µg/100g)
Flax seed	379380
Soy beans	103920
Soy nuts	68730.8
Tofu	27150.1
Tempeh	18307.9
Miso paste	11197.3
Soy yogurt	10275
Soy protein powder	8840.7
Sesame seed	8008.1
Flax bread	7540

Contd...

Table 6.1-Contd...

Phytoestrogen food sources	Phytoestrogens content (µg/100g)
Multigrain bread	4798.7
Soy milk	2957.2
Hummus	993
Garlic	603.6
Mung bean sprouts	495.1
Dried apricots	444.5
Alfalfa sprouts	441.4
Pistachios	382.5
Dried dates	329.5
Sunflower seed	216
Chestnuts	210.2
Olive oil	180.7
Almonds	131.1
Cashews	121.9
Green bean	105.8
Peanuts	34.5
Onion	32
Blueberry	17.5
Corn	9
Coffee, regular	6.3
Watermelon	2.9
Milk, cow	1.2

Table 6.2 : Total phytoestrogen and lignan content in vegetables, fruits, nuts and drinks

Food items	Lignan content (µg/100g)	Total phytoestrogen (µg/100g)
Vegetables		
Soy bean sprouts	2.2	789.6
Garlic	583.2	603.6
Winter squash	113.3	113.7
Green beans	66.8	105.8
Collards	97.8	101.3

Contd...

Table 6.2-Contd...

Food items	Lignan content (µg/100g)	Total phytoestrogen (µg/100g)
Broccoli	93.9	94.1
Cabbage	79.1	80
Fruits		
Dried prunes	177.5	183.5
Peaches	61.8	64.5
Strawberry	48.9	51.6
Raspberry	37.7	47.6
Watermelon	2.9	2.9
Nuts and other legume seeds		
Pistachios	198.9	382.5
Chestnuts	186.6	210.2
Walnuts	85.7	139.5
Cashews	99.4	121.9
Hazel nuts	77.1	107.5
Lentils	26.6	36.5
Beverages		
Wine, red	37.3	53.9
Tea, green	12	13
Wine, white	8	12.7
Tea, black	8.1	8.9
Coffee, decaf	4.8	5.5
Beer	1.1	2.7
Other		
Black bean souce	10.5	5330.3
Black licorice	415.1	862.7
Bread, rye	142.9	146.3

Types of Estrogen

The three major naturally occurring estrogens in women are estradiol, estriol, and estrone. In the body these are all produced from androgens through actions of enzymes.

- From menarche to menopause the primary estrogen is 17β-estradiol. In postmenopausal women more estrone is present than estradiol.
- Estradiol is produced from testosterone and estrone from androstenedione.
- Estrone is weaker than estradiol.

A range of synthetic and natural substances have been identified that also possess estrogenic activity. Synthetic substances of this kind are known as xenoestrogens, while natural plant products with estrogenic activity are called phytoestrogens.

Estrogen Production

Estrogen is produced primarily by developing follicles in the ovaries, the corpus luteum, and the placenta. Follicle-stimulating hormone (FSH) and luteinizing hormone (LH) stimulate the production of estrogen in the ovaries. Some estrogens are also produced in smaller amounts by other tissues such as the liver, adrenal glands, and the breasts. These secondary sources of estrogen are especially important in postmenopausal women.

Synthesis of estrogens starts in theca interna cells in the ovary, by the synthesis of androstenedione from cholesterol. Androstenedione is a substance of moderate androgenic activity. This compound crosses the basal membrane into the surrounding granulosa cells, where it is converted to estrone or estradiol, either immediately or through testosterone. The conversion of testosterone to estradiol, and of androstenedione to estrone, is catalyzed by the enzyme aromatase.

Estrogen Functions

While estrogens are present in both men and women, they are usually present at significantly higher levels in women of reproductive age. They promote the development of female secondary sex characteristics, such as breasts, and are also involved in the thickening of the endometrium and other aspects of regulating the menstrual cycle. In males estrogen regulates certain functions of the reproductive system important to the maturation of sperm and may be necessary for a healthy libido.

Estradiol levels vary through the menstrual cycle, with levels highest just before ovulation.

Structural

- promote formation of female secondary sex characteristics
- stimulate endometrial growth
- increase uterine growth
- maintenance of vessel and skin
- reduce bone resorption, increase bone formation

Protein synthesis

- increase hepatic production of binding proteins

Coagulation

- increase circulating level of factors 2,7,9,10, antithrombin III, plasminogen
- increase platelet adhesiveness

Lipid

- increase HDL, triglyceride, fat depositition
- decrease LDL

Fluid balance

- salt and water retention

Gastrointestinal tract

- reduce bowel motility
- increase cholesterol in bile

Cancer

- About 80% of breast cancers, once established, rely on supplies of the hormone estrogen to grow: they are known as hormone-sensitive or hormone-receptor-positive cancers. Suppression of production in the body of estrogen is a treatment for these cancers.

Studies have found better correlation between sexual desire and androgen levels than for estrogen levels.

In studies involving mice and rats, it was found that lung function may be improved by estrogen. In one study involving 16 animals, female mice that had their ovaries removed to deprive them of estrogen lost 45 percent of their working alveoli from their lungs. Upon receiving estrogen, the mice recovered full lung function.

Dietary Estrogens have Little Effect on Cancer Risk

Phytoestrogens are found in a wide range of foods including dairy products, soy foods, cereals, fruits, vegetables, nuts, seeds, coffee and tea. Previous studies have suggested dietary phytoestrogen intake is associated with increased breast cancer risk and reduced colorectal cancer risk in women. The results from earlier studies were hampered, however, by limited data about phytoestrogen content in food.

In a study, reported in the American Journal of Clinical Nutrition, researchers assigned phytoestrogen values to nearly 11,000 foods following chemical analyses. For the first time, phytoestrogen values were assigned to animal products.

Unlike plants, which themselves contain phytoestrogens, phytoestrogens are generated by the digestion of animal products like meat and dairy products by microbes in the gut, the researchers explain.

Phytoestrogen consumption was estimated for cancer-free adult participants in the European Prospective Investigation into Cancer and Nutrition - Norfolk

(EPIC-Norfolk). EPIC-Norfolk participants, recruited between 1993 and 1997, filled out a diet diary for a week and provided information about age, height, weight, smoking, aspirin use, menopausal status, and family history of cancer among other things.

Cancers that developed within 12 months of study recruitment were identified from a cancer registry totaling 244 breast cancers, 221 colorectal cancers, and 204 prostate cancers. The diets and other relevant information from those who developed cancer were compared to information from other participants (controls) who did not develop cancer.

The study concluded that phytoestrogen intake is not associated with incidence of breast or prostrate cancer. However, phytoestrogens found in some dairy products and egg may be associated with the risk of prostrate cancer and colon cancer in women.

"The results of the present study do not suggest that anyone should alter their phytoestrogen intake, in part because the majority of the associations between phytoestrogen intake and cancer risk were not significant," the doctoral candidate wrote in an email.

"It is worth noting that phytoestrogen intake within an Asian-style diet is more than ten-fold greater than in Western diets, without evidence of an increase in cancer risk," she added.

Because phytoestrogen consumption is on the rise in Britain, the authors urge further monitoring because "the relation between phytoestrogen and cancer may change over time."

Ten Ways to Lower Estrogen Toxic Load

High estrogen levels and problems eliminating it are well known to result in prostate and breast cancer. Estrogen is a problem for men as well as women due to multiple factors, especially the huge amounts of chemical estrogens we are exposed to in our daily lives in the form of cosmetics, shampoo, plastic containers and bottles, personal care products, pesticides and animal hormones.

Apart from these man-made environmenatal sources of estrogen our body also suffers from the deletrious effects of estrogen on account of ineffective metabolism in our body. This may lead to poor body conposition, inhibits weight loss and also aggravates the risk of prostrate and breast cancer. Over exposure to estrogen affects every human being regardless of age and gender.

Studies show that genetics and obesity contribute to about 30 percent of the cancers that affect the sex organs (breast, prostate, ovarian), but the cause of the remaining 70 percent is still unclear. It is likely due to chemical estrogen exposure and problems with metabolism due to diet and a sedentary lifestyle. The solution is to live a lifestyle that both detoxifies and minimizes exposure to chemical estrogens. Adopting certain changes in lifestyle may help in minimizing the exposure to chemical estrogen. These changes include:

1) Improve Gastrointestinal Health

2) Improve Diet

3) Decrease Body Fat

4) Use Phytoestrogens To ImproveEstrogen Detoxification

5) Stop Testosterone From Turning into Estrogen

6) Improve Estrogen Metabolism

7) Ensure Complete Elimination

8) Supplement With Essential Nutrients

9) Watch What You Drink

10) Limit Chemical Estrogen Exposure

Estrogen: The Basics

Estrogen is a hormone that is produced primarily in the ovaries in women and in the testes in men. For men, it plays an important role in sperm production and bone maintenance. Estrogen is also produced by other tissues in both men and women, including fat and the brain.

The amount of estrogen needed by men to support these functions is very small, and men tend to have excess estrogen in their systems for two reasons. First, an enzyme called aromatase that is found in tissues throughout the body will turn testosterone into estrogen. Aromatase is found in body fat meaning that men with more fat will produce more aromatase and therefore have higher estrogen levels and lower testosterone. The good news is you can block aromatase by eating or supplementing with nutrients that do this naturally. There are also drugs that inhibit aromatase that are used to prevent breast and prostate cancer, but it's best to take the natural route without consuming synthetic drugs.

Secondly, men have excess estrogen because of the chemical estrogens in the environment, such as BPA and phthalates. BPA is a petroleum based chemical that mimics estrogen in the body and studies have shown that it affects endocrine response in the body in humans and animals. For example, one study in the journal Toxicology Letters found that BPA exposure led to lower testosterone and poor sexual function in both men and rats because it inhibited the production of androstenedione—the hormone from which testosterone is produced.

Phthalates are another chemical estrogen that are used in plastics and many personal care products such as shampoo and lotion. They contribute to excess estrogen levels and need to be detoxified as safely and quickly as possible in order to minimize the damage they have on tissues in the body. Just as you can inhibit aromatase with proper nutrition, you can also give the body the nutrients it needs to detoxify excess estrogen safely from the body.

Foods and Supplements Essential to Lower Estrogen in Women

In women estrogenic hormones are responsible for the growth and development of female sexual characteristics. Estrogen is a group of chemical hormones that are abundant in women of reproductive age. It is produced in ovaries, adrenal glands, and fat tissue. In women estrogen functions by circulating in the bloodstream and binds to estrogen receptors on cells in targeted tissue affecting the breasts, uterus, brain, bone, liver, heart, and others. It also regulates various other metabolic processes, including bone growth and cholesterol levels. So as you can see estrogen is very important to the female body function. However as the female body changes, the estrogen level changes as well. It increases, which puts a woman's health and wellness at risk.

Improve Gastrointestinal Health

Poor gastrointestinal health can inhibit excretion of unwanted estrogen from the body and promote its reabsorption. A healthy gut with dietary fiber in the form lignan, such as flaxseeds, can bind to estrogen in the digestive tract so that it will be excreted from the body. Dietary fiber also reduces the amount of an enzyme (called B-glucouronidase) that uncouples or breaks apart bound estrogen that is on its way out of the body. When the estrogen breaks free in the large intestine, it re-enters circulation and is not removed from the body. This is a bad situation.

The solution is to eat adequate fiber and include lignans in the diet, including flax, leafy greens, and bran. Eat oat, rye, and barley if you are not on a gluten-free diet. A probiotic is essential because it will increase the good bacteria in the gut and support neurotransmitter function.

Improve Diet with Low Carb, High-Protein, Omega-3 Fats

A diet that is low in simple carbs and high in vegetable carb sources will help you detoxify estrogens and provide adequate fiber. To avoid excess estrogen, you need to manage insulin because doing so is better for body composition. A persistently high insulin produces a poor endocrine profile that can inhibit estrogen detoxification.

Getting your carbs from vegetable and fruit sources will provide the lignans and fiber needed for gut health and increase antioxidant levels, which can abolish free radicals that are produced by estrogen. Omega-3 fats, which are found in fish, is recommended for estrogen metabolism. This means it helps the body to metabolize estrogen.

A high protein diet will produce a better body composition for most people. Plus, low protein diets have been shown to decrease activity of something called cytochrome P450 that detoxifies estrogen. The amino acids lysine and threonine have been shown to support liver function and since estrogen is metabolized by the liver, it is thought that these proteins can help get rid of estrogen from the body. Lysine and threonine are found in meat, fish, beans, eggs, and some seeds (sesame, fenugreek). Sesame seeds also provide fiber and fenugreek helps lower the insulin response to carbs, making both good additions to your diet.

Decrease Body Fat

The more fat you have, the more estrogen you will have because fat tissue increases levels of the aromatase enzyme that turns testosterone to estrogen. Decreasing body fat and building lean mass are key to cancer prevention and estrogen detox.

Another way to protect the tissues from circulating estrogen is to keep it bound to sex hormone binding globulin (SHBG). When it is bound to SHBG, estrogen is not available to bind with cellular receptors and won't have its estrogenic impact. Flaxseed hulls are especially good at increasing SHBG, as well as inhibiting aromatase.

Use Phytoestrogens

Include foods with phytoestrogens in your diet because they will take natural and chemical estrogens out of play in the body. Phytoestrogens are plant-based compounds that can bind to estrogen receptors, but they have about 1/1000th of the effect on the body as real or chemical estrogen. When phytoestrogens bind to estrogen receptors they basically take up the parking sport of the true estrogen, and keep it from exerting its effect.

Lignans and isoflavones are the main phytoestrogens, and in addition to binding with estrogen receptors, they can increase SHBG levels, which protects the body by binding to estrogen. They decrease aromatase, which prevents testosterone turning into estrogen.

The best phytoestrogens to include in the diet are flax, sesame, leafy greens, kudzu, alfalfa, clover, licorice root, and legumes. Greens, flax, and sesame can be easily added to the diet, and the others can be supplemented to support estrogen detoxification.

Block Aromatase and Stop Testosterone from Turning into Estrogen

Blocking aromatase is key for getting rid of estrogen because it plays the main role in producing estrogen in men. If aromatase is present, there are two chances for estrogen to be produced in the body. First, the hormone androstenedione will be turned into testosterone unless aromatase is present in which case it will be turned into estrogen. Then, aromatase will turn testosterone into estrogen as well.

Nutrients that have a proven effect on aromatase include selenium, melatonin, zinc, green tea, and citrus flavonones-substances found in orange and grapefruit rinds along with tomato skins. You can include these in your diet and take a supplement for best results.

We know aromatase inhibitors work because there are numerous studies demonstrating their influence. One of the most illuminating is a review that found that women who took a combination of zinc, folic acid, acetyl-l-carnitine, and had adequate omega-3s improved fertility and sexual health. Flax and lignans were also part of the diet. This study tells us that estrogen detox is not a simple endeavor. Rather, it's a lifestyle that includes the ideal diet with additional nutrient supplementation to inhibit aromatase, boost SHBG, and reduce the ratio of estrogen.

Improve Estrogen Metabolism by Promoting the C-2 Pathway

Promoting the C-2 pathway of estrogen metabolism is probably the most important thing you can do to prevent cancer. The first step of estrogen elimination is for enzymes to initiate metabolism by joining the estrogen molecule. This will happen at either the 2-carbon position or the 16-carbon position of the molecule, which determines the pathway the estrogen will head down.

The C-2 pathway produces very weak estrogenic activity and is termed "good" estrogen. In contrast, the C-16 pathway produces robust estrogenic activity and promotes tissue damage that leads to cancer. There's also a C-4 pathway, that is not good, but its role is small and for simplicity sake you only need to know that you want to avoid it as well.

Research shows that women whose estrogen is metabolized down the C-16 pathway have significantly greater rates of breast cancer than those whose C-2 pathway dominates. In one large scale study of premenopausal women, those who metabolized estrogen predominantly via the C-2 pathway were 40 percent less likely to develop breast cancer during the five-year study.

Key nutrients for supporting the C-2 pathway are EPA fish oils, phytoestrogens, and of special importance, B vitamins and a substance called DIM. The B vitamins, particularly B6, B12, and folic acid promote the C-2 pathway. B6 is also known to decrease gene activity once estrogen is bound to a receptor, meaning this vitamin can inhibit cell damage and cancer development.

DIM is a compound found in cruciferous vegetables such as broccoli and cauliflower. It is often taken in supplement form because you would need to eat large quantities of these vegetables daily in order to provide sufficient DIM to have an effect on estrogen elimination.

Take note that most people need to supplement with a B vitamin and that trainees who take BCAAs will quickly become deficient in B vitamins, making it essential that you get extra. A high protein diet that provides adequate BCAA levels also requires extra B vitamins.

Ensure Complete Elimination of Estrogen

Once you shift your estrogen elimination to the C-2 pathway you have to make sure it gets excreted from the body. Two things can happen along the way out that cause big problems. First, estrogen that is heading down the C-2 pathway can be easily turned into something called quinones, which are highly reactive and can damage DNA and cause cancer.

In order to avoid the production of quinones you must have adequate amounts of two nutrients, magnesium and something called SAM. This process of metabolizing estrogen to avoid quinones is called methylation. It is the first place where things can go wrong on the estrogen detox pathway. Another notable antioxidant that can support damage to the body by estrogen quinones is alpha lipoic acid, which I mention here because it is one of my favorites and has many health benefits.

As estrogen is heading out of the intestine, it needs to be bound to glucuronic acid, but there is a bad intestinal bacteria that contains an enzyme that breaks estrogen apart from the glucuronic acid. This is the second place estrogen detoxification can go wrong. When the bad bacteria, secreting the enzyme called glucouronidase, uncouples the bond between estrogen and glucuronic acid, estrogen re-enters circulation, effectively raising estrogen levels in the body and damaging tissue. To avoid this, you need a healthy gut, which you can get by taking a probiotic, and eating lots of fiber and lignans.

Food and Supplement with Essential Nutrients

To review, the essential nutrients to help detoxify estrogen are the B vitamins, zinc, omega-3 fish oils, DIM (nutrient found in cruciferous vegetables), green tea, magnesium, selenium, and melatonin. The only nutrient I have not mentioned is vitamin E, which is a potent antioxidant.

Magnesium plays a role in methylation, or that final phase of estrogen excretion. I call your attention to it here because almost everyone needs to supplement with magnesium as most people are chronically deficient. Athletes and strength trainees are especially susceptible to low magnesium because this nutrient plays a role in muscle contractions. Low vitamin E is associated with elevated estrogen and it has been shown to inhibit the growth of breast cancer cells.

Watch What You Drink

Eliminate all alcohol besides certain red wines. Sardinian and Spanish wines are rich in antioxidants that help remove estrogens. Other good choices are Pinot and Merlot. Alcohol increases estrogen levels in women. Even moderate alcohol consumption other than Sardinian, Spanish, and certain French wines has been shown to increase the risk of breast cancer.

The one exception is wine that is rich in either resveratrol or trans-resveratrol, which has been shown to inhibit aromatase thereby lowering estrogen levels. For example, a study that was just published showed that red wine acted as an aromatase inhibitor and resulted in lower estrogen levels after one month in premenopausal women. The group of women that drank eight ounces of red wine daily had higher testosterone and lower estrogen levels than the group that drank white wine daily. Previous studies have shown that red wine appears to lower overall cancer risk, and it provides cardioprotective effects along with increasing insulin sensitivity.

Limit Chemical Estrogen Exposure

Avoiding chemical estrogens is one of the most important strategies for preventing cancer and protecting yourself. If you were able to have no contact with chemical estrogens, and you had good nutrition, a lean body composition, and a large proportion of muscle mass, it is very unlikely you would have excess estrogen or be at risk of cancer. But, chemical estrogens are everywhere. It is only recently that the mainstream medical community has started to seriously consider the connection between cancer and the toxic environment the industry has created with the lax regulation of toxic estrogenic chemicals.

There is even a movement in public health advocacy that government regulatory bodies and chemical companies need to take action to reduce environmental toxins. Although there is an awareness that the responsibility of reducing cancer risk should not be on the individual because we cannot completely avoid contact with chemical estrogens, the reality is that you have to take responsibility for eliminating estrogen from your body and the bodies of your loved ones.

Antiestrogen

An antiestrogen is a substance that blocks the production or utilization of estrogens, or inhibits their effects. (Estrogens are the family of hormones that promote the development and maintenance of female sex characteristics.)

Antiestrogens like tamoxifen can promote an invasive phenotype in estrogen receptor (ER)-positive breast cancer cells with deficient intercellular adhesion.

Although aromatase inhibitors could be considered antiestrogens by some definitions, they are often considered to be a distinct class. Aromatase inhibitors reduce the production of estrogen, while the term "antiestrogen" is usually reserved for agents reducing the response to estrogen.

Antiestrogens are a group of medications that block the effect that estrogen has on the growth of a tumor. For about 20 years, antiestrogens have been used mainly to help prevent and treat breast cancer. Since many breast cancer tumors use hormones to fuel their growth, blocking the hormones limits their ability to grow.

Antiestrogens refer to a group of drugs. Many breast cancer tumors grow due to normal levels of estrogen, a hormone found in the bloodstream. Some patients have tumors that are extra-sensitive to this normal estrogen level. The estrogen attaches to the area on the outside of the tumor cells and sends a signal to the cell that causes it to grow and multiply. Antiestrogens block the protein on the outside wall of the estrogen-sensitive breast cancer cell. By blocking this protein, known as the estrogen receptor, the free-floating estrogen cannot stimulate the cancer cells to grow and multiply any further.

The drug tamoxifen is a common antiestrogen that has proven to have a positive effect in breast cancer patients for both treatment and prevention. The drug raloxifene is a newer antiestrogen. Early research showed that raloxifene worked against breast cancer with fewer side effects than tamoxifene. In 2003, research also showed that raloxifene may be effective in decreasing new fractures among women with low bone mineral density. However, further clinical trials on raloxifene are needed.

Use of tamoxifen has been associated with a number of side effects, including vaginal bleeding, menstrual irregularities, and hypercalcemia (excess calcium in the blood). Most women also experience hot flashes while using the drug. Serious side effects include endometrial cancer and throm boem bolism (blocking of a blood vessel by a particle of ablood clot at the site the blood clot formed). In late 2003, cancer experts were beginning to recommend a new group of drugs called aromatase inhibitors (Arimidex, common name anastrozole or

Femara and Novartis, common name letrozole) as an alternative to tamoxifen or following tamoxifen therapy. These drugs fight breast cancer differently, but early research shows they fight it as effectively and with fewer side effects.

How Do Anti-Estrogens Work?

The average male has a testosterone level that is between 300 and 700 nanograms per deca-liter of blood (ng/dl). This broad range is affected by a variety of factors and aromatase is one of them. Most AI's have shown the ability to raise testosterone to levels approaching 1200ng/dl but this has never translated into muscle growth. You may have heard the term PCT on many of the steroid forums. After a cycle of pro-hormones and steroids, the male testes tend to shrink and lower natural production and the use of anti-estrogens helps reverse this effect faster than natural recovery alone. With anti-estrogens, there are two basic technologies that have similar effects.

The first are anti-aromatase agents, which limit the aromatase enzyme that converts testosterone to estrogen. The body has a feedback mechanism for estrogen that senses when estrogen levels get too low (the male body DOES need estrogen to function). If the estrogen levels get too low, then the body responds by making more testosterone which in theory converts to estrogen and corrects the problem. Estrogen (or lack of) is sensed by the pituitary gland and the testes are instructed via Luteinizing hormone to make more or less testosterone. So, by lowering estrogen artificially, the body is told to make more via increasing testosterone.Anti-aromatase agents temporarily lower estrogen to trick the body into producing more testosterone. This actually works really well, but there can be negative effects. Prescription Anti-Aromatase products are Arimidex(R), Letrozol(R) and Exemestane(R). These ingredients are illegal to sell to males except for special circumstances like breast cancer, but we have many natural agents that do the same thing which is great for the bodybuilder who is trying to increase natural testosterone levels or recover from a cycle of steroids.

Aromatase Inhibitor

These limit the conversion of testosterone to estrogen by binding and inactivating the aromatase enzyme, which has the downstream effect of raising testosterone via a feedback loop that is dependent on estrogen (estrogen is reduced, so the body creates more testosterone as a raw material) AI's have two methods of reduction. First, there is a suicide inhibitor, which locks up and deactivates the enzyme. The other method, competitive inhibition only temporarily blocks the enzyme from having activity. The items on the bodybuilding market are suicide inhibitors, which still work well enough to cause a major increase in testosterone for most males however these will not really work in females unless via some other pathway such as DHEA. Sadly in the current studies, this reduction in estrogen and the boost in testosterone doesn't translate into muscle gain, which is puzzling. I think if properly stacked with other items this could be a very good way to increase testosterone, but it seems that the body has many ways of reducing excess testosterone or the lab is seeing cross reaction which is the AI itself "looks" like testosterone on the test. The debate of whether to use AI's as a valid means to boost testosterone is one that is heated. Many experts and honestly most pharmaceutical steroid recovery agents are competitive ER inhibitors like Tamoxifen (NolvadexTM) which is interesting. The problem with any of the competitive receptor blockers on the market is that they suffer from rapid metabolic clearing via sulfation and glucoronidation.

This process is how the body removes anything that isn't food and there is a ton of it in the liver, making oral products very difficult design with any positive effect due to the rapid clearing of the ingredient. Ways around these metabolism routes are sublingual delivery (under the tongue), transdermal delivery (on the skin) or by blocking them with additional items that compete for the enzyme.

7

Toxicants in Food

A toxicant is any substance that can elicit a detrimental effect in a biological system. Any chemical may be regarded as toxicant at a given dose and route of administration. Food is a complex substance having unique characteristics owing to the diverse chemicals which make it. Some of these chemicals are beneficial to the consumer and are more commonly known as nutrients. These nutrients include the complex biomolecules such as carbohydrates, proteins, lipids, vitamins and minerals. In addition to the source of being nutrients essential for human survival food also serves as a source of numerous chemicals which may either be present in it inherently or produced (both biologically and synthetically) in it by external agents such as microorganisms and man himself. Many of these chemicals may be toxic when consumed. The capacity of the toxicants to pose a threat to the human life depends on the combination of various factors such as their concentration in food, the amount consumed and individual susceptibility One of the methods of classifying toxins in food is based on the origin of the toxin. Food toxicants can be divided into three categories:

1. Endogenous/Inherent Food plant Toxicants: These are substances produced by tissue cells in plants/food sources and other biological raw materials. These chemical substances often serve the purpose of protecting plant tissues from pests, as well as from pathogenic organisms. Transmission to man can be due to direct consumption of toxic plants or from animals who have consumed the plant that are then used for human foods. Examples include flavonoids, goitrogens, coumarins, cyanogenic compounds, herbal extracts etc.

2. Naturally occurring toxicants: They are produced by organisms that contaminate the food products. Microorganism such as dinoflagellates, fungi, and bacteria can produce toxicants that upon consumption can cause diseases. Some toxin-producing organisms produce toxins in the food matrix (which can cause intoxication if consumed), while others produce toxins inside the victim (intoxification). Some of these organisms are able to withstand heating temperature used in cooking, while others are able to tolerate extremes of pH without losing activity. Some of these

Micro organisms cause very serious diseases such as typhoid, dysentery, salmonellosis, cholera and food intoxications. They are generally specific depending upon the type of food and particular conditions of storage. e.g moulds (Aspergillus) are commonly associated with cereal product spoilage, Lactic acid bacteria (Lactobacillus) spoils raw milk and yeasts (Saccharomyces) spoil fruit juice when stored under unfavourable conditions.

3. Synthetic Toxicants: They are substances that are synthetically produced, which found their way into our food supply through contamination of the food processing environment. e.g pesticides, additives, preservatives. Pesticides include insecticides, herbicides, rodenticides, fungicides, fumigants etc. Amide herbicides (propanil) which is used extensively to control harmful weeds in rice crops could cause liver damage, central nervous system depression and death. The concentration of residues that can be found in foods produced from treated crops is being regulated (maximum residue levels-MRL) in such a manner that strict compliance is demanded. The synthetic toxicants also include the chemicals which enter into the food due to industrial pollution and food packaging contaminants.

The evolution of human eating patterns over several centuries, method of food preparation, selective breeding of crops have generally led to development of diets which are low in naturally occurring food toxicants. But the exponential growth in population has forced us to develop technologies which not only extend the shelf life of the food but also has the potential to develop novel foods. The drawback of this growth and modernization is the increased risk of complex toxicants that have invaded our food. These pose a severe threat to human health. The health hazards from different sources are ranked as follows:

1. Food borne microorganisms/ microbial contaminants.
2. Inappropriate eating habits
3. Environmental contaminants
4. Naturally occurring toxicants
5. Food additives

Some food toxins cannot be removed from foods and others may be created during processing or cooking. For decades now, the food industry has continually created new chemicals to manipulate, preserve, and transform our food. With the use of chemicals, scientists are able to mimic natural flavors, color foods to make them appear "natural" or "fresh," preserve foods for longer and longer periods of time. There are even foods products that are made entirely from chemicals. Coffee creamers, sugar substitutes, and candies consist almost completely of artificial ingredients. Such manipulation of our food can have a profound effect on our body's unique biochemical balance. The impact of food and related products on our daily life is so prominent that it is sometimes unavoidable to resist these chemicals associated with food.

This chapter tries to focus on the types of chemical hazards that are very common and can occur frequently in the food and related products used by the mankind today.

Origin of Toxicants in Foods

It is a well established principle in toxicology that all things are toxic at a high enough concentration. Majority of the toxins in food (almost 99%) are naturally occurring. It has been observed that many foods in raw form contain chemicals, which are deleterious to human health at high doses. Cooking and processing in general may help to remove or inactivate many chemicals (e.g. protease inhibitors, lectins) that are either directly toxic or inhibit digestion or absorption of nutrients. However, some chemicals have arisen as problems associated with food processing techniques developed in the last century, e.g. trans fatty acids resulting from chemical hydrogenation of unsaturated fats, or 3- monochloropropanediol from the chemical hydrolysis of proteins. One recently publicised example of a process derived toxicant in food is the formation of acrylamide in baked products. Although this has been occurring for centuries (e.g. in home baking of bread, potatoes and other starch-based foods), it was not discovered until 2002. A further area of concern is the migration of chemicals from packaging materials into foods, which has recently become a large problem for food manufacturers. Other toxicants are introduced in the foodstuffs by accident during the production of the products from food raw materials. Sometimes these are unavoidable and sometimes they are to a greater or lesser extent caused by poor growing, post-harvest or processing conditions. Mycotoxins produced by moulds on grain or nut products are one example; nitrate accumulation in leafy vegetables, and heavy metal accumulation in seafoods are others. Most difficult to predict or control are the chemical toxicants introduced deliberately, generally as a consequence of fraudulent trading (e.g. addition of melamine to milk to boost the apparent protein content).

Toxicants occurring in food can thus be divided into five broad categories:

- Inherent ('Natural') toxins
- Natural and environmental contaminants
- Process and storage-derived contaminants
- Deliberately added contaminants
- Pesticides and veterinary residues

i) Natural toxins

These chemicals occur as regular constituents of the food in question (e.g. lectins in kidney beans), or at increased levels as a response of the foodstuff to some sort of stress (e.g. glycoalkaloids in potatoes, an increased production of which can be stimulated when the tuber is exposed to light), and are inherent to the food raw material. There are also some instances of a processing regime potentially releasing a toxin from a nontoxic starting material (as occurs with cyanogenic glycosides in some canned stone fruits). The latter could be considered under the process-derived hazards category, but is essentially 'natural'. There are many types of natural toxins produced from many species of plants and the following examples serve to illustrate the importance of controlling the risk from these chemicals.

a) Lectins

Lectins are a group of glycoproteins that are present in high levels in legumes (e.g., black beans, soybeans, lima beans, kidney beans and lentils) and grain products. Lectins can reversibly bind to carbohydrates without altering their covalent structure. The ability of lectins to bind to and agglutinate red blood cells is well known and used for blood typing—hence the lectins are commonly called hemagglutinins. Lectins also can bind avidly to mucosal cells and interfere with nutrient absorption from the intestine. Because the ability of the lectins to cause intestinal malabsorption is dependent on the presence of enteric bacteria, it has been hypothesized that lectins may also produce toxicity by facilitating bacterial growth in the GI tract.

Lectins isolated from black beans can produce growth retardation when fed to rats at 0.5% of the diet, and lectin from kidney beans causes death within two weeks when fed to rats at 0.5% of the diet. Soybean lectin produces growth retardation when fed to rats at 1% of the diet. The castor bean lectin ricin (one of the most toxic natural substances known) is notorious for causing deaths of children, and has been used as an instrument of bioterrorism.

Phytohaemagglutinin (PHA) is a lectin found in significant quantities (as much as 2.4–5% of total protein) in legumes such as red or white kidney beans, green beans and fava beans. PHA has a number of different properties, including the ability to induce mitosis, affect membrane transport and permeability to proteins, and agglutinate red blood cells. Rats fed a diet containing 6% PHA exhibit weight loss, associated with malabsorption of lipid, nitrogen and vitamin B12. PHA from red kidney beans inhibits sodium and chloride absorption in the rabbit ileum, indicating that PHA can affect electrolyte transport in the gut. Symptoms of toxicity to PHA in humans such as nausea, vomiting, or diarrhea occur within three hours of ingestion. Recovery generally occurs within four or five hours of onset.

There are no FDA regulations or guidelines restricting the presence of lectins in food, but the FDA does provide recommended cooking practices prior to consuming legumes. Concentrations of PHA (and other lectins) are higher in uncooked than cooked beans. A raw, red kidney bean can contain up to 70,000 hemagluttinating units (hau). Most lectins are reduced by moist, but not dry heat. Therefore, steaming or boiling causes a significant reduction in concentrations of lectins in beans. Boiling for at least ten minutes has been shown to reduce hau in beans by 200-fold. Because cooking temperatures under 176 F do not destroy lectin, use of slow cooking and/or a crockpot is not advised for cooking beans.

b) Glycoalkaloids

Potato glycoalkaloids are the most common example of naturally occurring toxins that can and have caused problems when consumed in large quantities, but which we have learned to avoid without too much difficulty. Potatoes contain two main glycoalkaloids, α- solanine and α-chaconine, with α-chaconine being the more toxic. Symptoms of acute poisoning can range from abdominal pain, vomiting and diarrhoea (similar to bacterial food poisoning) to confusion, fever, hallucination, paralysis, convulsions and occasionally death. There is an unofficial, but widely accepted safety limit of 200 mg glycoalkaloid/kg fresh potato. Levels of glycoalkaloids in modern varieties are usually well below this value, but they can exceed the limit under certain circumstances. The associated bitterness that accompanies these increases means that the chances of ingesting a toxic dose are small unless the bitterness has been masked with other highly flavoured ingredients. Thus, although the chances of someone eating potatoes with high levels of glycoalkaloids are small, the possibility does exist, and hence the food industry must take precautions to eliminate the risk as far as is possible. Glycoalkaloids can only be made by the living potato tissue, and therefore will be halted by cooking and any other process that kills the tissue. However, they are heat stable and therefore preformed toxin will remain after processing. Glycoalkaloid levels in potatoes are highest in the flowers and in the sprouts on the tubers. Within the mass of the tuber itself, they are concentrated in the outer 2mm, so that unpeeled potato products are a higher risk than flesh-only products. Levels vary from one variety to another, and are generally higher in early varieties than in main crop varieties. Smaller potatoes tend to have higher levels than large potatoes, largely as a consequence of the increased surface area/volume ratio. Increased levels arise through various stress factors, such as pest and disease damage, drought, waterlogging, and extremes of temperature. During post-harvest handling, bruising, abrasion and other types of mechanical damage can all cause increases in levels, as can peeling (although the act of peeling will remove much of the glycoalkaoid content unless the peel is added back into the product). Light can also induce glycoalkaoid formation. Light also induces chlorophyll formation, causing the potatoes to turn green on the surface.

c) Oxalates

Oxalic acid and oxalates are widely distributed in plant foods, highest levels being found in spinach (0.3-1.2%), rhubarb (0.2-1.3%), tea (0.3-2.0%) and cocoa (0.5-0.9%). Although there is no question that the ingestion of sufficient oxalic acid as crystals or in solution can be fatal, there is considerable debate as to whether serious food poisoning from oxalate is usually due to food. The eating of rhubarb leaves has been a well-known cause of illness for centuries. Rhubarb leaves contain high amounts of oxalate. However, the levels of oxalate in rhubarb stalks are sufficiently high that consumption of normal levels of rhubarb stalks will result in at least as much oxalate intake as from small to moderate amounts of leaves. There is some debate as whether it is the oxalate in rhubarb leaves that is responsible for toxicity. Whatever the toxic principle, consumer perception is that rhubarb leaves are toxic, and hence consumer complaints about small fragments of leaves in canned rhubarb are well-known.

d) Cyanogenic glycosides

Many fruits and other plant foods contain compounds that have the potential to release cyanide. These compounds are usually glycosides - i.e. they consist of a sugar molecule linked to a cyanide group, usually indirectly through another component. The release of cyanide from these compounds occurs by enzymatic hydrolysis, usually when the plant tissue is crushed or otherwise disrupted (allowing the active enzyme to reach the substrate), but it can also occur in the digestive system after the food has been eaten. Some plants are toxic because of their high levels of these compounds. Other foods are considered safe to consume, despite their having moderate levels of cyanogenic glycosides. The most well-known of these compounds is amygdalin, a cyanogenic glycoside first identified in bitter almonds, which on hydrolysis by an enzyme complex known as emulsin yields glucose, benzaldehyde and hydrogen cyanide.

Cassava or manioc is a staple food for large numbers of the world's population. It is the world's seventh largest food crop in terms of production area. The toxic potential of cassava has been known for hundreds of years, and traditional methods of food preparation from cassava have been developed to reduce cyanide content. These include leaching out the linamarin precursor, washing in running water before cooking (bruising of the cassava root during harvesting often results in considerable cyanide release), and boiling in uncovered pots so that the cyanide can evaporate. Fermentation also significantly reduces cyanogenic potential.

Prussic acid (also known as hydrocyanic acid, hydrogen cyanide, or cyanide) is formed when cyanogenic glycosides found in leaves, cherry, apple and peach pits, oak moss and other plant tissues are damaged and come into contact with beta-glycosidase or emulsion enzymes. The enzymes release the cyanide from the glycoside, and the cyanide prevents the body's cells from utilizing oxygen, resulting in cellular necrosis and tissue damage. The mucous membranes and blood are bright red as they are oxygenated, but the cells in the tissues cannot utilize the oxygen. Clinical signs of prussic acid poisoning include rapid breathing, trembling, incoordination and in extreme cases, respiratory and/or cardiac arrest. Many fruit trees contain prussic acid glycosides in the leaves and seeds, but only negligible levels are present in the fleshy parts of the fruit. In the west African tropics, cassava is consumed as a dietary staple and inappropriate handling of the cassava prior to processing and consumption can result in a chronic form of cyanide poisoning termed "tropical ataxic neuropathy", the result of demyelinization of the optic, auditory, and peripheral nerve tracts.

Prussic acid as found in flavoring ingredients is limited to 25 ppm in cherry pits (*Prunus avium* L. or *P. cerasus* L.), cherry laurel leaves (*Prunus laurocerasus* L.), elder tree leaves (Sambucus nigra L.), and peach leaves (*Prunus persica* (L.) Batsch) (21 CFR 172.510); although the extract of bitter almond (*Prunus amygdalus* Batsch, *Prunus armeniaca* L., or *Prunus persica* (L.) Batsch) must be prussic acid free (21 CFR 182.20). There are no FDA regulations or guidelines restricting the presence of prussic acid in apple seed (Malus spp.), probably because extracts of these seeds have no economic value as flavor ingredients.

e) Trypsin inhibitors

There are substances which have the ability to inhibit the proteolytic activity of certain enzymes which are found throughout the plant kingdom. The most common of these are chemicals which inhibit the activity of the enzyme trypsin which is important for digestion of proteins in the stomach. Examples of plants containing trypsin inhibitors are Lima beans and soya beans. Most of the inhibitor molecules are proteins which are inactivated by heating; hence cooking is a key step to increasing the nutritional value of foods containing these inhibitors.

f) Bioactive amines

Pesticide-like action of bio-active amines (chemical compounds also belonging to the broader group of alkaloids) is based on their chemical structure resembling that of some of our hormones, such as adrenaline. Bio-active amines affect either blood vessels (vasoactive amines) - causing changes in blood pressure and related symptoms like migraine headaches - or the nervous system, by affecting the level and function of neurotransmitters (psychoactive amines).

For instance, the most widely consumed psychoactive amine, caffeine, causes a number of neurological effects from anxiety states and associated symptoms (including panic attacks), to "restless leg syndrome" and neurologically based migraines. Other pharmacological effects of caffeine include stimulating fluid elimination and dilating the airways.

In the nature, caffeine can be lethal to insects feeding on caffeine-containing herbs (it is chemically similar to strychnine, although not nearly as potent). It is much less of a threat to humans, but not necessarily harmless.

Most of caffeine's neurological effects are due to it acting as antagonist to neurotransmitter adenosine, hence affecting brain function. Apart from that, inside the cell, it inhibits conversion of cAMP (cyclic 3',5'-adenosine monophosphate) into its noncyclic form, thus lowering intracellular levels of this vary basic cellular metabolite. Specific consequences, again, depend on the intake level and individual biochemistry. In addition, caffeine affects hormonal function, effectively elevating important hormones, like adrenaline, noradrinaline, and catecholamine ("fight-or-flight" hormone).

The three primary metabolites of caffeine, paraxanthine, theobromine and theophylline, also have their specific, relatively minor effects.

The overall effect on health and wellbeing ranges from beneficial to harmful, mainly determined by the level of consumption and metabolic efficiency. Caffeine is absorbed from intestine within 45 minutes from ingestion; its half-life in an average healthy adult is 4.9 hours, but can vary significantly - especially toward slower metabolizing - from one individual to another.

Obviously, the worst possible combination is high caffeine consumption by a slow metabolizer; such individual is most exposed to the caffeine build-up and its toxic effects. Following table summarizes possible adverse effects of acute caffeine over dose (usually in excess of 300mg, or so, but can be significantly less for sensitive individuals).

Caffeine Toxicity (main symptoms)

Central nervous system irritability, anxiety, restlessness, insomnia, confusion, headache, delirium. Gastrointestinal nausea, abdominal pain, vomiting. Muscular trembling, twitching, overextension, seizures. Heart rapid and/or irregular heartbeat. Systemic dehydration, fever. Other visual flashes, ear ringing, rapid breathing, skin oversensitivity to touch/pain.

Chronic overuse of caffeine also may - and often does - cause adverse health effects. These are recognized as disorders: caffeine intoxication, as well as caffeine-induced sleep and/or anxiety disorder. Symptoms of the former are similar to those of caffeine overdose. For the latter, the symptoms can range from anxiety to panic attacks; they can mimic mental anxiety/panic disorders, including bipolar (manic depression), often leading into misdiagnosis and unnecessary long-term treatment with medications.

Separately from the overuse symptoms, but likely as frequent, are caffeine withdrawal symptoms, which may take place whenever a habitual caffeine intake is interrupted for more than 12 hours, or so. They vary individually, but typically are the result of the withdrawal of stimulatory effects of caffeine, combined with the increased sensitivity to adenosine (due to the increase in number of adenosine receptors, compensating for the caffeine obstructing their intended use). The symptoms persists for as long as it takes to the body to re-adjust, usually 1-5 days. They include headache, irritability, difficulty to concentrate, drowsiness, insomnia, stomachache, upper body and joint pain.

In all, habitual overuse of caffeine can take your health and wellbeing to a slippery slope. The main culprit of the overuse is usually coffee, in all forms, but some other dietary habits can also contribute. For comparison, 1 tablespoon (6g) of regular ground coffee (Folgers) contains 90mg of caffeine and 1 teaspoon (2.2g) of Folgers' instant coffee powder 75mg8. A standard 6 fl oz serving of brewed (percolated) coffee averages about 100mg (same as 2 fl oz of espresso, and some 20% less than 6 fl oz of drip coffee), most 12 fl oz regular sodas about half as much, and 6 fl oz of black tea about one third. Most chocolates have low caffeine content, but some chocolate products can have it comparable, per unit weight, to that in black tea and sodas.

Majority of people feel stimulating effect - increase in alertness and/or lowered fatigue - with caffeine intake of 25-50mg. Significantly higher doses - 5 to 10mg per kg of body weight - have been reported to increase endurance in competitive cycling by up to 50%. This dose is still safely bellow caffeine's LD50 (median lethal dose, a dose that kills half of subjects exposed), estimated for humans at 150-200mg per kg of body weight (equivalent of nearly 100 cups of regular coffee); obviously, regular consumption of caffeine at this level cannot be recommended.

Beside caffeine, the other two significant bio-active amines, histamine and tyramine, can be found in high amounts mostly in fermented foods: cheeses, yeast extracts, tuna, pickled herring, sausage, and others. Tyramine raises blood pressure by constricting blood vessels. Other possible symptoms include migraines, stomach pains and breathing difficulties.

Histamine, has the opposite effect - it dilates blood vessels, lowering blood pressure. Hence, in foods containing comparable levels of both, tyramine and histamine, one will likely tend to neutralize the effect of the other one (actual effect, as always, depends on individual biochemistry/sensitivities).

Table 7.1 : Some common foods with potentially high levels of tyramine and/or histamine.

Foods	TYRAMINE (mg/100g)	HISTAMINE (mg/100g)
Cheddar cheese	0-150	0-130
Camembert	2-200	0-50
Emmenthaler	20-100	n/a
Blue/Roquefort	3-110	0-230
Gouda	2-67	0-85
Mozzarella	0-41	0
Provolone	4-15	1-52
Swiss	0-180	0
Stilton blue	46-217	0
Yeast exctracts	0-226	21-283
Tuna	n/a	204-500
Pickled herring	300	0
Sausage	0-124	1-41
Meat extracts	10-30	0

g) Purines

When the body metabolizes purines - an aromatic organic compound whose derivatives are naturally occurring in foods as DNA/RNA constituents (nucleobases adenine and guanine) - inefficient enzyme action can result in the build up of their end metabolite, uric acid. It then crystallizes in joints, causing gout. Foods highest in purines are meats (including fish and chicken), and particularly organ meats.

Foods having over 400mg/100g of uric acid are very high; foods between 100-400mg/100g are moderately high, and those bellow 100mg/100g are considered low in purines.

Some plant foods – like soybean and some beans/legumes - have high nominal levels of purines, although generally lower than in meats.

h) Salicylates

Quite a few of fruits and vegetables have high salicylates content. Salicylic acid is phenolic compound (which include aspirin and aspirin-based pharmacological agents) to which some people - particularly children - can be sensitive. It can cause urticaria (hives) and/or angioedema, as well as mouth ulcers, irritability and hyperactivity in susceptible individuals.

There may also be some beneficial health effects of salicylates, resulting from their chemical similarity to aspirin. These are still being investigated and, obviously, have to be measured against their possible adverse effects.

Plant foods with highest salicylates level include raisins, canned prunes, raspberries, strawberries, honey (variable), most condiments, pickles, mint, licorice, sweet green pepper, endive, chicory, tomato sauce and pasta, zucchini, almonds and peanuts.

SALICYLATES, food content (mg/100g)

NEGLIGIBLE (<0.1) fruit: yellow apple, banana, pomegranate, green plum vegetables: brussels sprouts, cabbage, blackeyed/brown/garbanzo/lima/mung/ soy beans, celery, leeks, lettuce, lentils, peas, potato w/o peel, summer squash grains: barley, oats, rice, rye, wheat nuts: cashews animal: beef, cheese, chicken, egg, lamb, liver, pork, milk, yogurt, oysters, salmons, scallop, shrimp, tuna

LOW

(0.1-0.5) fruit: red apple, apple juice, apricot nectar, sour cherries, figs, light grapes, grapefruit juice, kiwi, lemon, mango, nectarine, orange juice, peach nectar, pear w/skin, pineapple juice, red plum, watermelon vegetables: asparagus, beet, carrot, cauliflower, corn, onion, potato w/peel, pumpkin, spinach (frozen), sweet potato (yellow), tomato, tomato juice, turnip, black olive nuts: brazil nut, coconut, hazelnut, peanut butter, pecans, sesame seed, sunflower seed, walnuts other: beer

MEDIUM (0.5-1) fruit: granny smith apple, canned apple, avocado, sweet cherry, dried figs, red grapes, grapefruit, mandarin, peach, tangelo vegetables: alfaalfa, broad beans, broccoli, cucumber w/o peel, eggplant w/peel, okra, spinach, squash, sweet potato (white), canned tomato nuts: macadamia, pine nuts, pistachios other: coffee, wine

HIGH (1-5) fruit: apricot, blackberries, blueberries, cantaloupe, cranberries, currants, dates, guava, sultana grapes, loganberries, orange, pineapple, dark red plum, strawberries, frozen raspberries vegetables: chicory, endive, radishes, sweet green pepper, zucchini, tomato paste/sauce, ginger root, green olives nuts: almonds, peanuts, water chestnuts other: white vinegar, teas (1 bag)

VERY HIGH (>5) fruit: raisins, raspberries, canned plum herbs: licorice, mustard powder (over 10mg/100g) other: pickles, honey

i)   Pyrrolizidine alkaloids

Pyrrolizidine alkaloids are found in quite a few herbs, some of them used occasionally for herbal preparations and teas. It includes Indian herb Heliotropium eichwaldii, with documented cases of toxicity when used internally, and some commonly used Chinese herbal preparations (zicao, kuandonghua, qianliguang and peilan).

The risk factor includes unknowingly substituted harmless herbs with those containing PAs. For instance, popular Mexican herbal tea, gordolobo yerba, usually obtained from Gnaphalium, has documented cases of liver poisoning when made of the similar in appearance Senecio longilobus.

j) Carrageenan

Algae often contain toxic substances. Carrageenan (undegraded, or natural type) is a substance extracted from seaweed, widely used as food additive (thickener and stabilizer). It has been found to cause ulcerative colon disease in laboratory animals.

While ulceration risk in humans is officially limited to the degraded (processed) version of carrageenan, it is prudent to make sure it is not on your menu on a regular basis in neither of the two forms.

k) β-Thujone

Thujone, a monoterpene ketone, is the primary constituent of essential oils derived from a variety of plants, including sage (*Salvia officinalis*), clary (*Salvia sclarea*), tansy (*Tanacetum vulgare*), wormwood (**Artemisia** spp. and white cedar (*Thuja occidentalis* L.). Essential oils from these plants are used in herbal medicines, as flavorings in alcoholic drinks and fragrances throughout the world. Thujone is potentially toxic and the presence of alpha- or beta-thujone in food and beverages is regulated by law in several countries. In the US, thujone as an isolated substance is banned as an ingredient to be added to food and many of the natural thujone-containing plant oils (e.g., wormwood, white cedar, oak moss (Evernia prunastri) and tansy) are used as flavorings in food under the condition that the finished food is thujone-free. Absinthe (made from wormwood) contains significant levels of thujone and is available in Spain, Denmark and Portugal. Wormwood itself is a popular flavoring for vodka in Sweden, while vermouth, chartreuse, and Benedictine all contain small levels of thujone. Sage oil is used to provide the characteristic flavor in sausages, meats, condiments and sauces, and contains approximately 20–30% thujone (alpha- and beta-). Both alpha- and beta-thujone act as noncompetitive blockers of the gamma-aminobutyric acid (GABA)-gated chloride channel. The essential oils of sage, hyssop (*Hyssopus officinalis* L.), and cedar all contain thujone and have been cited to have caused central nervous system effects characterized by tonic-clonic or solely clonic convulsions. Thujone is believed to be the toxic agent in absinthism, a syndrome produced by the chronic use of absinthe, made from the essence of wormwood. The syndrome is characterized by addiction, hyperexcitability and hallucinations. The debilitating illnesses suffered by Vincent Van Gogh and Henri de Toulouse-Lautrec have been linked to absinthism, while the toxicity of thujone was a major factor in banning absinthe in the early 1900s. A published case report detailed a male subject that drank about 10 mL of essential oil of wormwood (believing it was absinthe) and became agitated, incoherent and disoriented, subsequently developing renal failure. The no observable effect limit (NOEL) for convulsions in subchronic toxicity studies in female rats was 5 mg/kg bw/day. Detoxification of thujone is thought to occur via CYP450-dependent oxidation and subsequent glucuronidation and excretion. The FDA limits exposure to β-thujone from *Artemisia* spp., when used as a natural flavoring substance or natural substance used in conjunction with flavors (21 CFR 182.20).

l) Hypericin

St. John's wort (Hypericum perforatum;) is an herbal thought to alleviate symptoms of depression, and standardized extracts of St. John's wort are consumed typically in tablet or capsule form. The major active antidepressive constituents in St. John's wort are thought to be hyperforin and hypericin. The mechanism of action is not fully understood, but may involve inhibition of serotonin (5-HT) reuptake, similar to conventional antidepressive drugs. In this manner, hyperforin and hypericin taken in conjunction with other serotonin reuptake inhibitors may contribute to serotonin syndrome, a potentially life-threatening elevation of serotonin in the central nervous system. Hyperforin is also known to induce cytochrome P450 enzymes CYP3A4 and CYP2C9, which can lead to increased metabolism of certain drugs and decreased clinical response.

In large doses, St. John's wort is poisonous to grazing animals, with published cases of livestock poisoning characterized by general restlessness and skin irritation, hindlimb weakness, panting, confusion, depression and in some instances, mania and hyperactivity resulting in the animal running in circles until exhausted. In humans, consumption of St. John's wort may result in photosensitization, and at high continuous doses, some liver damage may occur. The FDA limits exposure to St. Johns wort (*Hypericum perforatum*), including the leaves, flowers, and caulis, by mandating that only hypericin-free alcohol distillate form may be used and then, only in alcoholic beverages.

m) Goitrogens (glucosinolates) in *Brassica* spp.

Certain raw foods have been found to contain substances that suppress the function of the thyroid gland by interfering with the uptake of iodine, an essential nutrient in growth, cognitive function, and hormonal balance. A lack of functional iodine is known to result in cognitive deficiencies (e.g., Cretinism). The decrease in iodine uptake causes the thyroid gland to enlarge, forming a goiter. Foods that have been identified as goitrogenic include spinach, cassava, peanuts, soybeans, strawberries, sweet potatoes, peaches, pears, and vegetables in the Brassica genus, which include broccoli, brussels sprouts, cabbage, canola, cauliflower, mustard greens, radishes, and rapeseed. Goiter has also been attributed to the consumption of large quantities of uncooked kale or cabbage.

High temperatures (*i.e.*, cooking) inactivate the goitrogenic substances, collectively termed glucosinolates. Cassava (Manihot esculenta) is an essential dietary source of energy in the tropics, but contains high levels of linamarin, a glucosinolate. Cassava must be properly processed-dried, soaked in water or baked to effectively reduce the linamarin content. Glucosinolates are sulfur-containing substances that are metabolized in the body by thioglucosidase to form thiocyanate, isothiocyanate, nitriles and sulfur. Under certain conditions the isothiocyanates undergo cyclization to form goitrins, increasing their potent goitrogenic activity. The oils from rapeseed (*Brassica napus*) must be analyzed for potential goitrins to circumvent potential goitrogenic activity when consuming these oils. No FDA regulations were located for permissible concentrations of glucosinolates in human food. Glucosinolates (calculated as epi-progoitrin) and goitrin are limited to not more than 4% and 0.1% (respectively) of the seed meal of Crambe abyssinica (Crambe meal) obtained after the removal of the oil and used as an animal feed ingredient.

n) Erucic acid in rape

Rape (*Brassica napus* L. or *Brassica campestris* L.) is an annual herb of the mustard family native to Europe and is grown in the United States because it produces oil-rich seeds for cooking oil. Rapeseed oil had been used for hundreds of years as oil for lamps and more recently as machine oil lubricant. Widespread use of rapeseed oil as a food ingredient was not considered until the late 1940s and 50s. However, early studies found that feeding high levels of rapeseed oil to rats significantly increased cholesterol levels in the adrenal glands and lipidosis in the cardiac tissue. This effect was also noted in chickens, ducks and turkeys fed high levels of rapeseed oil, resulting in growth retardation, mortality, and a thickening of the epicardium and increased fibrous tissue in different areas of the myocardium. Erucic acid was identified as the causative agent of these effects of rapeseed oil. Erucic acid is a long-chain fatty acid with one unsaturated carbon-carbon bond (C22:1). High levels of erucic acid have been liked to fatty deposit formation in heart muscle in animals. Erucic acid is poorly oxidized by the mitochondrial β-oxidation system, especially by the myocardial cells, which results in an accumulation of erucic acid, producing myocardial lipidosis which has been reported to reduce the contractile force of the heart. Although myocardial lipidosis due to erucic acid consumption has not been confirmed in humans, animal feeding studies confirmed the formation of myocardial lipidosis in a variety of animal species in a dose-dependent manner, which has been the standard assessment by government agencies of potential adverse effects in humans. Canola oil is obtained from Canola (Canadian oil, low acid), a rapeseed variety that was conventionally bred in the late 1970s in Canada to contain reduced levels of erucic acid and glucosinolates. The FDA limits the amount of erucic acid in Canola oil to no more than 2% of the component fatty acids.

o) Coumarins (tonka bean, woodruff, clover)

Coumarin (2H-1-benzopyran-2-one) is found in herb teas made from tonka beans (Dipteryx odorata), melilot (Melilotus officinalis or Melilotus arvensis) and woodruff (*Asperula odorata*), the flavoring oil of bergamot (from *Citrus bergamia*) and the spice cassia (Cinnamomum cassia; sometimes sold as cinnamon). Coumarin is liberated from the glycoside melilotoside (an ether of glucose bonded with an ester bond to coumarin) on drying coumarin-containing herb material.

Molds present in spoiled sweet (Melilotus) clover and other hay products can metabolize coumarin to dicoumarol, which is similar in structure to vitamin K. Vitamin K is necessary to activate prothrombin, which is converted to the blood clotting substance thrombin. By inhibiting vitamin K, dicoumarol promotes bleeding. Concentrations of dicoumarol in fodder >10 ppm have been responsible for fatalities by hemorrhaging in cattle.

The addition of coumarin to food in the United States was banned in 1954, based on reports of hepatoxicity in rats. However, because a number of foods contain coumarin, humans ingest approximately 0.02 mg coumarin/kg bw/day. The chronic administration of high doses of coumarin causes liver tumors in the rat and liver and lung tumors in the mouse. Overall, available data indicate that coumarin is not genotoxic. It is thought that the carcinogenicity of coumarin is caused by metabolism to toxic epoxides. Because doses of coumarin that cause toxicity and carcinogenicity in the lung and liver of experimental animals are more than 100 times the maximum human intake, exposure to coumarin from food poses no health risk to humans.

The addition of coumarin is prohibited. The regulation notes that coumarin is found in tonka beans and extract of tonka beans, among other natural sources, and is also synthesized. It has been used as a flavoring compound, therefore addressing not just natural products (which would include buffalo grass or sweetgrass (*Hierochloe odorata*) used in flavoring vodka and other natural sources (see above)), as well as synthesized coumarin. Further, according to the regulation, "(b) Food containing any added coumarin as such or as a constituent of tonka beans or tonka extract is deemed to be adulterated under the act, based upon an order published in the Federal Register of March 5, 1954 (19 Federal Register 1239)."

p) Furocoumarins

Furocoumarins represent a family of natural food constituents with phototoxic and photomutagenic properties. They are found mainly in plants belonging to the Rutaceae (e.g., citrus fruits) and Umbelliferae (e.g., parsnip, parsley, celery, carrots) families. Furocoumarins are produced in response to stress, to aid plants in defense against viruses, bacteria, fungi, insects and animals, and are regarded as natural pesticides. Concentrations may also increase after exposure to UV radiation, changes in temperature, prolonged storage, or treatment with hypochlorite or copper sulfate.

The three most active furocoumarins in producing photodermatitis are psoralen, 5-methoxypsoralen (5-MOP, bergapten), and 8-methoxypsoralen (8-MOP, xanthotoxin or methoxsalen). In the presence of near UV light (320–380 nm), these three linear furocoumarins can form adducts with DNA and DNA-crosslinks. The consequences of these photoadditions to cells are cell death, mutations and chromosome aberrations. In the presence of ultraviolet A radiation, 5-MOP and 8-MOP produce skin tumors in experimental animals. At a chronic dose of 37.5 mg/kg bw/day in the diet, 8-MOP produces increased incidences of tubular cell hyperplasia, adenomas, and adenocarcinomas of the kidney and carcinomas of the Zymbal gland in rats. Cases of skin cancer have been reported in patients treated with 8-MOP and long-wave ultraviolet light for treatment of psoriasis or mycosis fungoides. IARC has classified 5-MOP and 8-MOP plus ultraviolet radiation in group A (probably carcinogenic in humans) and in group 1 (carcinogenic to humans), respectively.

Citrus fruits, especially grapefruit, produce a variety of chemicals in their peels that may have adverse interactions with drugs. Typically, citrus fruit juice is produced utilizing the whole fruit, including the peel. One chemical found in the peel is bergamottin (also known as bergamot), a natural furanocoumarin that is known to inhibit some isoforms of the cytochrome P450 enzyme (CYP) 3A4. Inhibition of this enzyme prevents oxidative metabolism of certain drugs, resulting in an elevated concentration of a drug in the bloodstream. Bergamot and other chemicals in citrus (e.g., lime, grapefruit, orange, lemon) oils are also phototoxic, causing significant toxicity to the skin when exposed to sunlight. 5-Methoxypsoralen, the most phototoxic constituent of bergamot oil, showed mutagenic activity in bacterial assays and clastogenic effects in mammalian cells in culture when exposed to UV light.

Celery reportedly contains 100 ppb psoralens (100 micrograms/kg) and parsnips as much as 40 ppm (40 mg/kg). The estimated dietary intake of furocoumarins for people eating furocoumarin-containing foods (est. 80% of the population) is 1.31 mg/day, which is approximately 0.022 mg/kg bw/day for a 60 kg human. This is approximately 1000-fold lower than the 13-week dietary no observable adverse effect level for liver toxicity in the rat (25 mg 8-MOP/kg bw/ day) and 1700-fold lower than the dietary dose that has been shown to induce cancer in rats (37.5 mg/kg). Therefore, the risk of developing liver toxicity or cancer due to ingestion of psoralens in the diet is low.

In humans, the phototoxic threshold dose of furocoumarin mixtures after dietary exposure is of the order of 10 mg 8-MOP plus 10 mg 5-MOP, which is equivalent to about 15 mg 8-MOP per person. This phototoxic threshold dose is not reached by the consumption of celery roots and other conventional vegetables under normal dietary habits, which result in intake of approximately 2–8 mg furocoumarins per person. Therefore, ordinarily dietary exposure to psoralens is not considered to be a significant risk for development of photodermatitis, albeit the margin of safety is low. There are no FDA regulations or guidelines specific to the presence of furocoumarins in food.

q) Amylase inhibitors

Naturally occurring inhibitors of α-amylase are found in aqueous extracts of wheat, rye and kidney beans. The physiological role of α-amylase inhibitors in plants is not well understood, but may protect them against insect infestation. In mammals, some amylase inhibitors have been shown to attenuate the normal increase in blood glucose that occurs after ingestion of starch. However, since α-amylase inhibitors have been shown to be inactivated by gastric acid, pepsin or pancreatic proteinases, their potential as "starch blockers" is limited. α-Amylase inhibitors were once added to foods as "starch blockers" to limit carbohydrate absorption for the purpose of weight loss; however, the FDA later determined that at least this use of α-amylase inhibitors was as drug, and they were consequently taken off the market.

α-Amylase inhibitor protein is a major allergen (referred to as Asp o 2) that has been implicated in the development of occupational toxicity known as "baker's asthma disease". Although α-amylase inhibitor protein is naturally found in wheat flour, it is also found in flour in which α-amylase from Aspergillus oryzae has been added to enhance carbohydrate fermentation by yeast. Consequently, α-amylase inhibitor protein can be potentially found in baked products that are derived from sources other than wheat. Cases of food allergy have been reported in people ingesting bread containing α-amylase inhibitor protein. Symptoms of allergy include sneezing, rhinorrhea, oropharyngeal itching, hoarseness, cough and dyspnea.

High α-amylase inhibitor activity against human salivary α-amylase has been found in wheat flour (590 units/g), whole wheat flour (351 units/g) and whole rye flour (186 units/g). Bread baking reduces the activity by 80–100%, depending on type. The activity in uncooked spaghetti (248 units/g) is reduced more than 98% by 15 minutes of boiling. Boiling of red beans for 1.5 hours reduces activity to undetectable levels. However, α-amylase has been shown to retain some allergenic activity when heated to 200 C.

r) Anti-thiamine compounds

Substances that act on the availability of vitamins are commonly referred to as antivitamins. These include materials that can cause a deficiency of vitamins by competing with vitamins in various metabolic reactions as the result of similar chemical structure or destroying or decreasing the effects of a vitamin by modifying the molecular conformation or by forming a complex.

Thiaminase cleaves thiamine (vitamin B1) at the methylene linkage, rendering it biologically inactive. Activity of thiaminase requires a cosubstrate—usually an amine or sulfhydryl-containing protein such as proline or cysteine. Thiaminase is found in fish, crab, clams and in some fruits and vegetables such as blueberries, black currants, red beets, Brussels sprouts and red cabbage.

Thiamine is an essential vitamin involved in energy production. Thiamine deficiency is associated with impaired pyruvate utilization, resulting in a shortage of cellular ATP. In humans, thiamine deficiency may lead to weakness and weight loss. Severe thiamine deficiency produces "beri-beri", a disease characterized by anorexia, cardiac enlargement, and muscular weakness leading to ataxia. Cooking destroys thiaminases in fish and other sources. There are no FDA regulations or guidelines specific to the presence of thiaminase in food.

s) Zucchini and cucurbitacins

Members of the Cucurbitacea family (zucchini, cucumbers, pumpkins, squash, melons and gourds) produce cucurbitacins (oxygenated tetracyclic terpenes) that act as movement arresters and compulsive feeding stimulants for Diabriticine beetles (corn rootworms and cucumber beetles). Cucurbitacins are among the most bitter compounds known, and in nanogram quantities they deter most non-Diabrotic herbivores.

Because cucurbitacins act as feeding stimulants, they are added to insecticidal baits to increase efficacy. Therefore, dietary exposure to cucurbitacins could occur through ingesting plants that normally contain them or by ingesting plants to which cucurbitacin-containing pesticides have been applied.

Under normal circumstances, cucubitacins are produced at low enough concentrations that are not perceived as being bitter by humans. In response to stresses such as high temperatures, drought, low soil fertility and low soil pH, concentrations in fruits such as cucumbers may increase and cause the fruits to have a bitter taste. Occasional cases of stomach cramps and diarrhea have occurred in people ingesting bitter zucchini. Twenty–two cases of human poisoning from ingestion of as little as 3 grams of bitter zucchini were reported in Australia from 1981 to 1982, and in Alabama and California in 1984. The cultivar implicated in the Australia poisonings was "Blackjack". There are no FDA regulations or guidelines specific to the presence of cucurbitacins in food.

t) Phytates and phytic acid

Phytic acid (also referred to as phytate) is found in bran and germ of many plant seeds and in grains, legumes and nuts. Phytic acid is a simple sugar (myo-inositol) containing six phosphate sidechains, and as such, is a dietary source of phosphorus and an effective chelator of divalent cations such as zinc, copper, iron, magnesium and calcium. Studies indicate that phytate-mineral complexes are insoluble in the intestinal tract, reducing mineral bioavailability. Phytate also has been shown to inhibit digestive enzymes such as trypsin, pepsin, α-amylase and ß-glucosidase. Therefore, ingestion of foods containing high amounts of phytate could theoretically cause mineral deficiencies or decreased protein and starch digestibility. Vegetarians that consume large amounts of tofu and bean curd are particularly at risk of mineral deficiencies due to phytate consumption.

Due to the fact that phytate-rich foods are digested at a slower rate and produce lower blood glucose responses than foods that do not contain phytate, it has been hypothesized that phytate could have a therapeutic role in management of diabetes. It also may have utility as an antioxidant. However, because the beneficial effects of phytate are outweighed by its ability to cause essential mineral deficiencies, consumption of a diet containing high amounts of phytate is not recommended. Food manufacturers are developing methods to reduce phytate in foods, such as addition of the microbial phytase, which releases phosphates from the inositol backbone of phytate.

Phytate is fairly heat stable, but can be removed by soaking or fermentation. The soybean has one of the highest phytate levels of any grain or legume, and requires a long period of fermentation for reduction. In people who consume large amounts of soy products, mineral deficiencies can be prevented by consumption of meat or dairy products or use of supplemental vitamins. There are no FDA regulations or guidelines restricting the presence of phytates in food.

u) Hypoglycin in Ackee

Ackee (Blighia sapida;) is the national fruit of Jamaica and is also found in other Caribbean nations, Central America, South American and southern Florida. Consumers of the unripe fruit sometimes suffer from "Jamaican vomiting sickness syndrome" allegedly caused by the alkaloids hypoglycin A (HGA) and B. Levels of HGA in the opened, ripe fruit are undetectable, making opened fruit safe for consumption.

The hypoglycin toxin (L-methylenecyclopropylalanine) inactivates several flavoprotein acyl-CoA dehydrogenases, causing disturbances of the oxidation of fatty acids and amino acids. This leads to a secondary inhibition of gluconeogenesis which can precipitate an extreme, dangerous drop in blood-glucose levels (hypoglycemia) that can be fatal. Symptoms of poisoning from unripe ackee fruit occur within 6 to 48 hours of ingestion and include drowsiness, repeated vomiting, thirst, delirium, fever or loose bowels. Exhaustion of the muscular and nervous systems, collapse, coma, and death may ensue.

Dietary exposure to hypoglycin in Jamaicans ranges from 1.21–89.28 micrograms/gram ackee. Ingestion of one 100 gram fruit could therefore result in a dose of approximately 300 micrograms/kg bw in a 30 kg child. This dose is approximately one-fifth of the maximum tolerated dose of HGA in male and female rats of 1500 micrograms/kg bw/day, indicating that normal use levels of ackee do not have a large margin of safety.

The importation of canned ackee fruit into the United States is restricted to certain manufacturers to insure that only properly ripened ackees are used for canning, and the FDA routinely analyzes incoming shipments of ackee for hypoglycin levels that could be a health concern, having issued a recall of canned ackee fruit for this very reason in 2005. If hypoglycin poisoning is expected, glucose, fluids and electrolytes should be administered. Antiemetics may be used to control vomiting and benzodiazepines to control seizures. Endotracheal intubation should be performed in people exhibiting seizures or coma.

v) Safrole

Safrole (1-allyl-3,4-methylenedioxybenzene) is found in aromatic oils of nutmeg (*Myristica fragrans*), cinnamon (*Cinnamomum verum*) and camphor (*Cinnamomum camphora*) and is a major constituent of oil of sassafras (*Sassafras albidum*). Prior to being banned as a food additive in the United States in 1960, safrole was commonly used to flavor root beer and other foods. Most commercial "sassafras teas" and root beers are now artificially flavored as a result of the FDA ban.

At a concentration of 1% in the diet, safrole produces weight loss, testicular atrophy, bone marrow depletion and malignant liver tumors in rats. Based on sufficient evidence of carcinogenicity in experimental animals, safrole is reasonably anticipated to be a human carcinogen. The mechanism of carcinogenicity is thought to involve cytochrome P450 catalyzed hydroxylation of safrole to 1'-hydroxysafrole, and its subsequent metabolism to highly reactive electrophiles that bind to DNA.

Despite the FDA ban, sassafras is still a popular ingredient in herb teas and preparations. The hazardous dose of sassafras oil for humans (which typically contains 80% safrole) is considered to be 0.66 mg/kg. This may be exceeded by ingesting sassafras tea, which has been estimated by Segelman and Bisset to give a dose of 3 mg/kg for a 60 kg individual.

w) Myristicin

Myristicin is a naturally occurring insecticide and acaracide that is found in nutmeg and mace (*Myristica* spp.) at concentrations of 1.3% and 2.7%, respectively. It is also present in black pepper, carrot, celery parsley and dill. It is estimated that the average total intake of myristicin from dietary sources is "in the order of a few mg per person per day".

Myristicin is a weak inhibitor of monoamine oxidase, and is structurally related to mescaline. At a dose level of 6–7 mg/kg bw, it may cause psychotropic effects in man, such as increased alertness, and a feeling of irresponsibility, freedom and euphoria. Unpleasant symptoms, such as nausea, tremor, tachycardia, anxiety and fear have also been reported in humans ingesting this dose. Although the metabolism of myristicin resembles that of safrole, there is no evidence to suggest that myristicin is carcinogenic. There are no FDA regulations or guidelines specific to the presence of myristicin in food.

At the concentrations normally present in spices or food, the likelihood of toxicity arising from myristicin is low. However, ingestion of greater than 5 grams of nutmeg (corresponding to 1–2 mg/kg bw myristicin) has produced toxicological symptoms in humans that are similar to alcohol intoxication. Because the myristicin content of nutmeg is approximately 1–3%, it is likely that components of nutmeg in addition to myristicin contribute to nutmeg toxicity.

x) Japanese star anise

Chinese star anise (*Illicium verum*) is a common source of anethole, a popular flavoring ingredient. On the other hand, Japanese star anise (Illicium anisatum) is scientifically recognized as highly poisonous and not fit for human consumption. Japanese star anise contains the potent neurotoxins anisatin and neoanisatin, as well as the neurotoxic sesquiterpene lactone veranisatins that are normally found in other kinds of star anise, including Chinese star anise.

Brewed "teas" containing star anise have been associated with illnesses affecting about 40 individuals, including approximately 15 infants. The illnesses ranged from serious neurological effects, such as seizures, to vomiting, jitteriness and rapid eye movement. Due to the potential for adulteration, on September 10, 2003, the FDA issued an advisory to the public not to consume "teas" brewed from star anise, until the FDA is able to differentiate between the Japanese star anise and Chinese star anise, which does not contain anisatin.

ii) Natural and Environmental Contaminants

All plants and animals during their lifetime will accumulate various chemicals from their environment. Some of these chemicals, if they are accumulated at high enough levels, might be of toxicological significance to us when we eat the food. Specific examples that are of concern are nitrates in leafy vegetables, heavy metals in various foods, and specific toxins in shellfish. In many cases, the best way to control levels of these unwanted substances is to control the environment in which the food is produced. However, this is generally a long-term control measure and more immediate steps have to be taken to protect human health. As many of the toxins cannot be 'processed out', the short term controls are usually based around the setting of maximum permitted levels, and the removal from the supply chain of food that does not meet the required standard. These contaminants are divided below into 'natural' (of biological origin) and 'environmental', but they are linked in that the food plant or animal acquires them from its surroundings during its growth.

'Natural' Contaminants

A) Mycotoxins

Mycotoxins are a group of chemically diverse naturally occurring substances produced by a range of filamentous fungi or moulds. They have toxic effects on both humans and animals ranging from acute toxicity and death, through reduced egg and milk production, lack of weight gain, impairment or suppression of immune function to tumour formation, cancers and other chronic diseases The mycotoxins of greatest concern are produced by mould species from three main genera - Aspergillus, Penicillium and Fusarium. These are mainly storage moulds affecting commodities such as nuts, dried fruits and cereals. The moulds grow and produce toxins when commodities are stored incorrectly - usually at too high moisture levels. Specific mycotoxins of greatest concern are detailed below:

1.   Aflatoxins

Aflatoxins are produced mainly by some strains of Aspergillus flavus and most, if not all, strains of A. parasiticus. There are four main aflatoxins, B1, B2, G1 and G2, plus two additional ones that are significant, M1 and M2. The aflatoxins are potent liver toxins in most animals and carcinogens in some, with aflatoxin B1 being the most toxic and carcinogenic. Mould growth and aflatoxin production are greatest in warm temperatures and high humidity, particularly in tropical and sub-tropical regions, mainly on corn (maize), peanuts, cottonseed and tree nuts.

2.   Ochratoxins

Ochratoxins are a group of related compounds produced by Aspergillus ochraceus and related species, as well as Penicillium verrucosum. The main toxin in the group is Ochratoxin A, which causes liver damage in rats, dogs and pigs. Ochratoxins are also teratogenic to mice, rats and chicken embryos, and are now thought to be carcinogenic in humans.

3. Patulin

Patulin is produced by numerous Penicillium and Aspergillus species and by Byssochlamys nivea. However, the most common producer of patulin is Penicillium expansum, which occurs commonly in rotting apples, as a result of which patulin has frequently been found in commercial apple juice. Patulin is toxic to many biological systems, including bacteria, mammalian cell cultures, higher plants and animals. Its role in causing animal and human disease is unclear, but it is believed to be carcinogenic.

4. Cyclopiazonic acid (CPA)

Cyclopiazonic acid (CPA) is produced by several moulds which occur on agricultural products or are used in some food fermentations. It also occurs naturally in infected corn (maize) and peanuts. It affects rats, dogs, pigs and chickens, where it may cause anorexia, weight loss, diarrhoea, pyrexia, dehydration and other symptoms. Organs affected include liver, spleen, kidneys, and pancreas. It has the ability to chelate metal ions such as calcium, magnesium and iron, which may be an important mechanism of toxicity.

5. Zearalenone

Zearalenone (also known as F-2 toxin) is produced by several Fusarium species. It occurs naturally in high moisture corn (maize) in late autumn and winter, mainly from the growth of F. culmorum in Northern Europe and F. graminearum in North America. Production of this and other Fusarium toxins is favoured by high humidity and low temperatures, conditions which often occur in temperate regions during autumn harvest. It has been found in mouldy hay, high-moisture corn (maize), corn infected before harvest and pelleted feed rations, so it is an important contaminant of animal feed. The involvement of zearalenone in human disease is unconfirmed, but it is regarded as an endocrine disruptor and hence a potential hazard.

6. Tricothecenes

The tricothecenes are a group of over 20 chemically related toxins produced by several Fusarium species. These include deoxynivalenol (DON), T-2 toxin, diacetoxyscirpenal, neosolaniol, nivalenol, diacetylnivalenol, HT- 2 toxin and fusarenon X. The most commonly occurring of these is deoxynivalenol or DON, which causes vomiting in animals, hence its other name of vomitoxin. It may also be a teratogen and has been found in commodities such as corn (maize) and wheat as well as some processed food products.

7. Fumonisins

The fumonisins are a group of compounds mainly produced by Fusarium moniliforme and F. proliferatum. They have been linked to several diseases, including liver cancer and oesophagal cancer in humans.

8. Moniliformin

Moniliformin is so called because it was first thought to be produced by F. moniliforme isolated from corn (maize). However, it has since been shown to be produced mainly by other species of Fusarium. It has been shown to be highly toxic in experimental animals, causing rapid death without severe cellular damage.

9. Other mycotoxins

Other mycotoxins include sterigmatocystin, reported in green coffee, mouldy wheat and the rind of some hard cheese, citrinin, penicillic acid, mycophenolic acid, β-nitropropionioc acid, tremorgens (penitrem) and rubratoxin.

B) Shellfish toxins

There are several types of shellfish poisoning including neurotoxic (NSP), diarrhoetic (DSP), paralytic (PSP), amnesic (ASP), and ciguaterra fish poisoning (CFP). Shellfish toxins are not produced by the shellfish themselves, but are accumulated through the ingestion of planktonic dinoflagellates in the diet of the shellfish. The term shellfish generally refers to both marine crustaceans (lobsters, crab, shrimp etc), and molluscs. However, it is the bivalve molluscs – oysters, mussels, clams and scallops - which accumulate these algae by filter feeding, that are the major areas of concern. Paralytic shellfish poisoning is a global problem which has increased dramatically since the 1970s. The most significant toxins in PSP are saxitoxin and its derivatives, though the exact composition differs amongst algal species and amongst regions of occurrence. Generally the population density of such algae is not high enough to cause problems, but on occasion when environmental conditions (nutrients, temperature, sunlight etc) are favourable, population explosions called 'algal blooms' occur. Problems can arise if the algal bloom is of a species which produces toxins, such as the Alexandrium genus. Such toxins can then accumulate within the flesh of the filter-feeding bivalve at levels which cause disorder in humans after consumption. The toxins can persist within shellfish at dangerous levels for weeks or months after the algae are no longer present in the waters. Seafood containing saxitoxin looks and tastes normal, and cooking or steaming only partially destroys toxins. Therefore one of the most effective methods in preventing outbreaks of PSP is the detection of the toxins before the shellfish are harvested.

Amnesic shellfish poisoning is also caused by algae in the diet of shellfish; domoic acid is the principal toxin and is produced by various species, but the diatom Pseudo-nitzschia is the primary source. It can work its way up through the food chain, so illness can result from consumption of other contaminated seafood. As with PSP, decontamination of foodstuffs is not effective and detection of areas where the contamination exists is the best method of preventing problems.

Ciguatera fish poisoning is an intoxication caused by the consumption of coral reef fish which feed on certain marine plankton which contain specific toxins. It is one of the commonest marine food poisonings worldwide and a significant health problem with as many as 50,000 cases occurring each year. Toxins accumulate as they move up the food chain so that the larger carnivorous fish are more toxic. Symptoms are extremely varied and include gastrointestinal and cardiovascular problems, though most patients recover. The toxins are not easy to detect so the only effective control option is to avoid consumption of susceptible fish species.

'Environmental' contaminants

A) Dioxins/Polychlorinated biphenyls (PCBs)

PCBs and dioxins are persistent contaminants with a wide range of chemical structures. They have been found in soil, water, sediment, plants and animal tissue in all parts of the world. Dioxins and PCBs are heterocyclic organic molecules, with PCBs being chlorinated. They have long half-lives in the environment and many have been reported to have toxicological effects in humans. PCBs and dioxins are man-made chemicals used by industry and their release to the environment is generally through by-products of fires and by some manufacturing processes. Their widespread environmental occurrence means that PCBs and dioxins are present in virtually all foods, which is the main route to human exposure. The highest concentrations are in fatty foods such as oily fish and the main sources of dioxins in the diet are meat and milk. Levels accumulate as they move through the food chain.

Control options are based on prohibiting the use of dioxins and PCBs by industry and hence their release into the environment and the EU put into force a ban on the use of most PCBs from 1978. Legislative limits have been imposed within the EU for many foods (Regulation EC 1881/2006) as have methods for sampling (EC 1883/2006). No limits exist in the US although the FDA considers all detectable levels to be of concern.

B) Polycyclic aromatic hydrocarbons

Polycyclic aromatic hydrocarbons (PAHs) are a group of compounds comprising two or more fused aromatic rings. Many individual PAHs exist, the most simple of which is naphthalene. A variety of toxic properties have been related to PAH exposure, including the capacity to produce genotoxic and carcinogenic effects in mammals.

PAHs are found in petroleum and coal, and can also be formed by the incomplete combustion of these and other organic materials. These compounds have been detected in air, water, soil and foods. Foods may become contaminated through direct environmental exposure, migration from packaging material or during thermal processing of food, e.g., baking, grilling, frying and smoking.

The occurrence of PAHs in fruit, vegetables and cereals is primarily due to soil and air exposure. Although levels detected in foods of animal origin tend to be low, high levels have been recorded in smoked meats and animals farmed on contaminated land. Shellfish can accumulate PAHs from oils spilt by grounded tankers or from waste oils which have been incorrectly disposed of. PAHs can also be formed during the heating and drying processes which allow combustion products to come into contact with the food substance. Direct fire drying and heating processes used during the production of food oils can result in high levels of PAHs. The complexity and number of individual PAH compounds means that it is not easy to produce specific limits for regulation of levels. Benzo (a)pyrene has been used as a marker for PAH levels and limits for this have been set by the European Commission (EC 1881/2006) for a range of foods, although there is currently discussion about widening this to include other marker compounds.

Specific foods of concern are fish which are farmed in oil contaminated waters, fats and oils including coca butter, and smoked foods. Refining processes are generally ineffective in eliminating PAHs from foods so the main control measure is to limit their production during processing and to screen out foods known to contain high levels.

C) Heavy metals

Heavy metals are those with a high atomic mass, including, for example, mercury, cadmium, arsenic and lead, although other metals (e.g. tin) may also be included within this category of contaminant. They are natural components which originate from the earth's crust and are found all over the world. They are toxic in low amounts and have been recognised as a health hazard for many years. There are other routes for metal contamination of products such as migration from packaging (e.g. antimony from plastic bottles, and tin in canned food).

Metals can occur in a variety of foodstuffs of plant and animal origin. Mostly, they arise indirectly in foodstuffs from the environment – e.g. they are in soil that the crop is grown in, or on the grass that a cow is eating or in the water in which a fish is living. As such, once they become incorporated into the food they cannot be removed.

There is a risk to crops and animals themselves from metals in the environment (e.g. they can kill plants and reduce yields) and to humans from eating crop and livestock products. Metals which can be particularly harmful to animals and man include lead, cadmium, arsenic, mercury, copper, selenium and molybdenum. These elements can accumulate in primary products that are otherwise growing satisfactorily, but still affect animals and man.

Of particular relevance to crop products as food raw materials are lead and cadmium. Lead is a widespread environmental pollutant, deriving from such human activities as lead mining, smelting and processing, and burning of fossil fuels. The main route of crop contamination is via uptake from the soil. Soil contamination with both lead and cadmium is primarily from aerial deposition. Maximum levels for heavy metal contaminants have been established in many countries so it is important to be aware of the legislative limits which apply if exporting. Each metal has a specific limit which is food-type dependent and is a reflection on both the occurrence of the metal in that food and its toxicological effect. Control of raw materials is the only mechanism for ensuring that levels do not become unsafe. A particular problem has been lead and cadmium in cereals and close monitoring of levels in flour mills and maltings has been necessary to ensure that limits are not exceeded. The legislation in this area is constantly changing so food manufacturers need to keep abreast of proposed new limits and use horizon scanning methods to maintain vigilance for problems.

D) Nitrates

In general nitrates in agriculture are considered more of a hazard to the environment and water than in foods. However, nitrate intake from water and food has received considerable publicity because of its role in methaemoglobinaemia in infants and its reported implication in various types of cancer. Methaemoglobinaemia is caused by nitrate being reduced, under the conditions found in the infant stomach, to nitrite, which then combines with haemoglobin in the bloodstream. Methaemoglobinaemia, sometimes known as the "blue baby syndrome", can be fatal.

The possible involvement of nitrate in cancer is via its role in the generation of nitrosamines. Nitrosamines are known to be very potent carcinogens and are produced by the reaction of nitrate, when reduced to nitrite, with certain nitrogenous compounds found in proteinaceous substrates. Whilst nitrosamines can be formed in the body, the link between high nitrate exposure and the incidence of cancer is often not clear. Nitrates in food might, therefore, have some adverse health effect, but the levels in most crops are not generally considered a food safety hazard. However, green leafy vegetables usually contain higher levels of nitrate than most other foods, and maximum levels have been set in the EU and by Codex for nitrates in spinach and fresh lettuce. There are a number of factors which affect the levels of nitrates in these crops, including nitrate availability in the soil, seasonal variations, applications of nitrate fertilisers shortly before harvest and environmental influences.

E) Fluoride

Fluoride can be found dissolved in waters at high levels in certain parts of the world, and in some cases is above the WHO maximum limit. There is some controversy as to whether the presence of fluoride is a benefit or a threat to human health. The benefits for protection of dental health are well known and in fact fluoride is routinely added to water and/or toothpaste in many countries. There are also reports that fluoride can be a hazard to human health with links to cancer, bone health and endocrine disruption having been cited. There is no doubt that the debate regarding fluoridation of public water supplies will continue given the emotion regarding mass medication. Information regarding the hazardous effects of long term ingestion of fluorides is required to determine whether this policy is acceptable.

iii) Process-derived contaminants

The production of toxic chemicals in foodstuffs through processing is a recently discovered phenomenon, although historically these chemicals will have always been present. The first three examples below serve to show how unexpected contaminants may arise. In addition, the contamination of food with chemicals from packaging, pesticide and veterinary medicine applications could also loosely be described as process-derived.

A) Acrylamide

In 2002, Swedish scientists unexpectedly discovered acrylamide in food when they were carrying out a study into occupational acrylamide exposure. As part of the study, people who were not believed to have been exposed to acrylamide were included as controls and were also found to have significant acrylamide in their blood; further research determined that this unknown source was food. Subsequent research has now revealed that acrylamide is formed in food by traditional cooking methods such as baking, frying and roasting (i.e. high temperatures). It is formed at highest levels in starch containing foods and varies widely among different products and between production batches of the same foods. Examples of foods most at risk are potato products such as crisps and chips, coffee, savoury snacks such as cracker type biscuits, and bread and other cereal products.

Acrylamide is found in a number of starch-based foods that are fried or baked at temperatures greater than 120 C (248 F), including bread, bakery products, breakfast cereal, and potato products (e.g., chips, french fries). It also is found in cocoa-based products and coffee. Acrylamide is formed via a Maillard reaction, a reaction between the carbonyl group of a reducing sugar and the nucleophilic group of an amino acid. Although a number of carbohydrates can be used as the source of the carbonyl group, the amino acid required for the formation of acrylamide is asparagine.

Acrylamide is mutagenic and has been shown to be a neurotoxicant, reproductive toxicant and carcinogen in experimental animals and is classified by IARC as a probable human carcinogen. The main metabolite, glycidamide (an epoxide) is thought to be responsible for genotoxicity. In humans, the only toxicological effect that has been linked to acrylamide is neurotoxicity in individuals occupationally exposed to high levels. Epidemiological studies have failed to show an increased risk of cancer from either occupational or dietary exposure to acrylamide and reproductive toxicity has not been reported in humans exposed to acrylamide. Acrylamide is a unique substance that exemplifies the concept that the structure of the substance greatly influences the toxicity, as acrylamide is an animal feed ingredient (thickener and suspending agent) only when a part of a long-chain polymer having a minimum molecular weight of 3 million and a viscosity range of 3,000 to 6,000 centipoises at 77 F. The residual acrylamide cannot be more than 0.05% .

In 2005, JECFA estimated that average and high intake consumers ingest 1 or 4 µg/kg bw/day acrylamide from food, respectively. Using a NOAEL for neurotoxicity of 200 µg/kg bw/day in animals, margins of safety of 200 and 50 for the average and high intake groups were derived, respectively. Utilizing a benchmark dose of 0.3 mg/kg bw/day and a NOAEL of 2 mg/kg bw/day for development of mammary tumors or reproductive in rats (respectively), higher margins of safety were calculated for carcinogenicity (300 and 75, respectively) and reproductive toxicity (200 and 50, respectively).

Exposure to acrylamide can be reduced by avoiding deep-fried foods, soaking potato slices before cooking, cooking french fries at lower temperatures and to a lighter color, and toasting bread to a lighter color.

B) Chloropropanols

Chloropropanols are a group of chemical contaminants, the most notable of which is 3 monochloropropane-1,2- diol (3-MCPD). 3-MCPD can occur in foods and food ingredients at low levels as a result of processing, migration from packaging materials during storage, or domestic cooking. It has been found in a variety of foods, such as cooked/cured meats and fish, cheese, bread and toast, malt extracts and baked products, as well as in teabag paper, tissue and sausage casings. A major area of concern is its occurrence in food following the reaction between hydrochloric acid and lipids, particularly in foods processed at high temperatures such as soy sauce. In laboratory animal studies it has been shown that 3-MCPD is a carcinogen; it was originally classified as a genotoxic carcinogen, but more recent studies suggest that there is a lack of evidence of in vivo genotoxicity. However, the issue with 3-MCPD has meant that industry has looked to use enzymic methods of producing HVP rather than acid hydrolysis. Control of processing conditions and selection of ingredients is the main strategy being used by industry to control levels of chloropropanols. The level of 3-MCPD in the EU is prescribed by EC 1881/2006 though for other chloropropanols there are no limits and manufacturers are requested to reduce levels as far as is technically possible.

C) Furans

Furan is a colourless, volatile liquid used in some chemical manufacturing industries, which was occasionally found in foods. Recently, it has been discovered that furan is formed in some foods more commonly than previously thought. This discovery is probably a result of our ability to detect compounds at exceedingly low levels rather than a change in the presence of furan. It is believed that furan forms in food during traditional heat treatment techniques, such as cooking, bottling, and canning. Furan has been found in such canned or bottled foods as soups, sauces, beans, pasta meals, and baby foods.

D) Packaging migrants

There is a risk with any packaging material that its components may be transferred in some way to the food that it is surrounding. In most cases, the level of transfer is extremely slight and the components transferred are innocuous. However, there are instances where a realistic hazard exists and must be controlled. There are no official internationally agreed guidelines, but in the EU there is a general requirement that food packaging components must not be transferred into food during its normal shelf-life to the detriment of the food (i.e. to pose a health risk, or to adversely affect the quality of the food - its flavour, texture or appearance). Transfer of monomers and additives such as plasticizers in plastic packaging materials are the major area of concern. In the EU, there is a list of approved monomers and of additives that can be used in food contact plastic materials (this covers all contact with food, not just packaging materials) and also limits for the migration of these constituents into food. The general limit for containers and sealing devices is 60mg per kg of food. For other contact materials it is 10mg/dm2. To determine whether a particular plastic formulation meets these criteria, there are four model simulants that are used in laboratory trials to assess the plastic's properties. These are: distilled water; a 3% aqueous solution of acetic acid; 10% ethanol in water solution (or greater, if the alcoholic beverage in question has a higher alcohol content); and rectified olive oil. The regulations specify which simulants should be used for each category of food. In general, there are no simulants listed for dried foods, which can be considered to not take up plastics constituents from contact materials.

E) Tin

Tin can be considered to be a specific type of packaging-derived contaminant. Although there is no evidence that excess tin intake has any long-term health effects, some studies have shown that intake of high concentrations (above about 250ppm) may cause short-term gastrointestinal problems. For most foods, this is of no significance, but for foods packed in cans with some unlacquered tinplate, high levels can sometimes occur. Tin dissolution in unlacquered tinplate cans is essential in that it confers electrochemical protection to the iron, which makes up the structural component of the can and so maintains the can's integrity. Without it, the can would quickly become corroded by the contents of the can; this could cause serious discoloration and off-flavours in the product and swelling of the can. Tin is also involved in maintaining product quality (it helps prevent undesirable colour changes amongst other things, by mopping up any residual oxygen left in the headspace), so there is an advantage in some products of having some exposed (i.e. unlacquered) tinplate. As tin dissolution tends to be accelerated by oxygen, for products where exposed tin is considered to be beneficial, the base, lid and ends of the can may be lacquered, with the rest being unlacquered. Tin pick-up is normally relatively slow and does not give rise to excessive levels in the product within its shelf-life. However, certain natural variations within the product can cause problems.

F) Trans fatty acids

Trans fatty acids (also known as trans fat) are the sum of all unsaturated fatty acids that contain one or more isolated double bonds in a trans configuration. Trans fatty acids more closely resemble saturated fatty acids than cis unsaturated fatty acids because their trans configuration makes them rigid. Trans fatty acids in the diet originate from two sources. The first is from bacterial hydrogenation in the forestomach of ruminants, which produces trans fatty acids that are found in beef and mutton fat, milk and butter. Trans fatty acids are also produced from the hydrogenation of liquid oils (mainly of vegetable origin). This produces solid fats and partially hydrogenated oils such as margarines, spreads, shortenings and frying oil, which are more stable than liquid oils.

Biochemically, trans-fatty acids act similarly to saturated fatty acids, raising low density lipoprotein (LDL) cholesterol and decreasing high-density lipoprotein (HDL) cholesterol levels. High intakes of trans fatty acids have been associated with an increased risk of coronary heart disease (CHD) independent of other risk factors in large epidemiological studies. A tolerable upper limit of trans fatty acids has not been set because any incremental increase in the intake of trans fatty acids increases the risk of coronary heart disease.

In the US, the main sources of intake of trans fatty acids are baked goods (28%), fried foods (25%), margarine, spreads and shortenings (25%), savory snacks (10%), milk and butter (9%). In 1996, processed foods and oils accounted for 80% of the trans fat in the diet. In 1999, the FDA estimated that the average daily intake of trans fat in the United States is about 5.8 grams or 2.6% of calories per day. It has been hypothesized that replacing 2% energy from trans fatty acids with 2% energy from oleic acid would reduce mean plasma LDL cholesterol concentration by 0.08 mmol/L, and increase plasma HDL concentration by 0.08 mmol/L. These changes could reduce the incidence of CHD by 5–15%.

Due to increased efforts by food manufacturers to reduce or eliminate the use of partially hydrogenated vegetable fat in food production, it is estimated that trans fatty acid content of processed foods has decreased over the last decade.

G) Nitrosamines formed during drying, curing and preserving

Nitrosamines are formed from the interaction of nitrites or other nitrosating agents with amines in food (or in vivo), under acidic conditions. Nitrites may be directly added to food or can be formed from bacterial reduction of nitrate. Nitrites and nitrates may occur naturally in water or foods such as leafy vegetables due to the use of fertilizer, or may be added to foods to prevent growth of Clostridium botulinum, or to add color or flavor.

Nitrosamines have been found in a variety of different foods such as cheese, soybean oil, canned fruit, meat products, cured or smoked meats, fish and fish products, spices used for meat curing, and beer and other alcoholic beverages. Beer, meat products and fish are considered the main sources of exposure. Drying, kilning, salting, smoking or curing promotes formation of nitrosamines.

The nitrosamines most frequently found in food are nitrosodimethylamine (NDMA), N-nitrosopyrrolidine (NPYR), N-nitrosopiperidine (NPIP), and N-nitrosothiazolidine (NTHZ). NDMA, NPYR, NPIP are reasonably anticipated to be human carcinogens based on evidence of carcinogenicity in experimental animals. Evidence from case-control studies supports an association between nitrosamine intake with gastric cancer, but not esophageal cancer in humans. Levels of nitrosamines have been declining during the past three decades, concurrent with a lowering of the nitrite used in food, use of inhibitors such as ascorbic acid and use of lower operating temperatures and indirect heating during food processing. Based on an estimated exposure level of 3.3–5.0 ng/kg bw/day, the and the benchmark lower limit of 60 µg/kg bw/day, a margin of error associated with a low level of concern (12,000–18,2000) has been derived for NDMA, the most common nitrosamine in food.

Although current FDA regulations do not limit nitrosamine levels in foods, the FDA has provided an action level of 10 ppb for individual nitrosamines in both consumer and hospital rubber baby bottle nipples, while the FDA limits the approval of nitrites in curing mixes to the FDA-regulated food additive process (21 CFR 170.60), with the approval of sodium nitrite as a food additive (food preservative) (21 CFR 172.175). The USDA monitors finished meat products to insure that nitrite is not present in amounts exceeding 200 ppm (9 CFR 424.21).

H) Biogenic amines

Biogenic amines are normally formed in humans by normal cellular metabolism. In food, biogenic amines are mainly formed from microbial decarboxylation of amino acids. They are commonly found in fermented meat, beverages and dairy products, sauerkraut, and spoiled fish. The main biogenic amines in food are histamine, tyramine cadaverine, putrescine, spermidine and spermine. The two biogenic amines that have been associated with acute toxicity are histamine and tyramine. Putresine, spermine, sperimidine and cadaverine are not toxic in and of themselves, but may react with nitrite or nitrate to form nitrosamines. Scombrotoxicosis is a common seafood-borne disease associated with the consumption of toxic levels of histamine in spoiled scombroid fish such as tuna (*Thunnus* spp.), mackerel (*Scomber* spp.), saury (*Cololabis* saira) and bonito (*Sarda* spp.). Red wine may also contain relatively high levels of histamine. Symptoms of histamine intoxication from food are similar to allergies to other substances and include sneezing, nose congestion, breathing difficulties and urticaria.

Consumption of tyramine may precipitate migraine headache or a hypertensive crisis. The most serious case reports of tyramine toxicity have occurred in people consuming aged cheese. Because monoamine oxidase inhibitor (MAOI) drugs inhibit metabolism of amines, people taking these drugs may be particularly susceptible to tyramine toxicity. Whereas 200–800 mg of dietary tyramine induces only a mild rise in blood pressure in unmedicated adults, 10–25 mg may produce a serious adverse event in those taking MAOI drugs. Other potentiating factors for tyramine toxicity include alcohol consumption, gastrointestinal distress and exposure to other amines.

Efforts taken by food manufacturers to reduce biogenic amine concentrations in fermented foods include using amine-negative starter cultures, adding probiotic bacterial strains alone or in combination with starter cultures, high pressure processing or low-dose gamma radiation. FDA guidelines specify 50 mg/100 g as the toxic concentration of histamine in scombroid fish and the agency has published guidance on how to control levels.

iv) Deliberately added contaminants

There is no limit to what chemical contaminants might be deliberately added to foods during manufacture in order to cause harm to the consumer. In most cases, however, the aim is not to cause harm, but to defraud for financial gain. However, potential harm can still result, as evidenced from two of the examples given below.

A) Illegal or unauthorised dyes

The Sudan I-IV group of chemicals are synthetic azo dyes which have been historically used in industry to colour products such as shoe polish, automotive paints and petroleum derivatives. They are not permitted food colours. During the summer of 2003 it became apparent than chilli powder and related products in the European market, and originating from India, were contaminated with Sudan I-IV at levels between 2.8 and 3500 mg/kg. Although the Sudan dyes were deemed to be toxic, the levels at which they were found were probably not a major health concern because of the very low concentrations in which they were detected in final products. However, such dyes are not permitted for food use and were being added to the chilli powder in order to make it appear to be of better quality than it actually was. The chilli powder was incorporated into various sauces, which were themselves used as ingredients in a range of ready meals. With the significant dilution effect of this, analyzing the final food for Sudan dyes became a problem, as the levels involved were now very small. A major traceability program had to be launched to identify and remove all affected products. This involved the withdrawal of over 1000 products, at a very significant cost to the food industry. However, with laboratories now routinely testing for the presence of the Sudan dyes, the contamination spread progressively to a wide range of other dyes in order to avoid detection, including Para Red, Rhodamine B, Orange II, Red G, Butter Yellow and Metanil Yellow. As well as many dyes which were not permitted for any food use, these new colours included some, such as Bixin, which were permitted in some foods, but not in the spices to which they were being added.

B) Melamine

Melamine is an industrial chemical found in plastics. It can be combined with formaldehyde to produce melamine resin, a very durable thermosetting plastic used in Formica, and melamine foam, a polymeric cleaning product. The end products include countertops, dry erase boards, fabrics, glues, house wares, guitar saddles, guitar nuts, and flame retardants. Melamine is one of the major components in Pigment Yellow 150, a colorant in inks and plastics. It is also used in the manufacture of plasticizers for concrete.

In 2007 it was discovered in the US that melamine had been fraudulently added to wheat gluten and rice protein from China, which was subsequently used in pet foods. This was a widespread problem and resulted in a pet-food recall initiated by manufacturers who had found that their products had been contaminated. Further vegetable protein imported from China was later implicated. It was claimed that some of the animals that had eaten the contaminated food had become ill, although melamine was not previously believed to have been significantly toxic at low doses.

Melamine has no nutritional value but because it is high in nitrogen (66% by mass), its addition to food makes it appear to have more protein than it actually does and so meet required contractual obligations. Standard tests such as the Kjeldahl and Dumas tests estimate protein levels by measuring the nitrogen content, so values obtained can be increased by adding nitrogen-rich compounds such as melamine.

By early 2006, melamine production in mainland China was reported to be in "serious surplus". In September 2008, it was discovered that melamine was present in infant milk powder produced in China. Six infants are believed to have died as a result, and over 300,000 were reported to have been made ill. Traces of melamine were subsequently found in other dairy-based products in the region. Melamine has also been detected in other products, including eggs, originating in China. Actions taken in 2008 by the Government of China have reduced the practice of adulteration, with the goal of eliminating it. Court trials began in December 2008 for six people linked to the scandal and ended in January 2009 with those convicted being sentenced to death and executed.

Melamine is described as being "Harmful if swallowed, inhaled or absorbed through the skin. Chronic exposure may cause cancer or reproductive damage. It also acts as Eye, skin and respiratory irritant." However, the short-term lethal dose is on a par with common table salt with an LD50 of more than 3 grams per kilogram of bodyweight. However, it is thought that when melamine and cyanuric acid are absorbed together into the bloodstream, they concentrate and interact in the urine-filled microtubules in the kidneys, then crystallize and form large numbers of round, yellow crystals, which block and damage the renal cells that line the tubes, causing the kidneys to malfunction. Toxicology studies conducted after recalls of contaminated pet food concluded that the combination of melamine and cyanuric acid in the diet does lead to acute renal failure in cats and rats. The European Union set a standard for acceptable human consumption of melamine at 0.5 milligrams per kg of body mass (reduced to 0.2 mg per kg in April 2010). Member States of the European Union are required under Commission Decision 2008/757/EC to ensure that all composite products containing at least 15% of milk product, originating from China, are systematically tested before import into the Community and that all such products which are shown to contain melamine in excess of 2.5 mg/kg are immediately destroyed. More recently there has been concern about the migration of melamine from food contact materials. In addition, there have been reports of melamine residues as a result of the use of cyromazine, an insecticide derived from melamine.

C) Spanish Toxic Oil Syndrome

This incident started as a deliberate act of fraudulent adulteration. A large volume of rapeseed oil had been treated with aniline to downgrade it for industrial use. Some unscrupulous traders decided to refine, decolourise and deodorise this oil, mix it with other oils, package and label it as olive oil, and then illegally introduced it on to the Spanish market. Unfortunately, the oil contained a highly toxic substance formed in a reaction between the aniline and fatty acids in the oil, resulting in the deaths of up to 600 people and over 20,000 people affected by health problems.

v) Pesticides and veterinary residues

A) Pesticides

Pesticides include chemical and biological products specifically designed to control pests, weeds and diseases, particularly in the production of food. These include insecticides, fungicides, herbicides, rodenticides and molluscicides.

Pesticides are licensed for use against specific target organisms, and their use and application are strictly regulated to control the risks to the operator involved in applying them, and the surrounding environment, and to prevent significant residues being left in or on the food. Regulations include restrictions on the target organisms the chemical may be used against, the crops on which it may be used, the concentrations that may be applied and the number of applications permitted. There are strict limits on the levels of pesticide residues allowed in food and this is closely monitored by regulatory authorities worldwide. Pesticides can be classified by target organism, chemical structure, and physical state. They can be categorized as inorganic, synthetic, or biological (biopesticides). Biopesticides include microbial pesticides and biochemical pesticides. Plant-derived pesticides include the pyrethroids, rotenoids, and nicotinoids. Many pesticides can be grouped into chemical families. The main insecticide families include organochlorines, organophosphates and carbamates. These operate by disrupting the sodium/potassium balance of the nerve fibre, forcing the nerve to transmit continuously. Toxicities of these chemicals vary greatly, but they have been largely phased out because of their persistence and potential to bioaccumulate. The organochlorines have been largely replaced by the organophosphates and carbamates. Both of these operate through inhibiting the enzyme acetylcholinesterase, allowing acetylcholine to transfer nerve impulses indefinitely and causing a variety of symptoms such as weakness or paralysis. However, organophosphates are quite toxic to vertebrates, and they have in some cases been replaced by the less toxic carbamates. Prominent families of herbicides include phenoxy and benzoic acid herbicides (e.g. 2,4-D), triazines (e.g. atrazine), ureas (e.g. diuron), and chloroacetanilides (e.g. alachlor). Phenoxy compounds are designed as selective weedkillers to kill broadleaved weeds rather than grasses. The phenoxy and benzoic acid herbicides function in a similar way to plant growth hormones, and cause cells to grow without normal cell division, affecting the plant's nutrient transport system.

Triazines interfere with photosynthesis. Many commonly used pesticides such as glyphosate are not included in these families.

In the UK, there is a national monitoring programme overseen by the Pesticides Residues Committee, which measures the levels of pesticide residues in a wide range of foods, to check that they are within legal and safe limits. The limits apply both to food produced both in the UK and that imported from elsewhere. A number of different statutory bodies are involved in regulating which pesticides may be used and how. There are particularly strict limits on the levels of pesticides allowed in infant formulae and manufactured baby foods.

B) Veterinary residues

The use of medicines used to treat animals raised for food is regulated in a similar manner to that for pesticides used on food crops. There are a wide variety of chemicals for different uses, including:

- Antimicrobials such as sulphadiazine, enrofloxacin, ciprofloxacin, chlortetracycline, amoxicillin and oxytetracycline used to control bacterial diseases

- Pain-killers and anti-inflammatory medicines such as NSAIDs, including ibuprofen and phenylbutazone

- Dips to control external parasites, including organochlorine or organophosphorus insecticides

- Wormers to control internal parasites, such as ivermectin

- Coccidiostats to control protozoal diseases, particularly in poultry, such as nicarbazin

- Steroids such as boldenone

How are Maximum Limits Set?

As can be seen from the above examples, there are a variety of chemical hazards that could enter food. Some of these are unpredictable (e.g. those that are deliberately added), but most can be, and are, controlled. The main route for this is Good Manufacturing Practice and monitoring of environmental conditions and the quality of incoming ingredients and raw materials. However, part of the control at a national or international level may be in the form of the setting of maximum legal limits. What these limits are and how they are determined may vary from one part of the world to another, depending on specific circumstances, but in general three main areas are taken into consideration.

- Toxicity evidence: How toxic is the contaminant believed to be and how sound is the evidence for this belief?

- Good Manufacturing Practice: What is technologically achievable and how costly is it?

- Analytical capability: What are the limits of detection or quantification?

In all instances, safety is the primary concern, and maximum limits are usually set at about 100 times below the level at which a toxic effect is noted. However, maximum limits to control contaminant levels are only meaningful if they can be monitored by analysis (see below). In addition, even if a contaminant is only mildly toxic, it may be possible to reduce levels to well below the toxicity/100 threshold by Good Manufacturing Practice. This approach is taken with many pesticides, where good agricultural practice (including correct application regimes and suitable intervals between application and harvesting) will result in no remaining residues. Maximum levels are therefore set at the 'limit of detection' or 'limit of quantification'.

The maximum limit for a chemical will often be different for different food types - and there may well be a limited number of foods for which a maximum limit is set. It may be unnecessary to specify a maximum limit in cases where the chemical would not be expected to be found in the food. In contrast, it may very difficult to limit a chemical in some food types, and so higher limits are set, based on what is realistically achievable (bearing in mind that safety is still the over-riding factor). Nitrates provide a good example of this. In Europe, high nitrate levels are only a significant issue in leafy vegetables (spinach and lettuce), and it is these products for which limits have been set. However, levels will vary depending on growing conditions and season, and so different maxima have been set for different situations. These are typically in the range 2000-3000 ppm.

The Codex Alimentarius Commission has set maximum and guideline levels for the following chemical hazards that are an inherent risk in certain foods. The figures given are typical but may vary in some cases depending on product type and whether consumed raw or further processed. In particular the levels set for foods for infants and young children are often much lower than those for the general population.

The figures given are merely for illustration; for any individual contaminant in a particular foodstuff, the original text should be consulted.

- Mycotoxins
- Aflatoxins (15µg/kg in peanuts; 0.5µg/kg M1 in milk)
- Patulin (50µg/kg in apple juice)
- Heavy metals
- Arsenic (typically 0.1mg/kg)
- Cadmium (typically 0.05-0.2mg/kg)
- Lead (typically 0.1-1mg/kg)
- Mercury (0.001mg/kg in natural mineral water; 0.1mg/kg in food grade salt)
- Methylmercury (0.5mg/kg in fish - 1mg/kg in predatory fish)
- Tin (150mg/kg in canned beverages; 250mg/kg in canned fruit and vegetables)

Radionuclides (1-10,000 Bq/kg, depending on individual radionuclide - generally 10- fold lower in infant foods)

Others

Plastic monomers (typically 60mg/kg of food or 10mg/dm2 of package surface)

Acrylonitrile (0.02mg/kg)

Vinylchloride monomer (0.01mg/kg)

Asacomparison,intheEU,thefollowinghavebeenset(seehttp://eurlex.europa.eu/LexUriServ/LexUriServ.do?uri=CONSLEG:2006R1881:20090701:EN:PDF)

Nitrates (typically 2000-4500 mg/kg)

Mycotoxins

Aflatoxins (typically 4-15µg/kg in total; 0.05µg/kg M1 in milk)

Ochratoxin A (typically 2-10 µg/kg)

Patulin (50 µg/kg in apple juice; 25 µg/kg in solid apple products)

Deoxynivalenol (typically 500-1750µg/kg)

Zearalenone (typically 50-200 µg/kg)

Fumonisins (200-2000 µg/kg)

Metals

Lead (0.02-1.5mg/kg)

Cadmium (0.05-1mg/kg)

Mercury (0.5-1mg/kg)

Tin (100mg/kg in canned beverages; 200mg/kg in other canned foods)

3-MCPD (20 µg/kg in HVP and soy sauce)

Dioxins and PCBs (usually picogram levels per gram of fat)

Polycyclic aromatic hydrocarbons

Benzo[a]pyrene (1-10 µg/kg)

In addition, there are limits for many components of plastic packaging materials.

Analytical Approaches

As mentioned above, robust analytical methods are essential if the occurrence of chemical hazards in food is to be monitored and controlled. The type of method used will depend primarily on the chemical concerned, as well as the levels likely to be present and the food matrix.

Analysts have at their disposal a wider range of analytical techniques than ever before, and the sophistication of many of these would have been almost unimaginable just a few decades ago. This means that the analyst can now measure lower levels of a wide range of compounds in many different sample types. But it also means that the analyst has to be careful about the approach taken. Getting the right result requires the correct approach – and this includes using the right method of analysis.

A method of analysis typically involves several stages, and can involve a combination of techniques. Following sample receipt and the associated administrative requirements, the sample may need to be pre-treated (e.g. ground or blended), before the analyte is extracted (e.g. by solvent extraction). This latter stage may involve an initial crude extraction, followed by a purification stage (e.g. on an affinity chromatography column). Only then can the analyte be measured. Following analysis, the results have to be correctly interpreted and reported. In many cases, the extraction and/or purification stages are combined with the actual analytical stages, as happens with liquid or gas chromatography techniques linked with mass spectrometry.

Given the breadth of chemical hazards that might be present in food, the variability in their nature, and the many different types of food matrices, it is impossible to describe in any detail the types of analytical techniques that could be used. Some of the many generic techniques available are described in Jones (2005). In some cases it is possible to analyse many related chemicals in one sweep - screening. This is possible for a wide range of pesticides, for example, and for some of the illegal dyes. In many other cases targeted analysis is required, i.e. a specific procedure for an individual chemical.

When looking to analyse any chemical hazard in food (or indeed any chemical), there are a few basic points to note:

- Purpose of the analysis - it is important for those commissioning the analysis to be clear about the reasons for the analysis and how the result is to be used

- Sampling - samples should be representative of the product being analysed. Once taken, the samples should be handled, stored and prepared properly, so that they are not altered in any way that would affect the analysis

- Method suitability - the analytical method has to be fit for purpose - even if a method has been devised for the specific hazard in question, it may have to be adapted or modified for a particular foodstuff or to take into account other chemicals present that may interfere with the analysis

- Validation - following on from the above, the method, if it is new or modified, will have to be validated - i.e. tested to show that it works

- Quality control and standardisation - although the method itself has been shown to be fit for purpose, there needs to be evidence that it can produce consistent results over a period of time and in the hands of different analysts.

- Measurement uncertainty - no method will ever give exactly the right result all the time - in fact, in any analysis the result obtained will only ever be an approximation (adequately close, if the method is suitable) to the 'true' answer. It is important to understand where the potential sources of error might arise, and which are the most significant, when interpreting the results.

PREVENTING CHEMICAL SAFETY BREAKDOWNS IN THE FOOD CHAIN

HACCP

The most effective and efficient way of minimising the chances of chemical (and any other) safety issues arising in the food chain is through the use of HACCP (Hazard Analysis and Critical Control Points) systems. In the EU, it is a requirement throughout the industry to use HACCP-based systems to ensure food safety. In essence this means identifying which chemicals may be a problem in a particular food, and the measures to limit (or eliminate) their occurrence or remove them. It is then a case of monitoring and documenting what is being done and sampling the final product from time to time to ensure that the protocol is working.

The HACCP approach is based on seven internationally recognized simple principles:

1. Conduct a hazard analysis: prepare a flow diagram of the steps in the process; identify and list the hazards associated with the process and specify how they are going to be controlled.

2. Determine the critical control points (CCPs), i.e. those stages at which hazard control is essential for the production of a safe end-product.

3. Establish critical limits for each hazard at each CCP, i.e. the levels for each individual hazard that must not be exceeded if a safe product is going to be achieved. This may, for example, be a requirement to boil red kidney beans vigorously for 10 minutes in order to eliminate haemagglutinin (lectin) activity.

4. Set up a system to monitor control of each CCP by scheduled testing and observations, to ensure that the hazard remains within critical limits.

5. Establish what corrective action needs to be taken if monitoring indicates that a particular CCP is not under control or is moving out of control, i.e. is going beyond critical limits – this means stopping something going wrong before it happens, if at all possible.

6. Set up procedures to make sure that the overall HACCP plan is working as desired; this may include some end-product testing and a regular review of the system.

7. Establish thorough documentation of the system, process and procedures, and of all measurementstaken relating to the monitoring of the process.

Surveillance

General monitoring of levels of specific chemicals in foods is part of the HACCP process, but in addition to this there are general government-initiated surveillance programmes for specific chemicals. These may be long-term studies to determine trends in levels of well-known hazards in the environment, such as dioxins or nitrates, or may be as a result of a specific problem that arise. As an example, both the UK's Food Standards Agency (FSA) and the EU's European Food Safety Authority (EFSA) publish reports of surveillance exercises. In addition, there are also systems in place to inform the industry of specific incidents as they arise.

Traceability

Maintaining adequate traceability in the food supply chain is a prerequisite to controlling the hazards which may be present in many food ingredients. This is a mandatory requirement in many countries and should include robust supplier assurance programmes as well as full records of all transactions as food is traded, processed and placed on sale. In the event of a recall due to the identification of a food hazard it will be necessary to identify through the records all possible products implicated and to remove them from sale and/or consumption.

8

Genetically Modified Foods: Risk Perceptions and Safety Issues

Genetically modified foods (GM foods, or biotech foods) are foods derived from genetically modified organisms (GMOs), specifically, genetically modified crops. GMOs have had specific changes introduced into their DNA by genetic engineering techniques. These techniques are much more precise than mutagenesis (mutation breeding) where an organism is exposed to radiation or chemicals to create a non-specific but stable change. Other techniques by which humans modify food organisms include selective breeding and somaclonal variation.

Commercial sale of genetically modified foods began in 1994, when Calgene first marketed its Flavr Savr delayed ripening tomato.Typically, genetically modified foods are transgenic plant products: soybean, corn, canola, and cotton seed oil. These may have been engineered for faster growth, resistance to pathogens, production of extra nutrients, or any other beneficial purpose. GM livestock have also been experimentally developed, although as of July 2010 none are currently on the market. While there is broad scientific consensus that food on the market derived from GM crops pose no greater risk to human health than conventional food.

Method of Production

Genetically engineered plants are generated in a laboratory by altering their genetic makeup and are tested in the laboratory for desired qualities. This is usually done by adding one or more genesto a plant's genome using genetic engineering techniques. Most genetically modified plants are generated by the biolistic method (particle gun) or by *Agrobacterium tumefaciens* mediated transformation.

Once satisfactory plants are produced, sufficient seeds are gathered, and the companies producing the seed need to apply for regulatory approval to field-test the seeds. If these field tests are successful, the company must seek regulatory approval for the crop to be marketed. Once that approval is obtained, the seeds are mass-produced, and sold to farmers. The farmers produce genetically modified crops, which also contain the inserted gene and its protein product. The farmers then sell their crops as commodities into the food supply market, in countries where such sales are permitted.

History

Scientists first discovered that DNA can transfer between organisms in 1946. The first genetically modified plant was produced in 1983, using an antibiotic-resistant tobacco plant. In 1994, the transgenic Flavr Savr tomato was approved by the FDA for marketing in the US - the modification allowed the tomato to delay ripening after picking. In the early 1990s, recombinant chymosin was approved for use in several countries, replacing rennet in cheese-making. In the US in 1995, the following transgenic crops received marketing approval: canola with modified oil composition (Calgene), *Bacillus thuringiensis* (Bt) corn/maize (Ciba-Geigy), cotton resistant to the herbicide bromoxynil (Calgene), Bt cotton (Monsanto), *Bt* potatoes (Monsanto), soybeans resistant to the herbicide glyphosate (Monsanto), virus-resistant squash (Monsanto-Asgrow), and additional delayed ripening tomatoes (DNAP, Zeneca/Peto, and Monsanto). In 2000, with the creation of golden rice, scientists genetically modified food to increase its nutrient value for the first time. As of 2011, the U.S. leads a list of multiple countries in the production of GM crops, and 25 GM crops had received regulatory approval to be grown commercially. As of 2013, roughly 85% of corn, 91% of soybeans, and 88% of cotton produced in the United States are genetically modified.

Foods with Protein or DNA Remaining from GMOs

Currently, there are several GM crops that are food sources. In some cases, the product is directly consumed as food, but in most cases, crops that have been genetically modified are sold as commodities, which are further processed into food ingredients.

Fruits and Vegetables

Papaya has been genetically modified to resist the ringspot virus. 'SunUp' is a transgenic red-fleshed Sunset cultivar that is homozygous for the coat protein gene of PRV; 'Rainbow' is a yellow-fleshed F1 hybrid developed by crossing 'SunUp' and nontransgenic yellow-fleshed 'Kapoho'. The New York Times stated that "in the early 1990s, Hawaii's papaya industry was facing disaster because of the deadly papaya ringspot virus. Its single-handed savior was a breed engineered to be resistant to the virus. Without it, the state's papaya industry would have collapsed. Today, 80% of Hawaiian papaya is genetically engineered, and there is still no conventional or organic method to control ringspot virus."

The New Leaf potato, brought to market by Monsanto in the late 1990s, was developed for the fast food market, but was withdrawn from the market in 2001[18] after fast food retailers did not pick it up and food processors ran into export problems. There are currently no transgenic potatoes marketed for human consumption. However, in October 2011 BASF requested cultivation and marketing approval as a feed and food from the EFSA for its Fortuna potato, which was made resistant to late blight by adding two resistance genes, blb1 and blb2, which originate from the Mexican wild potato *Solanum bulbocastanum.*

As of 2005, about 13% of the zucchini grown in the US was genetically modified to resist three viruses; the zucchini is also grown in Canada.

As of 2012, an apple that has been genetically modified to resist browning, known as the Nonbrowning Arctic apple produced by Okanagan Specialty Fruits, is awaiting regulatory approval in the US and Canada. A gene in the fruit has been modified such that the apple produces lesspolyphenol oxidase, a chemical that manifests the browning.

Milled Corn Products

Human-grade corn can be processed into grits, meal, and flour. Grits are the coarsest product from the corn dry milling process. Grits vary in texture and are generally used in corn flakes, breakfast cereals, and snack foods. Brewers' grits are used in the beer manufacturing process.

Corn meal is an ingredient in several products including cornbread, muffins, fritters, cereals, bakery mixes, pancake mixes, and snacks. The finest grade corn meal is often used to coat English muffins and pizzas. Cornmeal is also sold as a packaged good.

Corn flour is one of the finest textured corn products generated in the dry milling process. Some of the products containing corn flour include mixes for pancakes, muffins, doughnuts, breadings, and batters, as well as baby foods, meat products, cereals, and some fermented products. Masa flour is another finely textured corn product. It is produced using the alkaline-cooked process. A related product, masa dough, can be made using corn flour and water. Masa flour and masa dough are used in the production of taco shells, corn chips, and tortillas.

Milled Soy Products

Soybean seed contains about 19% oil. To extract soybean oil from seed, the soybeans are cracked, adjusted for moisture content, rolled into flakes and solvent-extracted with commercial hexane. The remaining soybean meal has a 50% soy protein content. The meal is 'toasted' (a misnomer because the heat treatment is with moist steam) and ground in a hammer mill. Ninety-eight percent of the U.S. soybean crop is used for livestock feed. Part of the remaining 2% of soybean meal is processed further into high protein soy products that are used in a variety of foods, such as salad dressings, soups, meat analogues, beverage powders, cheeses, nondairy creamer, frozen desserts, whipped topping, infant formulas, breads, breakfast cereals, pastas, and pet foods.

Soy Protein Isolates

Food-grade soy protein isolate first became available on October 2, 1959 with the dedication of Central Soya's edible soy isolate, Promine D, production facility on the Glidden Company industrial site in Chicago. Soy protein isolate is a highly refined or purified form of soy protein with a minimum protein content of 90% on a moisture-free basis. It is made from soybean meal which has had most of the nonprotein components, fats and carbohydrates removed. Soy isolates are mainly used to improve the texture of processed meat products, but are also used to increase protein content, to enhance moisture retention, and are used as an emulsifier.

Soy Protein Concentrates

Soy protein concentrate is about 70% soy protein and is basically soybean meal without the water-soluble carbohydrates. Soy protein concentrate retains most of the fiber of the original soybean. It is widely used as a functional or nutritional ingredient in a wide variety of food products, mainly in baked foods, breakfast cereals, and in some meat products. Soy protein concentrate is used in meat and poultry products to increase water and fat retention and to improve nutritional values (more protein, less fat).

Flours

Soy flour is made by grinding soybeans into a fine powder. It comes in three forms: natural or full-fat (contains natural oils); defatted (oils removed) with 50% protein content and with either high water solubility or low water solubility; and lecithinated (lecithin added). As soy flour is gluten-free, yeast-raised breads made with soy flour are dense in texture. Soy grits are similar to soy flour except the soybeans have been toasted and cracked into coarse pieces. *Kinako* is a soy flour used in Japanese cuisine.

Textured Soy Protein

Textured soy protein (TSP) is made by forming a dough from soybean meal with water in a screw-type extruder, and heating with or without steam. The dough is extruded through a die into various possible shapes and dried in an oven. The extrusion technology changes the structure of the soy protein, resulting in a fibrous, spongy matrix similar in texture to meat. TSP is used as a low-cost substitute in meat and poultry products.

Highly Processed Derivatives Containing Little to No DNA or Protein

Lecithin

Corn oil and soy oil, already free of protein and DNA, are sources of lecithin, which is widely used in processed food as an emulsifier. Lecithin is highly processed. Therefore, GM protein or DNA from the original GM crop from which it is derived is often undetectable with standard testing practices - in other words, it is not substantially different from lecithin derived from non-GM crops. Nonetheless, consumer concerns about genetically modified food have extended to highly purified derivatives from GM food, like lecithin. This concern led to policy and regulatory changes in Europe in 2000, when Regulation (EC) 50/2000 was passed which required labelling of food containing additives derived from GMOs, including lecithin. Because it is nearly impossible to detect the origin of derivatives like lecithin with current testing practices, the European regulations require those who wish to sell lecithin in Europe to use a meticulous system of Identity preservation (IP).

Vegetable Oil

Most vegetable oil used in the US is produced from several crops, including the GM crops canola, corn, cotton, and soybeans. Vegetable oil is sold directly to consumers as cooking oil, shortening, and margarine, and is used in prepared foods.

There is no, or a vanishingly small amount of, protein or DNA from the original GM crop in vegetable oil. Vegetable oil is made of triglycerides extracted from plants or seeds and then refined, and may be further processed via hydrogenation to turn liquid oils into solids. The refining process removes all, or nearly all non-triglyceride ingredients.

Corn Starch and Starch Sugars, Including Syrups

Starch or amylum is a carbohydrate consisting of a large number of glucose units joined by glycosidic bonds. This polysaccharide is produced by all green plants as an energy store. Pure starch is a white, tasteless and odourless powder that is insoluble in cold water or alcohol. It consists of two types of molecules: the linear and helical amylose and the branched amylopectin. Depending on the plant, starch generally contains 20 to 25% amylose and 75 to 80% amylopectin by weight.

To make corn starch, corn is steeped for 30 to 48 hours, which ferments it slightly. The germ is separated from the endosperm and those two components are ground separately (still soaked). Next the starch is removed from each by washing. The starch is separated from the corn steep liquor, the cereal germ, the fibers and the corn gluten mostly in hydrocyclones and centrifuges, and then dried. This process is called wet milling and results in pure starch. The products of that pure starch contain no GM DNA or protein.

Starch can further modified to create modified starch for specific purposes, including creation of many of the sugars in processed foods. They include:

- Maltodextrin, a lightly hydrolyzed starch product used as a bland-tasting filler and thickener.

- Various glucose syrups, also called corn syrups in the US, viscous solutions used as sweeteners and thickeners in many kinds of processed foods.

- Dextrose, commercial glucose, prepared by the complete hydrolysis of starch.

- High fructose syrup, made by treating dextrose solutions with the enzyme glucose isomerase, until a substantial fraction of the glucose has been converted to fructose. In the United States, high fructose corn syrup is the principal sweetener used in sweetened beverages because fructose has better handling characteristics, such as microbiological stability, and more consistent sweetness/flavor. One kind of high fructose corn syrup, HFCS-

55, is typically sweeter than regular sucrose because it is made with more fructose, while the sweetness of HFCS-42 is on par with sucrose.

- Sugar alcohols, such as maltitol, erythritol, sorbitol, mannitol and hydrogenated starch hydrolysate, are sweeteners made by reducing sugars.

Sugar

The United States imports 10% of its sugar from other countries, while the remaining 90% is extracted from domestically grown sugar beet and sugarcane. Of the domestically grown sugar crops, half of the extracted sugar is derived from sugar beet, and the other half is from sugarcane.

After deregulation in 2005, glyphosate-resistant sugar beet was extensively adopted in the United States. 95% of sugar beet acres in the US were planted with glyphosate-resistant seed in 2011. Sugar beets that are herbicide-tolerant have been approved in Australia, Canada, Colombia, EU, Japan, Korea, Mexico, New Zealand, Philippines, Russian Federation, Singapore, and USA.

The food products of sugar beets are refined sugar and molasses. Pulp remaining from the refining process is used as animal feed. The sugar produced from GM sugarbeets is highly refined and contains no DNA or protein—it is just sucrose, the same as sugar produced from non-GM sugarbeets.

Foods Processed Using Genetically Engineered Products

Cheese

Rennet is a mixture of enzymes used to coagulate cheese. Originally it was available only from the fourth stomach of calves, and was scarce and expensive, or was available from microbial sources, which often suffered from bad tastes. With the development of genetic engineering, it became possible to extract rennet-producing genes from animal stomach and insert them into certain bacteria, fungi or yeasts to make them produce chymosin, the key enzyme in rennet. The genetically modified microorganism is killed after fermentation and chymosin isolated from the fermentation broth, so that the Fermentation-Produced Chymosin (FPC) used by cheese producers is identical in amino acid sequence to the animal source. The majority of the applied chymosin is retained in the whey and, at most, may be present in cheese in trace quantities. In ripe cheese, the type and provenance of chymosin used in production cannot be determined.

FPC was the first artificially produced enzyme to be registered and allowed by the US Food and Drug Administration. FPC products have been on the market since 1990 and have been considered in the last 20 years the ideal milk-clotting enzyme. In 1999, about 60% of US hard cheese was made with FPC and it has up to 80% of the global market share for rennet. By 2008, approximately 80% to 90% of commercially made cheeses in the US and Britain were made using FPC. Today, the most widely used Fermentation-Produced Chymosin (FPC) is produced either by the fungus *Aspergillus niger* and commercialized under the trademark CHY-MAX® by the Danish company Chr. Hansen, or produced by *Kluyveromyces lactis* and commercialized under the trademark MAXIREN® by the Dutch company DSM.

Foods Made from Animals Fed with GM Crops or Treated with Bovine Growth Hormone

Livestock and poultry are raised on animal feed, much of which is composed of the leftovers from processing crops, including GM crops. For example, approximately 43% of a canola seed is oil. What remains is a canola meal that is used as an ingredient in animal feed and contains protein from the canola. Likewise, the bulk of the soybean crop is grown for oil production and soy meal, with the high-protein defatted and toasted soy meal used as livestock feed and dog food. 98% of the U.S. soybean crop is used for livestock feed. As for corn, in 2011, 49% of the total maize harvest was used for livestock feed (including the percentage of waste from distillers grains). "Despite methods that are becoming more and more sensitive, tests have not yet been able to establish a difference in the meat, milk, or eggs of animals depending on the type of feed they are fed. It is impossible to tell if an animal was fed GM soy just by looking at the resulting meat, dairy, or egg products. The only way to verify the presence of GMOs in animal feed is to analyze the origin of the feed itself."

In some countries, recombinant bovine somatotropin (also called rBST, or bovine growth hormone or BGH) is approved for administration to dairy cows in order to increase milk production. rBST may be present in milk from rBST treated cows, but it is destroyed in the digestive system and even if directly injected, has no direct affect on humans. The Food and Drug Administration,World Health Organization, American Medical Association, American Dietetic Association, and the National Institute of Health have independently stated that dairy products and meat from BST treated cows are safe for human consumption. However, on 30 September 2010, the United States Court of Appeals, Sixth Circuit, analyzing evidence submitted in briefs, found that there is a "compositional difference" between milk from rBGH-treated cows and milk from untreated cows. The court stated that milk from rBGH-treated cows has: increased levels of the hormoneInsulin-like growth factor 1 (IGF-1); higher fat content and lower protein content when produced at certain points in the cow's lactation cycle; and more somatic cell counts, which may "make the milk turn sour more quickly."

Foods Made from GM Animals

As of December 2012 there were no genetically modified animals approved for use as food, but a GM salmon was near FDA approval at that time.

Animals (e.g. goat,) usually used for food production (e.g. milk,) have already been genetically modified and approved by the FDA and EMA to produce non-food products (for example, recombinant antithrombin, an anticoagulant protein drug.)

Detection

Testing on GMOs in food and feed is routinely done using molecular techniques like DNA microarrays or qPCR. These tests can be based on screening genetic elements (like p35S, tNos, pat, or bar) or event-specific markers for the official GMOs (like Mon810, Bt11, or GT73). The array-based method combines multiplex PCR and array technology to screen samples for different potential GMOs, combining different approaches (screening elements, plant-specific markers, and event-specific markers).

The qPCR is used to detect specific GMO events by usage of specific primers for screening elements or event-specific markers. Controls are necessary to avoid false positive or false negative results. For example, a test for CaMV is used to avoid a false positive in the event of virus contaminated sample.

In a January 2010 paper, the extraction and detection of DNA along a complete industrial soybean oil processing chain was described to monitor the presence of Roundup Ready (RR) soybean: "The amplification of soybean lectin gene by end-point polymerase chain reaction (PCR) was successfully achieved in all the steps of extraction and refining processes, until the fully refined soybean oil. The amplification of RR soybean by PCR assays using event-specific primers was also achieved for all the extraction and refining steps, except for the intermediate steps of refining (neutralisation, washing and bleaching) possibly due to sample instability. The real-time PCR assays using specific probes confirmed all the results and proved that it is possible to detect and quantify genetically modified organisms in the fully refined soybean oil. To our knowledge, this has never been reported before and represents an important accomplishment regarding the traceability of genetically modified organisms in refined oils."

Regulation of the Release of Genetic Modified Organisms

The regulation of genetic engineering concerns the approaches taken by governments to assess and manage the risks associated with the use of genetic engineering technology and the development and release of genetically modified organisms (GMO), including genetically modified crops and genetically modified fish. There are differences in the regulation of GMOs between countries, with some of the most marked differences occurring between the USA and Europe. Regulation varies in a given country depending on the intended use of the products of the genetic engineering. For example, a crop not intended for food use is generally not reviewed by authorities responsible for food safety.

One of the key issues concerning regulators is whether GM products should be labeled. Labeling can be mandatory up to a threshold GM content level (which varies between countries) or voluntary. A study investigating voluntary labeling in South Africa found that 31% of products labeled as GMO-free had a GM content above 1.0%. In Canada and the USA labeling of GM food is voluntary, while in Europe all food (including processed food) or feed which contains greater than 0.9% of approved GMOs must be labelled.

Although there is now broad scientific consensus that GE crops on the market are safe to eat, ((OECD, 2000) some scientists who work at institutions such as the University of Texas and Cornell University, and advocacy groups such as Greenpeace and World Wildlife Fund have called for additional and more rigorous testing for GM food.

History

The development of a regulatory framework concerning genetic engineering began in 1975, at Asilomar, California. The first use of Recombinant DNA (rDNA) technology had just been successfully accomplished by Stanley Cohen and Herbert Boyer two years previously and the scientific community recognized that as well as benefits this technology could also pose some risks. TheAsilomar meeting recommended a set of guidelines regarding the cautious use of recombinant technology and any products resulting from that technology. The Asilomar recommendations were voluntary, but in 1976 the US National Institute of Health (NIH) formed a rDNA advisory committee. (Hutt, 1978)This was followed by other regulatory offices (the United States Department of Agriculture(USDA), Environmental Protection Agency (EPA) and Food and Drug Administration (FDA)), effectively making all rDNA research tightly regulated in the USA. In 1982 the Organization for Economic Co-operation and Development (OECD) released a report into the potential hazards of releasing genetically modified organisms into the environment as the first transgenic plants were being developed. As the technology improved and genetically organisms moved from model organisms to potential commercial products the USA established a committee at the Office of Science and Technology (OSTP) to develop mechanisms to regulate the developing technology. In 1986 the OSTP assigned regulatory approval of genetically modified plants in the US to the USDA, FDA and EPA.

The basic concepts for the safety assessment of foods derived from GMOs have been developed in close collaboration under the auspices of the Organisation for Economic Co-operation and Development (OECD) and the United Nations' World Health Organisation (WHO) and Food and Agricultural Organisation (FAO). A first joint FAO/WHO consultation in 1990 resulted in the publication of the report 'Strategies for Assessing the Safety of Foods Produced by Biotechnology' in 1991. Building on that, an international consensus was reached by the OECD's Group of National Experts on Safety in Biotechnology, for assessing biotechnology in general, including field testing GM crops. That Group met again in Bergen, Norway in 1992 and reached consensus on principles for evaluating the safety of GM food; its report, 'The safety evaluation of foods derived by modern technology – concepts and principles' was published in 1993. That report recommends conducting the safety assessment of a GM food on a case-by-case basis through comparison to an existing food with a long history of safe use. This basic concept has been refined in subsequent workshops and consultations organized by the OECD, WHO, and FAO, and the OECD in particular has taken the lead in acquiring data and developing standards for conventional foods to be used in assessing substantial equivalence. In 2003 the Codex Alimentarius Commission of the FAO/WHO adopted a set of "Principles and Guidelines on foods derived from biotechnology" to help countries coordinate and standardize regulation of GM food to help ensure public safety and facilitate international trade and updated its guidelines for import and export of food in 2004.

Substantial Equivalence

"Substantial equivalence" is a starting point for the safety assessment for GM foods that is widely used by national and international agencies - including the Canadian Food Inspection Agency, Japan's Ministry of Health and Welfare and the U.S. Food and Drug Administration, the United Nation's Food and Agriculture Organization, the World Health Organization and the OECD.

A quote from FAO, one of the agencies that developed the concept, is useful for defining it: "Substantial equivalence embodies the concept that if a new food or food component is found to be substantially equivalent to an existing food or food component, it can be treated in the same manner with respect to safety (i.e., the food or food component can be concluded to be as safe as the conventional food or food component)". The concept of substantial equivalence also recognises the fact that existing foods often contain toxic components (usually called antinutrients) and are still able to be consumed safely - in practice there is some tolerable chemical risk taken with all foods, so a comparative method for assessing safety needs to be adopted. For instance, potatoes and tomatoes can contain toxic levels of respectively, solanine and alpha-tomatine alkaloids.

To decide if a modified product is substantially equivalent, the product is tested by the manufacturer for unexpected changes in a limited set of components such as toxins, nutrients, or allergens that are present in the unmodified food. The manufacturer's data is then assessed by a regulatory agency, such as the U.S. Food and Drug Administration. That data, along with data on the genetic modification itself and resulting proteins (or lack of protein), is submitted to regulators. If regulators determine that the submitted data show no significant difference between the modified and unmodified products, then the regulators will generally not require further food safety testing. However, if the product has no natural equivalent, or shows significant differences from the unmodified food, or for other reasons that regulators may have (for instance, if a gene produces a protein that had not been a food component before), the regulators may require that further safety testing be carried out.

A 2003 review in *Trends in Biotechnology* identified seven main parts of a standard safety test:

- Study of the introduced DNA and the new proteins or metabolites that it produces;
- Analysis of the chemical composition of the relevant plant parts, measuring nutrients, anti-nutrients as well as any natural toxins or known allergens;
- Assess the risk of gene transfer from the food to microorganisms in the human gut;

- Study the possibility that any new components in the food might be allergens;

- Estimate how much of a normal diet the food will make up;

- Estimate any toxicological or nutritional problems revealed by this data in light of data on equivalent foods;

- Additional animal toxicity tests if there is the possibility that the food might pose a risk.

There has been discussion about applying new biochemical concepts and methods in evaluating substantial equivalence, such as metabolic profiling and protein profiling. These concepts refer, respectively, to the complete measured biochemical spectrum (total fingerprint) of compounds (metabolites) or of proteins present in a food or crop. The goal would be to compare overall the biochemical profile of a new food to an existing food to see if the new food's profile falls within the range of natural variation already exhibited by the profile of existing foods or crops. However, these techniques are not considered sufficiently evaluated, and standards have not yet been developed, to apply them.

There are controversies over the definition and application of substantial equivalence.

By Continent

Africa

In 2010, after nine years of talks, the Common Market for Eastern and Southern Africa (COMESA) produced a draft policy on GM technology, which was sent to all 19 national governments for consultation in September 2010. Under the proposed policy, new GM crops would be scientifically assessed by COMESA. If the GM crop was deemed safe for the environmental and human health, permission would be granted for the crop to be grown in all 19 member countries, although the final decision would be left to each individual country. South Africa is the major grower of Genetically Modified crops in Africa, with smaller amounts grown in Burkina Faso and Egypt. The National Assembly of Burkina Faso passed a biosafety law in early 2006, which established a National Biosafety Agency that would regulate GM products with the advice of various governmental and non-governmental advisory committees. In Burkina Faso, the African Biosafety Network of Expertise school, set up by the African Union and funded by the Bill and Melinda Gates Foundation, opened in April 2010. Its aim is to train and develop African regulators to approve, monitor and track genetically modified crops. Kenya passed laws in 2011(Denge and Gachenge, 2011), and Ghana and Nigeria passed laws in 2012 which allowed the production and importation of GM crops. A study investigating voluntary labeling in South Africa found that 31% of products labeled as GMO-free had a GM content above 1.0%.

In 2002, Zambia cut off the flow of genetically modified food (mostly maize) from UN's World Food Programme on the basis of the Cartagena Protocol. This left the population without food aid during a famine. In December 2005 the Zambian government changed its mind in the face of further famine and allowed the import of GM maize. However, the Zambian Minister for Agriculture Mundia Sikatana has insisted that the ban on genetically modified maize remains, saying "We do not want GM (genetically modified) foods and our hope is that all of us can continue to produce non-GM foods."

Asia

India and China are the two largest producers of genetically modified products in Asia. India currently only grows GM cotton, while China produces GM varieties of cotton, poplar, petunia, tomato, papaya and sweet pepper. Cost of enforcement of regulations in India are generally higher, possibly due to the greater influence farmers and small seed firms have on policy makers, while the enforcement of regulations was more effective in China.

GM crops in China go through three phases of field trials (pilot field testing, environmental release testing, and preproduction testing) before they are submitted to the Office of Agricultural Genetic Engineering Biosafety Administration (OAGEBA) for assessment. Producers must apply to OAGEBA at each stage of the field tests. The Chinese Ministry of Science and Technology developed the first biosafety regulations for GM products in 1993 and they were updated in 2001. The 75 member National Biosafety Committee evaluates all applications, although OAGEBA has the final decision. Most of the National Biosafety Committee are involved in biotechnology leading to criticisms that they do not represent a wide enough range of public concerns.

The release of transgenic crops in India is governed by the Indian Environment Protection Act, which was enacted in 1986. The Institutional Biosafety Committee (IBSC), Review Committee on Genetic Manipulation (RCGM) and Genetic Engineering Approval Committee (GEAC) all review any genetically modified organism to be released, with transgenic crops also needing permission from the Ministry of Agriculture.[43] India regulators cleared the Bt brinjal, a genetically modified eggplant, for commercialisation in October 2009. Following opposition from some scientists, farmers and environmental groups a moratorium was imposed on its release in February 2010.

Other Asian countries that grew GM crops in 2011 were Pakistan, the Philippines and Myanmar. Japan requires labeling so consumers can exercise choice between foods that have genetically modified, conventional or organic origins.

South America

Brazil and Argentina are the 2nd and 3rd largest producers of GM food behind the USA. The Argentine government was one of the first to accept GM food. Assessment of GM products for release is provided by the National Agricultural Biotechnology Advisory Committee (environmental impact), the National Service of Health and Agrifood Quality (food safety) and the National Agribusiness

Direction (effect on trade), with the final decision made by the Secretariat of Agriculture, Livestock, Fishery and Food. The government is looking to tighten the current law which allows farmers to keep seed without paying royalties in a bid to encourage more private investment.

In Brazil the National Biosafety Technical Commission is responsible for assessing environmental and food safety and prepares guidelines for transport, importation and field experiments involving GM products. The Council of Ministers evaluates the commercial and economical issues with release. The National Biosafety Technical Commission has 27 members and includes 12 scientists, 9 ministerial representatives and 6 other specialists.

In April 2004 Hugo Chávez announced a total ban on genetically modified seeds in Venezuela. On September 28, 2008, Ecuador prohibited genetically engineered crops and seeds in its 2008 Constitution, approved by 64% of the population in a referendum (Article 15). Honduras, Costa Rica, Colombia, Bolivia, Paraguay, Chile, and Uruguay also allow GM crops to be grown.

Europe

Until the 1990s, Europe's regulation was less strict than in the United States, one turning point being cited as the export of the United States' first GM-containing soy harvest in 1996. The GM soy made up about 2% of the total harvest at the time, and EuroCommerce and European food retailers required that it be separated. In 1998, the use of MON810, a Bt expressing maize conferring resistance to the European corn borer, was approved for commercial cultivation in Europe. Shortly thereafter, the EU enacted a *de facto* moratorium on new approvals of GMOs pending new regulatory laws passed in 2003.

Those new laws provided the European Union (EU) with possibly the most stringent GMO regulations in the world. All GMOs, along with irradiated food, are considered "new food" and subject to extensive, case-by-case, science based food evaluation by the European Food Safety Authority (EFSA). The criteria for authorization fall in four broad categories: "safety," "freedom of choice," "labelling," and "traceability." The EFSA reports to the European Commission who then draft a proposal for granting or refusing the authorisation. This proposal is submitted to the Section on GM Food and Feed of the Standing Committee on the Food Chain and Animal Health and if accepted it will be adopted by the EC or passed on to the Council of Agricultural Ministers. Once in the Council it has three months to reach a qualified majority for or against the proposal, if no majority is reached the proposal is passed back to the EC who will then adopt the proposal. However, even after authorization, individual EU member states can ban individual varieties under a 'safeguard clause' if there are "justifiable reasons" that the variety may cause harm to humans or the environment. The member state must then supply sufficient evidence that this is the case. The Commission is obliged to investigate these cases and either overturn the original registrations or request the country to withdraw its temporary restriction. The laws of the EU also stipulated that member nations establish minimum distances between fields of GM crops and non-GM crops. The distances for GM maize from non-GM maize for the six largest biotechnology countries are; France: 50 meters, Britain: 110 meters for grain maize and 80 for silage maize, Netherlands: 25 meters in general and 250 for organic or GM-free fields, Sweden: 15–50 meters, Finland: data not available, and Germany: 150 meters and 300 from organic fields.

In 2006, the World Trade Organization concluded that the EU moratorium, which had been in effect from 1998 to 2004, had violated international trade rules. The moratorium had not affected previously approved crops. The only crop authorised for cultivation before the moratorium was Monsanto's MON 810. The next approval for cultivation was the Amflora potato for industrial applications in 2010 which was grown in Germany, Sweden and the Czech Republic that year.

The slow pace of approval has been criticized as endangering European food safety although as of 2012, the EU has authorized the use of 48 genetically modified organisms. Most of these were for use in animal feed (it was reported in 2012 that the EU imports about 30 million tons a year of GM crops for animal consumption., food or food additives. 26 of these were varieties of maize. In July 2012 the EU gave approval for an Irish trial cultivation of potatoes resistant to the blight that caused the Great Irish Famine.

The safeguard clause mentioned above has been applied by many member states in various circumstances, and in April 2011 there were 22 active bans in place across six member states:Austria, France, Germany, Luxembourg, Greece, and Hungary. However, on review many of these have been considered scientifically unjustified.

In January 2005, the Hungarian government announced a ban on importing and planting of genetic modified maize seeds, which was subsequently authorized by the EU.

- In February 2008 the French government used the safeguard clause to ban the cultivation of MON810 after Senator Jean-François Le Grand, chairman of a committee set up to evaluate biotechnology, said there were "serious doubts" about the safety of the product (although this ban was declared illegal in 2011 by the European Court of Justice and the French Conseil d'État. The French farm ministry reinstated the ban in 2012, but this was rejected by the EFSA.

- In 2009 German Federal Minister Ilse Aigner announced an immediate halt to cultivation and marketing of MON810 maize under the safeguard clause.

- In March 2010, Bulgaria imposed a complete ban on genetically modified crop growing either commercially or for trials. The cabinet of Boyko Borisov initially imposed a 5-year moratorium, but later extended it to a permanent ban after widespread public protests against the introduction of genetically modified crops in the country. And in recent years, France and several other European countries banned cultivation of Monsanto's MON-810 corn and similar genetically modified food crops.

In 2012, the European Food Safety Authority (EFSA) Panel on Genetically Modified Organisms (GMO) released a "Scientific opinion addressing the safety assessment of plants developed through cisgenesis and intragenesis" in a response to a request from the European Commission. The opinion was, that while "the frequency of unintended changes may differ between breeding techniques and their occurrence cannot be predicted and needs to be assessed case by case," "similar hazards can be associated with cisgenic and conventionally bred plants, while novel hazards can be associated with intragenic and transgenic plants." In other words, cisgenic genetic engineering approaches should be considered similar in risk to conventional breeding approaches, each of which are more risky than transgenic approaches.

Labeling and Traceability

The regulations concerning the import and sale of GMOs for human and animal consumption grown outside the EU involve providing freedom of choice to the farmers and consumers. All food (including processed food) or feed which contains greater than 0.9% of approved GMOs must be labelled. Twice GMOs unapproved by the EC have arrived in the EU and been forced to return to their port of origin. (John, 2010) The first was in 2006 when a shipment of rice from America containing an experimental GMO variety (LLRice601) not meant for commercialisation arrived at Rotterdam. The second in 2009 when trace amounts of a GMO maize approved in the US were found in a "non-GM" soy flour cargo.

The coexistence has raised significant concern in many European countries and so EU law also requires that all GM food be traceable to its origin, and that all food with GM content greater than 0.9% be labelled. Due to high demand from European consumers for freedom of choice between GM and non-GM foods. EU regulations require measures to avoid mixing of foods and feed produced from GM crops and conventional or organic crops, which can be done via isolation distances or biological containment strategies. (Unlike the US, European countries require labeling of GM food.) European research programs such as Co-Extra, Transcontainer, and SIGMEA are investigating appropriate tools and rules for traceability. The OECD has introduced a "unique identifier" which is given to any GMO when it is approved, which must be forwarded at every stage of processing. Such measures are generally not used in North America because they are very costly and the industry admits of no safety-related reasons to employ them. The EC has issued guidelines to allow the co-existence of GM and non-GM crops through buffer zones (where no GM crops are grown). These are regulated by individual countries and vary from 15 meters in Sweden to 800 meters in Luxembourg. All food (including processed food) or feedwhich contains greater than 0.9% of approved GMOs must be labelled.

A 5-digit Price Look-Up code beginning with the digit *8* indicates genetically modified food. However the absence of the "8" does not necessarily indicate the food is not genetically modified since no retailer to date has elected to use the digit in voluntarily labeling genetically modified foods.

North America

The United States and Canada do not require labeling of genetically modified foods. The USA is the largest commercial grower of genetically modified crops in the world. United States regulatory policy is governed by the Coordinated Framework for Regulation of Biotechnology This regulatory policy framework that was developed under the Presidency of Ronald Reagan to ensure safety of the public and to ensure the continuing development of the fledgling biotechnology industry without overly burdensome regulation. The policy as it developed had three tenets: "(1) U.S. policy would focus on the product of genetic modification (GM) techniques, not the process itself, (2) only regulation grounded in verifiable scientific risks would be tolerated, and (3) GM products are on a continuum with existing products and, therefore, existing statutes are sufficient to review the products."

For a genetically modified organism to be approved for release, it must be assessed by the Animal and Plant Health Inspection Service (APHIS) agency within the US Department of Agriculture(USDA) and may also be assessed by the Food and Drug Administration (FDA) and the Environmental protection agency (EPA), depending on the intended use of the organism. The USDA evaluates the plant's potential to become a weed, and the FDA reviews plants that could enter or alter the food supply, and the EPA regulates genetically modified plants with pesticide properties, as well as agrochemical residues. Most genetically modified plants are reviewed by at least two of the agencies, with many subject to all three. Within the organization are departments that regulate different areas of GM food including, the Center for Food Safety and Applied Nutrition (CFSAN,) and the Center for Biologics Evaluation and Research (CBER). Final approval can still be denied by individual counties within each state. In 2004, Mendocino County, California became the first and only county to impose a ban on the "Propagation, Cultivation, Raising, and Growing of Genetically Modified Organisms", the measure passing with a 57% majority.

Several laws govern the US regulatory agencies. These laws are statutes the agencies review when determining the safety of a particular GM food. These laws include:

- The Federal Insecticide, Fungicide, and Rodenticide Act (FIFRA) (EPA);
- The Toxic Substances Control Act (TSCA) (EPA);
- The Federal Food, Drug, and Cosmetic Act (FFDCA) (FDA and EPA);
- The Plant Protection Act (PPA) (USDA);
- The Virus-Serum-Toxin Act (VSTA) (USDA);
- The Public Health Service Act (PHSA)(FDA);
- The Dietary Supplement Health and Education Act (DSHEA) (FDA)
- The Meat Inspection Act (MIA)(USDA);
- The Poultry Products Inspection Act (PPIA) (USDA);

- The Egg Products Inspection Act (EPIA) (USDA); and

- The National Environmental Protection Act (NEPA).

Mainland Canada is one of the world's largest producers of GM canola and also grows GM maize, soybean and sugarbeet. Health Canada, under the Food and Drugs Act, and the Canadian Food Inspection Agency are responsible for evaluating the safety and nutritional value of genetically modified foods. The Canadian regulatory system is based on whether a product has novel features regardless of method of origin. In other words, a product is regulated as GM if it carries some trait not previously found in the species whether it was generated using traditional breeding methods (e.g selective breeding, cell fusion, mutation breeding) or genetic engineering. Canadian law requires that manufacturers and importers submit detailed scientific data to Health Canada for safety assessments for approval. This data includes: information on how the GM plant was developed; nucleic acid data that characterizes the genetic change; composition and nutritional data of the novel food compared to the original non-modified food' potential for new toxins; and potential for being an allergen. A decision is then made whether to approve the product for release along with any restrictions or requirements. Labeling of foods as products of Genetic Engineering or not products of Genetic Engineering is voluntary. The Canadian regulations were reviewed by the Canadian Biotechnology Advisory Committee between 1999 and 2003, with the conclusion that the current level of regulation was satisfactory. The committee was accused by environmental and citizen groups of not representing the full spectrum of public interests by only having one member of the board of 20 representing non-governmental organisations and for being too closely aligned to industry groups.

On the 15 February 2005, after consulting the Mexican Academy of Sciences, Mexico's senate passed a law allowing planting and selling of genetically modified cotton and soybean. The law requires all genetically modified products to be labelled according to guidelines issued by the Mexican Ministry of Health. In 2009 the government enacted statutory provisions for the regulation of genetically modified maize. Mexico is the center of diversity for maize and concerns have been raised about the impact genetically modified maize could have on local strains.

Oceania

Malaysia, New Zealand, and Australia require labeling so consumers can exercise choice between foods that have genetically modified, conventional or organic origins.

Food Standards Australia New Zealand must approve any food produced from GM crops, or made using genetically engineered enzymes, before it can be marketed in Australia or New Zealand. FSANZ makes a list of such approvals available on its website.

Genetic engineering in Australia was originally (since 1987) overseen by the Genetic Manipulation Advisory Committee, before the Office of the Gene Technology Regulator (OGTR) and Food Standards Australia New Zealand took over in 2001. The OTGR is a Commonwealth Government Authority within the Department of Health and Ageing and reports directly to Parliament through a Ministerial Council on Gene Technology and has legislative powers. It was established as part of the Gene Technology Act 2003 and operates according to the Gene Technology Regulations 2001. The OGTR reports directly to Parliament through a Ministerial Council on Gene Technology and has legislative powers. The OGTR decides on license applications for the release of all genetically modified organisms, while regulation is provided by the Therapeutic Goods Administration for GM medicines or Food Standards Australia New Zealand for GM food. The individual state governments are then able to assess the impact of release on markets and trade and apply further legislation to control approved genetically modified products.

Genetically modified cotton, canola, and carnations are grown in Australia. Genetically modified cotton has been grown commercially in New South Wales and Queensland since 1996. GM canola was approved in 2003 and was first grown in 2008.

In 2011 genetically modified plants were grown in all states except South Australia and Tasmania, who have extended their moratoriums until 2019 and 2014. The Queensland and Northern Territory Governments have not implemented any further legislation beyond the national level, but several other states placed bans on planting certain GM crops. In 2007 the New South Wales government extended a blanket moratorium on GM food crops until 2011, but allowed groups to apply for exemptions. New South Wales approved GM Canola for commercial cultivation in 2008, while the Victorian government let the moratorium on GM Canola expire in 2007. Western Australia passed the Genetically Modified Crops Free Areas Act in 2003 and was declared a GM free area in 2004. In 2008 an exception was made for the commercial cultivation of GM cotton in the Ord River Irrigation Areas. Trials of GM canola were carried out in 2003 and in 2010 the Western Australian government allowed the commercialisation of GM canola.

In New Zealand, no genetically modified food is grown and no medicines containing live genetically modified organisms have been approved for use. However, medicines manufactured using genetically modified organisms that do not contain live organisms have been approved for sale, and imported foods with genetically modified components are sold. In 2000 the Government appointed a Royal Commission to report on issues relating to genetically modified organisms (GMOs). The Report of the Royal Commission on Genetic Modification, released in July 2001, concluded that New Zealand should keep its options open with regard to genetic engineering and to proceed carefully in order to minimise and manage any risks. Field trials have been carried out with GM pine trees and brassicas.

Genetically Modified Food Controversies

The genetically modified foods controversy is a dispute over the relative advantages and disadvantages of food derived from genetically modified organisms, genetically modified crops used to produce food and other goods, and other uses of genetically modified organisms in food production. The dispute involves consumers, biotechnology companies, governmental regulators, non-governmental organizations and scientists. The key areas of controversy related to genetically modified (GM) food are: risk of harm from GM food, whether GM food should be labeled, the role of government regulators, the effect of GM crops on the environment, the impact of GM crops for farmers, including farmers in developing countries, the role of GM crops in feeding the growing world population, and GM crops as part of the industrial agriculture system.

There is broad scientific consensus that food on the market derived from GM crops pose no greater risk than conventional food. No reports of ill effects have been documented in the human population from GM food. Supporters of food derived from GMOs hold that food is as safe as other foods and that labels send a message to consumers that GM food is somehow dangerous. They trust that regulators and the regulatory process are sufficiently objective and rigorous, and that risks of contamination of the non-GM food supply and of the environment can be managed. They trust that there is sufficient law and regulation to maintain competition in the market for seeds, believe that GM technology is key to feeding a growing world population, and view GM technology as a continuation of the manipulation of plants that humans have conducted for millennia.

Advocacy groups such as Greenpeace and World Wildlife Fund have concerns that risks of GM food have not been adequately identified and managed, and have questioned the objectivity of regulatory authorities. Opponents of food derived from GMOs are concerned about the safety of the food itself and wish it banned, or at least labeled. They have concerns about the objectivity of regulators and rigor of the regulatory process, about contamination of the non-GM food supply, about effects of GMOs on the environment, about industrial agriculture in general, and about the consolidation of control of the food supply in companies that make and sell GMOs, especially in the developing world. Some are concerned that GM technology tampers too deeply with nature.

Public Perception

Social science surveys have documented that individuals are more risk averse about food than institutions. There is widespread concern within the public about the risks of biotechnology, a desire for more information about the risks themselves and a desire for choice in being exposed to risk. The introduction of so-called *"wonder-products"* such as DDT and PCBs and their subsequent withdrawal after unforeseen problems were discovered, has undermined public trust in companies that introduce products that are pervasively used, and in the government agencies meant to regulate them. There is also a widespread sense that social and technological change is speeding up and people feel powerless to affect this change; diffuse anxiety driven by this context becomes focused when it is food that is being changed.

In 2006, the Pew Initiative on Food and Biotechnology made public a review of U.S. survey results from 2001-2006. The review showed that Americans' knowledge of genetically modified foods and animals was low through the period. During this period there were protests against Calgene's Flavr Savr transgenic tomato that described the GM tomato as being made with fish genes, confusing it with DNA

Plant Technology's Fish tomato experimental transgenic organism, which was never commercialized.

A 2010 Deloitte survey found that 34% of U.S. consumers were very or extremely concerned about GM food, a 3% reduction from 2008. The same survey found a strong gender difference in opinion: 10% of men were extremely concerned, compared with 16% of women, and 16% of women were unconcerned, compared with 27% of men. A 2009 review article of European consumer polls concluded that opposition to GMOs in Europe has been gradually decreasing. Approximately half of European consumers accepted gene technology, particularly when benefits for consumers and for the environment could be linked to GMO products. 80% of respondents did not cite the application of GMOs in agriculture as a significant environmental problem. Many consumers seem unafraid of health risks from GMO products and most European consumers did not actively avoid GMO products while shopping. The 2010 "Eurobarometer" survey, which assesses public attitudes about biotech and the life sciences in Europe, found that "cisgenics, GM crops produced by adding only genes from the same species or from plants that are crossable by conventional breeding," evokes a different reaction than transgenic methods, where "genes are taken from other species or bacteria that are taxonomically very different from the gene recipient and transferred into plants." A 2007 survey by the Food Standards Australia and New Zealand found that in Australia where labeling is mandatory, 27% of Australians looked at the label to see if it contained GM material when purchasing a grocery product for the first time.

There is a concerted and organised effort from many environmental and other advocacy groups to impose moratoriums or ban GMO products from being commercialised. International organisations like Greenpeace and Friends of the Earth include genetic engineering as part of their environmental and political concerns. Other groups like GMWatch and The Institute of Science in Society concentrate mostly or solely on opposing genetically modified crops.

Opponents of GM food have been labelled "the Climate Skeptics of the Left" by Keith Kloor of Slate Magazine. Others have labelled the anti-GM ideologies as conspiracy theories.

Health

Governments worldwide assess and manage the risks associated with the release of genetically modified organisms and the marketing of genetically modified food. There are differences in the risk assessment of GM food, and therefore in the regulation of GMOs, between countries. Some of the most marked differences occur between the USA and Europe. Crops not intended for food use are generally not reviewed by authorities responsible for food safety. Food derived from GMOs is not tested in humans before it is marketed as it is not a single chemical, nor is it intended to be ingested in specific doses and times, which makes it difficult to design meaningful clinical studies. Regulators examine the genetic modification, its protein products, and any intended changes that those proteins make to the food. Regulators also check to see whether the food derived from a GMO is "substantially equivalent" to its non-GM-derived counterpart, which provides a way to detect any negative non-intended consequences of the genetic engineering. If the newly incorporated protein is not similar to that of other proteins found in food or if anomalies arise in the substantial equivalence comparison, further toxicological testing is required.

There is broad scientific consensus that food on the market derived from GM crops is safe enough to eat. In 2012, the American Association for the Advancement of Science stated "Foods containing ingredients from genetically modified (GM) crops pose no greater risk than the same foods made from crops modified by conventional plant breeding techniques." TheAmerican Medical Association, the National Academies of Sciences and the Royal Society of Medicine have stated that no adverse health effects on the human population related to GM food have been reported and/or substantiated in peer-reviewed literature to date. The European Commission Directorate-General for Research and Innovation 2010 report on GMOs noted that "The main conclusion to be drawn from the efforts of more than 130 research projects, covering a period of more than 25 years of research, and involving more than 500 independent research groups, is that biotechnology, and in particular GMOs, are not *per se* more risky than e.g. conventional plant breeding technologies." A 2004 report by Working Group 1 of the ENTRANSFOOD project, a group of scientists funded by the European Commission to identify prerequisites for introducing agricultural biotechnology products in a way that is largely acceptable to European society, (CORDIS, 2005) concluded that "the combination of existing test methods provides a sound test-regime to assess the safety of GM crops."

There is a view from many of the scientists and regulators who support GM food that there is a continuing need for improved testing technologies and protocols to identify and manage risk better. A consensus document released by the OECD in 2010 says that molecular characterisation by itself is not the best way to predict the safety of GM plants, but can focus the other safety assessment procedures. They also suggest that new technologies will develop that will aid in the "food, feed and environmental risk/safety assessments." While generally transgenic and cisgenic organisms are treated similarly when assessed, in 2012 the European Food Safety Authority (EFSA) Panel on Genetically Modified Organisms (GMO) has said that "novel hazards" could be associated with transgenic crops that will not be present in cisgenic ones. Advocacy groups such as Greenpeace, World Wildlife Fund, Organic Consumers Association, and Center for Food Safety have concerns that potential risks to health and the environment relating to GM have not yet been adequately investigated. In Japan, the Consumers Union of Japan say that truly independent research in these areas is systematically blocked by the GM corporations which own the GM seeds and reference materials. Independence in research has been studied by a 2011 analysis into conflicts of interest which found a significant correlation between author affiliation to industry and study outcome in scientific work published on health risks or nutritional assessment studies of genetically modified products.

Substantial Equivalence

The starting point for the safety assessment of genetically engineered food products by regulatory bodies is to assess if the food is "substantially equivalent" to their counterparts, which themselves are the products of genetic manipulation via traditional methods of cross-breeding and hybridization. The application of substantial equivalence has been criticized. In 1999, Andrew Chesson of the University of Aberdeen warned that substantial equivalence testing "could be flawed in some cases" and that some current safety tests could allow harmful substances to enter the human food chain. The same year Erik Millstone, Eric Brunner and Sue Mayer argued in a commentary in *Nature* that the substantial equivalence standard was pseudo-scientific and was the product of politics and business lobbying—they claimed it was created primarily to reassure consumers and to aid biotechnology companies in avoiding the time and cost of more rigorous safety testing. They suggested that all GM foods should have extensive biological, toxicological and immunological tests and that the concept of substantial equivalence should be abandoned. This commentary was criticized for providing a misleading presentation of history, for distorting existing data and applying bad logic. Retired scientist Harry Kuiper said it presented an oversimplified version of safety assessments and that equivalence testing involves more than chemical tests and may include toxicity testing. An opinion piece in the Los Angeles Times in 2001 by Barbara Keeler and Marc Lappe supported legislation in the US Congress to set aside the substantial equivalence standard and instead mandate that safety studies be performed.

This process was examined further in a 2002 which stated that substantial equivalence does not measure risks, but instead identifies differences between existing products and new foods, which might pose dangers to health. If differences do exist, identifying these differences is a starting point for a full safety assessment, rather than an end point. It concluded that "The concept of substantial equivalence is an adequate tool in order to identify safety issues related to genetically modified products that have a traditional counterpart". The review also noted difficulties in applying this standard in practice, including the fact that traditional foods contain many chemicals that have toxic or carcinogenic effects and that our existing diets therefore have not been proven to be safe. This lack of knowledge on unmodified food poses a problem, as GM foods may have differences in anti-nutrients and natural toxins that have never been identified in the original plant, raising the possibility that harmful changes could be missed. The possibility also exists that positive modifications may be missed. For example, corn damaged by insects often contains high levels of fumonisins, carcinongic toxins made by fungi that are carried on the backs of insects and that grow in the wounds of the damaged corn. Studies show that most Bt corn has lower levels of fumonisins than conventional corn damaged by insects. Regulators are aware of these issues and workshops and consultations organized by the OECD, WHO, and FAO have worked to acquire data and develop standards for conventional foods, for use in assessing substantial equivalence.

A survey of publications describing comparisons between the intrinsic qualities of GM and non-GM reference crop lines (comparing genomes, proteomes, and metabolomes of the plants themselves, not the plants' effects on an organism eating them) indicates that transgenic modification of crops has less impact on gene expression or on protein and metabolite levels than the variability generated by conventional breeding.

In a 2013 review published in the Journal of Agricultural and Food Chemistry, Rod A. Herman (Dow AgroSciences) and William D. Price (retired from FDA) argue that transgenesis is less disruptive of composition compared with traditional breeding techniques which routinely involve genetic mutations, deletions, insertions, and rearrangements. The FDA found all of the 148 transgenic events that they evaluated to be substantially equivalent to their conventional counterparts, as have the Japanese regulators for 189 submissions including combined-trait products. This equivalence is confirmed by over 80 peer-reviewed publications. Hence, the authors argue, compositional equivalence studies uniquely required for GM crops may no longer be justified on the basis of scientific uncertainty.

Allergenicity

Regulatory authorities require that new GM foods be tested for allergenicity before they are marketed.

Some environmental organizations, such as the European Green Party and Greenpeace, have suggested that GM food might trigger food allergies. A 2005 review in the journal *Allergy* of the results from allergen testing of current GM foods stated that "no biotech proteins in foods have been documented to cause allergic reactions".

The development of GM products which have been found to cause allergic reactions have been halted by the companies developing them before they were brought to market. In the early 1990s, Pioneer Hi-Bred attempted to improve the nutrition content of soybeans intended for animal feed by adding a gene from the Brazil nut. Because they knew that people have allergies to nuts, Pioneer ran both in vitro tests for allergy, in which they tested whether serum from people with nut allergies reacted to the transgenic soy; they also did skin prick tests with protein from the transgenic soy. The tests showed that the transgenic soy was allergenic. Pioneer Hi-Bred therefore discontinued further development. In 2005, a pest-resistant field pea developed by the Australian Commonwealth Scientific and Industrial Research Organisation for use as a pasture crop was shown to cause an allergic reaction in mice. Work on this variety was immediately halted. These cases of products that failed safety testing have been viewed as evidence that genetic modification can produce unexpected and dangerous changes in foods, and as evidence that the current tests are effective at identifying safety problems before foods come on the market.

Genetic modification can also be used to remove allergens from foods, potentially reducing the risk of food allergies. A hypo-allergenic strain of soybean was tested in 2003 and shown to lack the major allergen that is found in the beans. A similar approach has been tried in ryegrass, which produces pollen that is a major cause of hay fever: here a fertile GM grass was produced that lacked the main pollen allergen, demonstrating that the production of hypoallergenic grass is also possible.

Horizontal Gene Transfer from Plants to Animals

One concern raised has been the possibility of the transgenes transferring from plants used as feed to animals that are used for food, or from plants as used as food, to humans. See below for environmental risks of gene flow among plants.

The risk of horizontal gene transfer between plants and animals is very low and in most cases with GM crops this is expected to be lower than background rates. Two studies on the possible effects of giving genetically modified feed to animals found no residues of recombinant DNA or novel proteins in any organ or tissue samples obtained from animals fed with GMP plants. Studies have found DNA from the M13 virus, Green fluorescent protein and Rubisco genes in the blood and tissue of animals and in 2012 a paper showed that a specific microRNA from rice could be found at very low quantities in human and animal serum.

Of particular concern is that the antibiotic resistance gene commonly used as a genetic marker in transgenic crops could be transferred to harmful bacteria, creating superbugs that are resistant to multiple antibiotics. In 2004 a study involving human volunteers was conducted to see if the transgene from GM soy would transfer to the bacteria that naturally lives in the human gut. As of 2012 it is the only human feeding study conducted with genetically modified food. The transgene was only detected in three volunteers, part of seven who had previously had their large intestines removed for medical reasons. As this gene transfer did not increase after the consumption of GM soy, the researchers concluded that gene transfer did not occur during the experiment. In volunteers with complete digestive tracts, the transgene did not survive passage through intact gastrointestinal tract. The antibiotic genes used in genetic engineering are already found in many natural pathogens, commonly used during animal husbandry and not widely used prescribed.

Animal Feeding Studies

A 2012 review of more than 24 long-term animal feeding studies conducted by public research laboratories, concluded that none of these studies discovered any safety problem linked to long-term consumption of GM food. A 2009 review found that although most studies concluded that GM foods do not differ in nutrition or cause any detectable toxic effects in animals, some studies did report adverse changes at a cellular level caused by some GM foods, concluding that "More scientific effort and investigation is needed to ensure that consumption of GM foods is not likely to provoke any form of health problem". A review published in 2009 concluded that "results of most studies with GM foods indicate that they may cause some common toxic effects such as hepatic, pancreatic, renal, or reproductive effects and may alter the hematological, biochemical, and immunologic parameters". However responses to this review in 2009 and 2010 note that concentrated on articles with an anti-GM bias that have been refuted by scientists in peer-reviewed articles elsewhere - for example the 35S promoter, stability of transgenes, antibiotic marker genes and the claims for toxic effects of GM foods. It is concluded in a 2005 review that the current GM food with only a single gene modification are similar in nutrition and safety to non-GM foods, but noted that food with multiple gene modifications would be more difficult to test, and would require further animal studies. A 2004 review of animal feeding trials found no differences among animals eating genetically modified plants.

Human Studies and Obstacles

While some groups and individuals have called for more human testing of GM food, there are several obstacles to such studies. Both the US General Accounting Office (in a review of FDA procedures requested by Congress) and the FAO/WHO have confirmed that long term studies of the effect of GM food on humans are not feasible, for reasons including: there is no plausible hypothesis to test; very little is known about the potential long-term effects of any foods; identification of such effects is further confounded by the great variability in the way people react to foods; and epidemiological studies are not likely to differentiate the health effects of GM foods from the many undesirable effects of conventional foods. Additionally, there are strong ethics that guide the conduct of research on human subjects, which mandate that the intervention being tested must have a potential benefit for the human subjects, such as treatment for a disease or nutritional benefit (ruling out toxicity testing on humans). In this context, scientists and regulators discussing clinical studies of GM food have written that the "ethical and technical constraints of conducting human trials, and the necessity of doing so, is a subject that requires considerable attention." Golden rice has been tested in humans to see if the rice provides a nutritional benefit, namely, increased levels of Vitamin A. However the authors of a study in Chinese children published in 2012 have come under fire for not obtaining the consent of the parents of the children nor the Chinese government.

Individual Studies

There have been some individual studies published in journals that have suggested negative impacts from eating GM food. The first such peer reviewed paper to be published in 1998 was in 1999. Pusztai had fed rats GM potatoes transformed with the Galanthus nivalis agglutinin (GNA) gene from the Galanthus (snowdrop) plant, allowing the GNA lectin protein to be synthesised. (Ewen and Purztai, 1999) Lectin is known to be toxic, especially to gut epithelium, and while some companies were considering making GM crops expressing lectin, GNA was an unlikely candidate. On June 22, 1998 a short interview was shown on Granada Television's current affairs programme World in Action, with Pusztai saying that rats fed the potatoes had stunted growth and a repressed immune system. A media frenzy resulted and Pusztai was suspended from the Rowett Institute with misconduct procedures used to seize his data and ban him from speaking publicly. The Rowett Institute and the Royal Society reviewed Pusztai's work and concluded that the data did not support his conclusions. When his work was eventually published in *The Lancet* it reported significant differences in the thickness of the gut epithelium of rats fed genetically modified potatoes (compared to those fed the control diet), but no differences in growth or immune system function were suggested. The published paper was criticised on the grounds that the unmodified potatoes were not a fair control diet, and that any rats fed only on potatoes will suffer from a protein deficiency. Pusztai responded to these criticisms by stating that all the diets had the same protein and energy content and that the food intake of all rats was the same. The incident became known as the Pusztai affair.

In 2007, 2009, and 2011 published re-analysis studies that used data from Monsanto rat feeding experiments for three GM maize varieties (insect resistant MON 863 and MON 810, and the glyphosate resistance NK603). It concluded that they had actually caused liver, kidney, and heart damage in the rats. The European Food Safety Authority (EFSA) reviewed the data and concluded that the small differences were all within the normal range for control rats. The EFSA review also stated that the statistical methods used were incorrect. The EFSA conclusions were supported by Food Standards Australia New Zealand (FSANZ), a panel of toxicologists funded by Monsanto and the French High Council of Biotechnologies Scientific Committee (HCB).

In 2012 the Séralini lab published a paper that looked at the long term effects of feeding rats various levels of GM roundup resistance maize, maize spiked with the roundup chemical and a mixture of the two. The paper concluded that rats fed GM maize had an increased incidence of cancer. Once published, there was widespread criticism of the study. Séralini held a press conference just before the paper was released; he allowed reporters access to the paper before his press conference only if they signed a confidentiality agreement under which they could not get other scientists' responses to the paper. This method of announcing the research met with strong criticism from scientists and some journalists as it excluded critical commentary in the breaking stories. Many claimed that Séralini's conclusions were impossible to justify given the statistical power of the study and that Sprague-Dawley rats were not appropriate for a lifetime study (as opposed to a shorter toxicity study) because these rats have a high tendency to get cancer over their lifespan (one study found over 80% got cancer under normal conditions). For a similar study the Organisation for Economic Co-operation and Development guidelines recommend using 65 rats per experiment, not 10. Questions were also raised about the statistical method chosen to analyse the data and the lack of data regarding the amount of food fed to the rats and their growth rates. Other criticisms included the lack of a dose–response relationship (females fed three times the dose showed a decreased number of tumours) and no identifiable mechanism for the increase in tumours. Six French national academies of science issued an unprecedented joint statement condemning the study and the journal that published it. *Food and Chemical Toxicology* published 17 letters to the editor that expressed strong criticism of the Seralini paper. National food safety and regulatory agencies also reviewed the paper and dismissed it.

A 2011 study, the first to evaluate the correlation between maternal and fetal exposure to Bt toxin produced in genetically modified maize and to determine exposure levels of the pesticides and their metabolites, reported the presence of pesticides associated with GM foods in both non-pregnant women and pregnant women and their fetuses. The paper and the media reports around it were criticized for overstating the results. FSANZ took the unusual step of posting a direct response, saying that the suitability of the ELISA assay method for detecting the Cry1Ab protein was not validated and that there was no evidence that GM food was the source of the protein. They also suggested that even if the protein was detected it was more likely to come from conventional or organic sources.

Environment

Genetically modified crops are planted in fields much like regular crops. There they interact directly with organisms that feed on the crops, and indirectly with other organisms in the wider food chain. The pollen from the plants behaves like the pollen of any other crop. This has led to concerns about effects of genetically-engineered crops on non-target species, and about gene flow to other plants, animals and bacteria. Some supporters of GM crops see these crops as providing benefits to the environment through a reduction in the use of pesticides (Conner et al., 2003; Wolfenbarger and Phifer, 2000) and a reduction in greenhouse gas emissions.

Non Target Organisms

One of the major uses of GM crops is in insect pest control through the expression of the *cry* (crystal delta-endotoxins) and *cyt* (cytolysins) genes from *Bacillus thuringiensis* (Bt). There are concerns that these toxins could target predatory and other beneficial or harmless insects as well as the targeted pest insect. The proteins produced by Bt have been used as organic sprays for insect control in France since 1938 and the USA since 1958 with no ill effects on the environment reported. While *cyt* proteins are toxic towards the insect orders Coleoptera (beetles) and Diptera (flies), *cry* proteins selectively target Lepidopterans (moths and butterflies). As a toxic mechanism, *cry* proteins bind to specific receptors on the membranes of mid-gut (epithelial) cells resulting in rupture of those cells. Any organism that lacks the appropriate receptors in its gut cannot be affected by the *cry* protein, and therefore Bt. Regulatory agencies assess the potential for the transgenic plant to impact non target organisms before approving their commercial release.

In 1999 a paper was published in *Nature* showing that in a lab environment pollen from Bt maize dusted onto milkweed could harm the monarch butterfly. A collaborative research exercise was carried out over the next two years by several groups of scientists in the US and Canada, looking at the effects of Bt pollen in both the field and the laboratory. This resulted in a risk assessment that concluded that any risk posed by the corn to butterfly populations under real-world conditions was negligible. A 2002 review of the scientific literature concluded that "the commercial large-scale cultivation of current Bt–maize hybrids did not pose a significant risk to the monarch population" and noted that despite large-scale planting of GM crops, the butterfly's population is increasing.

An analysis of laboratory settings found that Bt toxins can affect nontarget organisms, usually organisms closely related to the intended targets. Typically, exposure occurs through the consumption of plant parts, such as pollen or plant debris, or through Bt ingestion by their predatory food choices. The methodology used has been called into question by a group of academic scientists who wrote "We are deeply concerned about the inappropriate methods used in their paper, the lack of ecological context, and the authors' advocacy of how laboratory studies on non-target arthropods should be conducted and interpreted".

Biodiversity

There are concerns that the genetic diversity of various crops will decrease (as the development of GM varieties will lead to less cultivars being used overall) or that they will indirectly affect the diversity of other organisms. Also, there are concerns that the widespread use of GM crops designed to resist agrochemicals, leads to increased use of those agrochemicals, which in turn causes damage to the environment and to biodiversity.

Studies comparing the genetic diversity of cotton have found that in the USA the diversity has either increased or stayed the same, while in India it has reduced. This has been put down to the larger number of breeding varieties the technology was used on in the USA compared to India. A review of the effects of Bt crops on soil ecosystems found that in general they "appear to have no consistent, significant, and long-term effects on the microbiota and their activities in soil". The diversity and number of weed populations has been shown to decrease in farm-scale trials in the UK and Denmark when comparing herbicide resistant crops to their conventional counterparts. The UK trial suggested that the diversity of birds could be impacted by the decrease in weed seeds available for feeding. Published data from farms involved in the trials showed that seed eating birds were more abundant on conventional maize after the application of the herbicide, but that there were no significant differences in any other crop or prior to herbicide treatment. A 2012 study found a correlation between the reduction of milkweed in farms that grew glyphosate-resistant crops and the decline in adult monarch butterfly populations in Mexico. The New York Times reported that the study "raises the somewhat radical notion that perhaps weeds on farms should be protected.

A scientific study published in 2005 designed to "simulate the impact of a direct overspray on a wetland" with four different agrochemicals (carbaryl (Sevin), malathion, 2,4-Dichlorophenoxyacetic acid, and glyphosate in a Roundup formulation) by creating artificial ecosystems in tanks and then applying "each chemical at the manufacturer's maximum recommended application rates", found that "species richness was reduced by 15% with Sevin, 30% with malathion, and 22% with Roundup, whereas 2,4-D had no effect". The study has been used by environmental groups to argue that use of agrochemicals causes unintended harm to the environment and to biodiversity.

Emergence of Secondary Pests

Several studies have documented surges in secondary pests (which are not affected by Bt toxins) within a few years of adoption of Bt cotton. In China, the main problem has been with mirids, which have in some cases "completely eroded all benefits from Bt cotton cultivation".A 2009 study in China concluded that the increase in secondary pests depended on local temperature and rainfall conditions and increased in half the villages studied. The increase in insecticide use for the control of these secondary insects was far smaller than the reduction in total insecticide use due to Bt cotton adoption. Another study published in 2011 was based on a survey of 1,000 randomly selected farm households in five provinces in China and found that the reduction in pesticide use in Bt cotton cultivars is significantly lower than that reported in research elsewhere, consistent with the hypothesis suggested by recent studies that more pesticide sprayings are needed over time to control emerging secondary pests, such as aphids, spider mites, and lygus bugs. Similar problems have been reported in India, with both mealy bugs and aphids.

Gene Flow

Genes from a genetically modified organism may pass to another organism just like an endogenous gene. The process is known as outcrossing and can occur in any new open-pollinated crop variety, with newly introduced traits potentially crossing into neighboring crop plants of the same or sometimes closely related species. There are concerns that the spread of genes from modified organisms to unmodified relatives could produce species of weeds resistant to herbicides or could disrupt the ecosystem. This is primarily a concern if the transgenic organism has a significant survival capacity and can increase in frequency and persist in natural populations.

In most countries environmental studies are required prior to the approval of a GM plant for commercial purposes, and a monitoring plan must be presented to identify potential effects which have not been anticipated prior to the approval. In 2009 the government of Mexico created a regulatory pathway for approval of genetically modified maize, but because Mexico is the center of diversity for maize, concerns have been raised about the effect that genetically modified maize could have on local strains. A 2001 report in *Nature* presented evidence that Bt maize was cross-breeding with unmodified maize in Mexico, although the data in this paper was later described as originating from an artifact and *Nature* stated that "the evidence available is not sufficient to justify the publication of the original paper". A subsequent large-scale study, in 2005, failed to find any evidence of contamination in Oaxaca. However, other authors have stated that they also found evidence of cross-breeding between natural maize and transgenic maize.

As one of the major genetically modified traits is resistance to herbicides there have been concerns raised about the development of "super weeds".

In 2005, scientists at the UK Centre for Ecology and Hydrology reported the first evidence of horizontal gene transfer of pesticide resistance to weeds, in a few plants from a single season; they found no evidence that any of the hybrids had survived in subsequent seasons.

A study published in 2010 by scientists at the University of Arkansas, North Dakota State University, California State University and the US Environmental Protection Agency showed that about 83 percent of wild or weedy canola tested contained genetically modified herbicide resistance genes. According to the researchers, the lack of reports in the US suggests inadequate oversight and monitoring protocols are in place in the US. The development of weeds resistant to glyphosate, the most commonly applied herbicide, could mean that farmers must return to more labour intensive methods to control weeds, use more dangerous herbicides or till the soil (so increasing the risk of erosion). A 2010 report by the National Academy of Sciences stated that the advent of glyphosate-herbicide resistant weeds could cause the genetically engineered crops to lose their effectiveness unless farmers also use other established weed management strategies.

Another problem is that the gene can get into conventional or organic crops, affecting the trade of these crops as GE-free. Most countries have co-exixtence regulations to try and prevent cross-contamination of GM and non-GM crops. There have also been cases where genes from unapproved crops have escaped. In 2006, American exports of rice to Europe were interrupted when much of the US crop was confirmed to be contaminated with unapproved engineered genes. An investigation by the USDA's Animal and Plant Health Inspection Service (APHIS) was unable to determine the cause of the contamination. In 2007, the U.S. Department of Agriculture fined Scotts Miracle-Gro $500,000 when modified genetic material from creeping bentgrass, a new golf-course grass Scotts had been testing, was found within close relatives of the same genus (*Agrostis*) as well as in native grasses up to 21 km (13 mi) away from the test sites, released when freshly cut grass was blown by the wind.

One means that has been explored to avoid environmental contamination is Genetic use of restriction technology, also dubbed 'Terminator'. This uncommercialized technology would allow the production of crops with sterile seeds, which would prevent the escape of genetically modified traits. Groups concerned with control of the food supply had expressed concern that the technology would be used to limit access to viable seeds. Another similar hypothetical trait-specific technology known as 'Traitor' or 'T-GURT', requires application of a chemical to genetically modified crops to reactivate engineered traits. These technologies have also caused controversy, as there are fears the technology itself, and the patents on them, would allow companies to further control the market for seeds.

Chemical Use

One of the major environmental benefits from using GM crops is the reduction in the use of pesticides. Insect-resistant Bt-expressing crops will reduce the number of pest insects feeding on these plants without the farmers having to apply as much insecticides. A study published by the UK consultancy PG Economics, concluded that globally pesticide spraying was reduced by 286,000 tons in 2006, decreasing the environmental impact of herbicides and pesticides by 15%. A survey of small Indian farms between 2002 and 2008 concluded that Bt cotton adoption has led to higher yields and lower pesticide use. One study concluded insecticide use on cotton and corn during the years 1996 to 2005 fell by 35.6 million kg of insecticide active ingredient, which is roughly equal to the amount of pesticide applied to arable crops in the EU in one year. A study on the effects of using Bt cotton in six northern provinces of China from 1990 to 2010 concluded that Bt cotton halved the use of pesticides and doubled the level of ladybirds, lacewings and spiders, with the environmental benefits extended to neighbouring crops of maize, peanuts and soybeans. (Lu et al., 2012) The development of glyphosphate resistant plants has changed the herbicide use profile away from atrazine, metribuzin, and alachlor, which reduced the dangers of herbicide runoff into drinking water.

Resistant Insect Pests

Resistance evolves naturally after a population has been subjected to intense selection pressure in the form of repeated use of a single herbicide or insecticide. In November 2009, Monsanto scientists found the pink bollworm had become resistant to the first generation Bt cotton in parts of Gujarat, India - that generation expresses one Bt gene, $Cry1Ac$. This was the first instance of Bt resistance confirmed by Monsanto anywhere in the world. Bollworm resistance to first generation Bt cotton has also been identified in the Australia, China, Spain and the United States. The strategy to delay the emergence of Bt resistant pests has been to have non-GM refuges within the GM crops to dilute any resistant genes that may arise or more recently to develop GM crops that have multiple Bt genes that target different receptors within the insect.

Economics

The economic value derived from growing genetically modified food has been a major selling point for the technology. One of the key reasons for the widespread adoption is the perceived economic benefit the technology brings to farmers, including those in developing nations. A 2010 study by US scientists, found that the economic benefit of Bt corn to farmers in five mid-west states was $6.9 billion over the previous 14 years. They were surprised that the majority ($4.3 billion) of the benefit accrued to non-Bt corn. This was speculated to be because the European Corn Borers that attack the Bt corn die and there are fewer left to attack the non-GM corn nearby. Agriculture economists have calculated that "world surplus [increased by] $240.3 million for 1996. Of this total, the largest share (59%) went to U.S. farmers. The gene developer, Monsanto, received the next largest share (21%), followed by U.S. consumers (9%), the rest of the world (6%), and the germplasm supplier, Delta and Pine Land Company (5%)." A comprehensive 2012 study by PG Economics, a UK company, concluded that GM crops increased farm incomes worldwide by $14 billion in 2010, with over half this total going to farmers in developing countries.

Claims of major benefits to farmers, including poor farmers in developing countries, have been challenged by opponents. The task of isolating impacts of the technology is complicated by the prevalence of biased observers, and by the rarity of controlled comparisons (such as identical seeds, differing only in the presence or absence of the Bt trait, being grown in identical situations). The main Bt crop being grown by small farmers in developing countries is cotton, and a 2006 exhaustive review of findings on Bt cotton by agricultural economists concluded, "the overall balance sheet, though promising, is mixed. Economic returns are highly variable over years, farm type, and geographical location" Mark Lynas, an environmental activist, believes that an outright rejection of the technology is "illogical and potentially harmful to the interests of poorer peoples and the environment".

Impoverished Nations

The effect that genetically modified food may have on developing nations is debated. There is agreement that there is a food supply issue, although there is disagreement on the best ways to solve this. Some scientists suggest that a second Green Revolution with increased use of GM crops is needed to meet the demand for food in the developing world. Others say that there is more than enough food in the world and that the hunger crisis is caused by problems in food distribution and politics, not production. The potential for genetically modified food to help impoverished nations was recognised by the International Assessment of Agricultural Science and Technology for Development, but as of 2008 they found no conclusive evidence that they have offered a solution.

Constraints to the deployment of this technology to impoverished nations are the lack of easy access, expense of modern agricultural equipment, and that certain aspects of the system revolving around intellectual property rights are unfair to "undeveloped countries". Consultative Group on International Agricultural Research (CGIAR), an aid and research organization, was praised by the World Bank for its efforts but suggested they shift to genetics research and productivity enhancement. This plan has several obstacles such as patents, commercial licenses, and the difficulty that third world countries have in accessing the international collection of genetic resources and other intellectual property rights that would educate them about modern technology. The International Treaty on Plant Genetic Resources for Food and Agriculture has attempted to remedy this problem, but results have been inconsistent. As a result, "orphan crops", such as teff, millets, cowpeas, and indigenous plants, which are important in these countries receive little investment.

Yield

There is also debate over whether the use of genetically modified crops increases or decreases yield. The currently commercialised varieties have traits that reduce yield loss from insect pressure or weed interference. There are however crops and animals being developed with traits aimed at directly increasing the yield, with the closest to commercialisation being salmon with an added growth hormone gene.

A 2010 article supported by Crop Life International summarised the results of 49 peer reviewed studies on GM crops worldwide. (Carpenter, 2010) On average, farmers in developed countries experienced increase in yield of 6% and in underdeveloped countries of 29%. Tillage was decreased by 25–58% on herbicide resistant soybeans, insecticide applications on Bt crops were reduced by 14–76% and 72% of farmers worldwide experienced positive economic results. Another yield gain can be seen with the planting of glyphosate-resistant crops. It allowed farmers to plant rows closer together as they did not have to control post-emergent weeds with mechanical tillage.

Critics of genetic engineered crops disagree that they result in increased yield. In 2009 the Union of Concerned Scientists summarized peer-reviewed studies on the yield contribution of genetic engineered crops—soybeans and maize in the United States. The report concluded that in the United States, other agricultural methods have made a greater contribution to national crop yield increases in recent years than genetic engineering.

Intellectual Property

Traditionally, farmers in all nations saved their own seed from year to year. However since the early 1900s hybrid crops have been widely used in the developed world and seeds to grow these crops must be purchased each year from seed producers. The offspring of the hybrid corn, while still viable, lose the beneficial traits of the parents, resulting in the loss of hybrid vigor. In these cases, the use of hybrid plants has been the primary reason for growers not saving seed, not intellectual property issues. However, for non-hybrid biotech crops, such as transgenic soybeans, seed companies use intellectual property law and tangible property common law, each expressed in contracts, to forbid farmers from saving seed. For example, Monsanto's typical bailment license (covering transfer of the seeds themselves) forbids saving seeds, and also requires that purchasers sign a separate patent license agreement.

Corporations say that they need product control in order to prevent seed piracy, to fulfill financial obligations to shareholders, and to invest in further GM development. DuPont spent approximately half its $2 billion R&D budget on agriculture in 2011, while Monsanto spends 9-10% of their sales in their research and development effort every year.

Detractors such as Greenpeace say that patent rights give corporations a dangerous amount of control over their product. Others claim that "patenting seeds gives companies excessive power over something that is vital for everyone." Regarding the issues of intellectual property and patent law, an international report from the year 2000 states: "If the rights to these tools are strongly and universally enforced - and not extensively licensed or provided *pro bono* in the developing world - then the potential applications of GM technologies described previously are unlikely to benefit the less developed nations of the world for a long time (i.e. until after the restrictions conveyed by these rights have expired).

Monsanto has filed patent infringement suits against 145 farmers, but has proceeded to trial with only 11. Although in some of those 11 cases, a defense of unintentional contamination bygene flow was used, Monsanto won all 11 cases. Monsanto Canada's Director of Public Affairs has stated that "It is not, nor has it ever been Monsanto Canada's policy to enforce its patent on Roundup Ready crops when they are present on a farmer's field by accident. Only when there has been a knowing and deliberate violation of its patent rights will Monsanto act."

One example of such litigation is the Monsanto v. Schmeiser case. This case is widely misunderstood: "The fear about a company claiming ownership of a farmer's crop based on the inadvertent presence of GM pollen grain or seed is widespread and unfounded." In 1997, Percy Schmeiser, a canola breeder and grower in Bruno, Saskatchewan, discovered that a section of one of his fields contained canola that was resistant to herbicide Roundup by spraying it with Roundup, leaving only the resistant plants. He had not purchased roundup-resistant canola; it was apparently sown from seed blown onto his land from neighboring fields. He later harvested and saved the seed from this area, and replanted the saved seed in 1998. During the 1998 growing season, Monsanto approached Schmeiser and asked him to take a license to the patent covering the transgenic seed he had planted; Schmeiser refused, claiming that he owned the physical seeds he had harvested in 1997 and had the right to do with them as he wished. Monsanto sued Schmeiser for patent infringement and prevailed in the initial case. Schmeiser appealed and lost, and appealed again to the Canadian Supreme Court, which in 2004 ruled 5 to 4 in Monsanto's favor.

Market Dynamics

The seed industry is dominated by several seed and biotechnology firms. Firms have engaged in vertical integration, causing structural changes in the seed industry. It is reported that in 2011, 73% of the global market is controlled by 10 companies.

In 2001, the USDA published an article showing that the concentration of market power in the seed industry has led to economies of scale that facilitated market efficiency because production costs have decreased, however, the move by some companies to divest their seed operations calls into question the long-term viability of these conglomerates. Two economists, guest speakers on the AgBio Forum cite that the huge market power possessed by the small number of biotechnology companies in crop biotechnology could be beneficial in raising welfare despite the pricing strategies they practice because "even though price discrimination is often considered to be an unwanted market distortion, it may increase total welfare by increasing total output and by making goods available to markets where they would not appear otherwise."

Market power gives seed and biotechnology firms the ability to set or influence price, dictate terms, and act as a barrier to entry into the industry. It also gives firms the bargaining power over governments in policy making. In March 2010, the US Justice Department and the U.S. Department of Agriculture held a meeting in Ankeny, Iowa to look at the competitive dynamics in the seed industry. Christine Varney, who heads the antitrust division in the Justice Department, said that her team was investigating whether biotech-seed patents are being abused to extend or maintain companies' dominance in the industry. A key issue is how Monsanto sells and licenses its patented trait that allows farmers to kill weeds with Roundup herbicide while leaving crops unharmed - the gene was in 93 percent of U.S. soybeans grown in 2009. About 250 family farmers, consumers and other critics of corporate agriculture held a town meeting prior to the governmental meeting to protest Monsanto for what they see as manipulation of the market by buying up independent seed companies, patenting the seeds and then raising seed prices.

International Trade

Europe

GM food and GM crops have been the subject of international trade disputes. Such a dispute arose between the US and Europe in the early 2000s. Until the 1990s, Europe's regulation was less strict than in the United States. In 1998, the use of MON810, a Bt expressing maize conferring resistance to the European corn borer, was approved for commercial cultivation in Europe. However, in the 1990s, a series of unrelated food crises created consumer apprehension about food safety in general and eroded public trust in government oversight of the food industry - most importantly, the infection of cows with bovine spongiform encephalopathy and the mishandling of food safety by European authorities. In 1998, a *de facto* moratorium led to the suspension of approvals of new genetically modified organisms (GMO) in the European Union pending the adoption of revised rules to govern the approval, marketing and labelling of biotech products.

The approval of GM crops in the US in the mid-1990s precipitated strong public concern in Europe and led to a dramatic decrease in US exports to the EU. "Prior to 1997, corn exports to Europe represented about 4% of total U.S. corn exports, generating about $300 million in sales. Starting in 1997, however, the U.S. largely stopped shipping bulk commodity corn to the EU because such shipments typically coming led corn from many farms, including genetically modified varieties not approved by the EU. The change was dramatic. For example, before 1997, the U.S. sold about 1.75 million tons of corn annually to Spain and Portugal, the two largest importers of U.S. corn in the EU. But in the 1998–99 crop year, Spain bought less than a tenth of the previous year's amount and Portugal bought none at all."

In May 2003, the United States and twelve other countries filed a formal complaint with the World Trade Organization that the European Union was violating international trade agreements, in blocking imports of U.S. farm products through its long-standing ban on genetically modified food. The countries argued that the EU's regulatory process was far too slow and its standards were unreasonable given the overwhelming body of scientific evidence showing that the crops were safe. The case was also lobbied by U.S. biotechnology giant Monsanto and France's Aventis, as well as by US agricultural groups such as the National Corn Growers Association. In response, in June 2003, the European Parliament ratified a U.N. biosafety protocol regulating international trade in genetically modified food, and in July agreed to new regulations requiring labeling and traceability, as well as an opt-out provision for individual countries. Following this, the approval of new GMOs began again in May 2004. While a number of other GMOs have been approved since then, approvals remain controversial and various countries have utilized the opt-out provisions. In 2006, the WTO ruled that the pre-2004 restrictions had been violations, although the ruling had little immediate effect since the moratorium had already been lifted.

In late 2007, the U.S. ambassador to France recommended "moving to retaliation" to cause "some pain" against France and the European Union in an attempt to fight the French ban and changes in European policy toward genetically modified crops, according to a U.S. government diplomatic cable obtained by WikiLeaks.

20. Questions on Genetically Modified Foods (WHO, 2013)

Q. 1. What are genetically modified (GM) organisms and GM foods?

Ans. These questions and answers have been prepared by WHO in response to questions and concerns by a number of WHO Member State Governments with regard to the nature and safety of genetically modified food.

Genetically modified organisms (GMOs) can be defined as organisms in which the genetic material (DNA) has been altered in a way that does not occur naturally. The technology is often called "modern biotechnology" or "gene technology", sometimes also "recombinant DNA technology" or "genetic engineering". It allows selected individual genes to be transferred from one organism into another, also between non-related species.

Such methods are used to create GM plants – which are then used to grow GM food crops.

Q.2. Why are GM foods produced?

Ans. GM foods are developed – and marketed – because there is some perceived advantage either to the producer or consumer of these foods. This is meant to translate into a product with a lower price, greater benefit (in terms of durability or nutritional value) or both. Initially GM seed developers wanted their products to be accepted by producers so have concentrated on innovations that farmers (and the food industry more generally) would appreciate.

The initial objective for developing plants based on GM organisms was to improve crop protection. The GM crops currently on the market are mainly aimed at an increased level of crop protection through the introduction of resistance against plant diseases caused by insects or viruses or through increased tolerance towards herbicides.

Insect resistance is achieved by incorporating into the food plant the gene for toxin production from the bacterium Bacillus thuringiensis (BT). This toxin is currently used as a conventional insecticide in agriculture and is safe for human consumption. GM crops that permanently produce this toxin have been shown to require lower quantities of insecticides in specific situations, e.g. where pest pressure is high.

Virus resistance is achieved through the introduction of a gene from certain viruses which cause disease in plants. Virus resistance makes plants less susceptible to diseases caused by such viruses, resulting in higher crop yields.

Herbicide tolerance is achieved through the introduction of a gene from a bacterium conveying resistance to some herbicides. In situations where weed pressure is high, the use of such crops has resulted in a reduction in the quantity of the herbicides used.

Q.3. Are GM foods assessed differently from traditional foods?

Ans. Generally consumers consider that traditional foods (that have often been eaten for thousands of years) are safe. When new foods are developed by natural methods, some of the existing characteristics of foods can be altered, either in a positive or a negative way National food authorities may be called upon to examine traditional foods, but this is not always the case. Indeed, new plants developed through traditional breeding techniques may not be evaluated rigorously using risk assessment techniques.

With GM foods most national authorities consider that specific assessments are necessary. Specific systems have been set up for the rigorous evaluation of GM organisms and GM foods relative to both human health and the environment. Similar evaluations are generally not performed for traditional foods. Hence there is a significant difference in the evaluation process prior to marketing for these two groups of food.

One of the objectives of the WHO Food Safety Programme is to assist national authorities in the identification of foods that should be subject to risk assessment, including GM foods, and to recommend the correct assessments.

Q.4. How are the potential risks to human health determined?

Ans. The safety assessment of GM foods generally investigates: (a) direct health effects (toxicity), (b) tendencies to provoke allergic reaction (allergenicity); (c) specific components thought to have nutritional or toxic properties; (d) the stability of the inserted gene; (e) nutritional effects associated with genetic modification; and (f) any unintended effects which could result from the gene insertion.

Q.5. What are the main issues of concern for human health?

Ans. While theoretical discussions have covered a broad range of aspects, the three main issues debated are tendencies to provoke allergic reaction (allergenicity), gene transfer and outcrossing.

Allergenicity : As a matter of principle, the transfer of genes from commonly allergenic foods is discouraged unless it can be demonstrated that the protein product of the transferred gene is not allergenic. While traditionally developed foods are not generally tested for allergenicity, protocols for tests for GM foods have been evaluated by the Food and Agriculture Organization of the United Nations (FAO) and WHO. No allergic effects have been found relative to GM foods currently on the market.

Gene transfer : Gene transfer from GM foods to cells of the body or to bacteria in the gastrointestinal tract would cause concern if the transferred genetic material adversely affects human health. This would be particularly relevant if antibiotic resistance genes, used in creating GMOs, were to be transferred. Although the probability of transfer is low, the use of technology without antibiotic resistance genes has been encouraged by a recent FAO/ WHO expert panel.

Outcrossing : The movement of genes from GM plants into conventional crops or related species in the wild (referred to as "outcrossing"), as well as the mixing of crops derived from conventional seeds with those grown using GM crops, may have an indirect effect on food safety and food security. This risk is real, as was shown when traces of a maize type which was only approved for feed use appeared in maize products for human consumption in the United States of America. Several countries have adopted strategies to reduce mixing, including a clear separation of the fields within which GM crops and conventional crops are grown.

Feasibility and methods for post-marketing monitoring of GM food products, for the continued surveillance of the safety of GM food products, are under discussion.

Q.6. How is a risk assessment for the environment performed?

Ans. Environmental risk assessments cover both the GMO concerned and the potential receiving environment. The assessment process includes evaluation of the characteristics of the GMO and its effect and stability in the environment, combined with ecological characteristics of the environment in which the introduction will take place. The assessment also includes unintended effects which could result from the insertion of the new gene.

Q.7. What are the issues of concern for the environment?

Ans. **Issues of concern include:** the capability of the GMO to escape and potentially introduce the engineered genes into wild populations; the persistence of the gene after the GMO has been harvested; the susceptibility of non-target organisms (e.g. insects which are not pests) to the gene product; the stability of the gene; the reduction in the spectrum of other plants including loss of biodiversity; and increased use of chemicals in agriculture. The environmental safety aspects of GM crops vary considerably according to local conditions.

Current investigations focus on: the potentially detrimental effect on beneficial insects or a faster induction of resistant insects; the potential generation of new plant pathogens; the potential detrimental consequences for plant biodiversity and wildlife, and a decreased use of the important practice of crop rotation in certain local situations; and the movement of herbicide resistance genes to other plants.

Q.8. Are GM foods safe?

Ans. Different GM organisms include different genes inserted in different ways. This means that individual GM foods and their safety should be assessed on a case-by-case basis and that it is not possible to make general statements on the safety of all GM foods.

GM foods currently available on the international market have passed risk assessments and are not likely to present risks for human health. In addition, no effects on human health have been shown as a result of the consumption of such foods by the general population in the countries where they have been approved. Continuous use of risk assessments based on the Codex principles and, where appropriate, including post market monitoring, should form the basis for evaluating the safety of GM foods.

Q.9. How are GM foods regulated nationally?

Ans. The way governments have regulated GM foods varies. In some countries GM foods are not yet regulated. Countries which have legislation in place focus primarily on assessment of risks for consumer health. Countries which have provisions for GM foods usually also regulate GMOs in general, taking into account health and environmental risks, as well as control- and trade-related issues (such as potential testing and labelling regimes). In view of the dynamics of the debate on GM foods, legislation is likely to continue to evolve.

Q.10. What kind of GM foods are on the market internationally?

Ans. All GM crops available on the international market today have been designed using one of three basic traits: resistance to insect damage; resistance to viral infections; and tolerance towards certain herbicides. All the genes used to modify crops are derived from microorganisms.

Q.11. What happens when GM foods are traded internationally?

Ans. No specific international regulatory systems are currently in place. However, several international organizations are involved in developing protocols for GMOs.

The Codex Alimentarius Commission (Codex) is the joint FAO/WHO body responsible for compiling the standards, codes of practice, guidelines and recommendations that constitute the Codex Alimentarius: the international food code. Codex is developing principles for the human health risk analysis of GM foods. The premise of these principles dictates a premarket assessment, performed on a case-by-case basis and including an evaluation of both direct effects (from the inserted gene) and unintended effects (that may arise as a consequence of insertion of the new gene). The principles are at an advanced stage of development and are expected to be adopted in July 2003. Codex principles do not have a binding effect on national legislation, but are referred to specifically in the Sanitary and Phytosanitary Agreement of the World Trade Organization (SPS Agreement), and can be used as a reference in case of trade disputes.

The Cartagena Protocol on Biosafety (CPB), an environmental treaty legally binding for its Parties, regulates transboundary movements of living modified organisms (LMOs). GM foods are within the scope of the Protocol only if they contain LMOs that are capable of transferring or replicating genetic material. The cornerstone of the CPB is a requirement that exporters seek consent from importers before the first shipment of LMOs intended for release into the environment. The Protocol will enter into force 90 days after the 50th country has ratified it, which may be in early 2003 in view of the accelerated depositions registered since June 2002.

Q.12. Have GM products on the international market passed a risk assessment?

Ans. The GM products that are currently on the international market have all passed risk assessments conducted by national authorities. These different assessments in general follow the same basic principles, including an assessment of environmental and human health risk. These assessments are thorough, they have not indicated any risk to human health.

Q. 13. Why has there been concern about GM foods among some politicians, public interest groups and consumers, especially in Europe?

Ans. Since the first introduction on the market in the mid-1990s of a major GM food (herbicide-resistant soybeans), there has been increasing concern about such food among politicians, activists and consumers, especially in Europe. Several factors are involved.

In the late 1980s – early 1990s, the results of decades of molecular research reached the public domain. Until that time, consumers were generally not very aware of the potential of this research. In the case of food, consumers started to wonder about safety because they perceive that modern biotechnology is leading to the creation of new species.

Consumers frequently ask, "what is in it for me?". Where medicines are concerned, many consumers more readily accept biotechnology as beneficial for their health (e.g. medicines with improved treatment potential). In the case of the first GM foods introduced onto the European market, the products were of no apparent direct benefit to consumers (not cheaper, no increased shelf-life, no better taste). The potential for GM seeds to result in bigger yields per cultivated area should lead to lower prices. However, public attention has focused on the risk side of the risk-benefit equation.

Consumer confidence in the safety of food supplies in Europe has decreased significantly as a result of a number of food scares that took place in the second half of the 1990s that are unrelated to GM foods. This has also had an impact on discussions about the acceptability of GM foods. Consumers have questioned the validity of risk assessments, both with regard to consumer health and environmental risks, focusing in particular on long-term effects. Other topics for debate by consumer organizations have included allergenicity and antimicrobial resistance. Consumer concerns have triggered a discussion on the desirability of labelling GM foods, allowing an informed choice. At the same time, it has proved difficult to detect traces of GMOs in foods: this means that very low concentrations often cannot be detected.

Q.14. How has this concern affected the marketing of GM foods in the European Union?

Ans. The public concerns about GM food and GMOs in general have had a significant impact on the marketing of GM products in the European Union (EU). In fact, they have resulted in the so-called moratorium on approval of

GM products to be placed on the market. Marketing of GM food and GMOs in general are the subject of extensive legislation. Community legislation has been in place since the early 1990s. The procedure for approval of the release of GMOs into the environment is rather complex and basically requires agreement between the Member States and the European Commission. Between 1991 and 1998, the marketing of 18 GMOs was authorized in the EU by a Commission decision.

As of October 1998, no further authorizations have been granted and there are currently 12 applications pending. Some Member States have invoked a safeguard clause to temporarily ban the placing on the market in their country of GM maize and oilseed rape products. There are currently nine ongoing cases. Eight of these have been examined by the Scientific Committee on Plants, which in all cases deemed that the information submitted by Member States did not justify their bans.

During the 1990s, the regulatory framework was further extended and refined in response to the legitimate concerns of citizens, consumer organizations and economic operators (described under Question 13). A revised directive will come into force in October 2002. It will update and strengthen the existing rules concerning the process of risk assessment, risk management and decision-making with regard to the release of GMOs into the environment. The new directive also foresees mandatory monitoring of long-term effects associated with the interaction between GMOs and the environment.

Labelling in the EU is mandatory for products derived from modern biotechnology or products containing GM organisms. Legislation also addresses the problem of accidental contamination of conventional food by GM material. It introduces a 1% minimum threshold for DNA or protein resulting from genetic modification, below which labelling is not required.

In 2001, the European Commission adopted two new legislative proposals on GMOs concerning traceability, reinforcing current labelling rules and streamlining the authorization procedure for GMOs in food and feed and for their deliberate release into the environment.

The European Commission is of the opinion that these new proposals, building on existing legislation, aim to address the concerns of Member States and to build consumer confidence in the authorization of GM products. The Commission expects that adoption of these proposals will pave the way for resuming the authorization of new GM products in the EU.

Q.15. What is the state of public debate on GM foods in other regions of the world?

Ans. The release of GMOs into the environment and the marketing of GM foods have resulted in a public debate in many parts of the world. This debate is likely to continue, probably in the broader context of other uses of biotechnology (e.g. in human medicine) and their consequences for human societies. Even though the issues under debate are usually very similar (costs and benefits, safety issues), the outcome of the debate differs from country to country. On issues such as labelling and traceability of GM foods as a way to address consumer concerns, there is no consensus to date. This has become apparent during discussions within the Codex Alimentarius Commission over the past few years. Despite the lack of consensus on these topics, significant progress has been made on the harmonization of views concerning risk assessment. The Codex Alimentarius Commission is about to adopt principles on premarket risk assessment, and the provisions of the Cartegena Protocol on Biosafety also reveal a growing understanding at the international level.

Most recently, the humanitarian crisis in southern Africa has drawn attention to the use of GM food as food aid in emergency situations. A number of governments in the region raised concerns relating to environmental and food safety fears. Although workable solutions have been found for distribution of milled grain in some countries, others have restricted the use of GM food aid and obtained commodities which do not contain GMOs.

Q.16. Are people's reactions related to the different attitudes to food in various regions of the world?

Ans. Depending on the region of the world, people often have different attitudes to food. In addition to nutritional value, food often has societal and historical connotations, and in some instances may have religious importance. Technological modification of food and food production can evoke a negative response among consumers, especially in the absence of good communication on risk assessment efforts and cost/benefit evaluations.

Q.17. Are there implications for the rights of farmers to own their crops?

Ans. Yes, intellectual property rights are likely to be an element in the debate on GM foods, with an impact on the rights of farmers. Intellectual property rights (IPRs), especially patenting obligations of the TRIPS Agreement (an agreement under the World Trade Organization concerning trade-related aspects of intellectual property rights) have been discussed in the light of their consequences on the further availability of a diversity of crops. In the context of the related subject of the use of gene technology in medicine, WHO has reviewed the conflict between IPRs and an equal access to genetic resources and the sharing of benefits. The review has considered potential problems of monopolization and doubts about new patent regulations in the field of genetic sequences in human medicine. Such considerations are likely to also affect the debate on GM foods.

Q.18. Why are certain groups concerned about the growing influence of the chemical industry on agriculture?

Ans. Certain groups are concerned about what they consider to be an undesirable level of control of seed markets by a few chemical companies. Sustainable agriculture and biodiversity benefit most from the use of a rich variety of crops, both in terms of good crop protection practices as well as from the perspective of society at large and the values attached to food. These groups fear that as a result of the interest of the chemical industry in seed markets, the range of varieties used by farmers may be reduced mainly to GM crops. This would impact on the food basket of a society as well as in the long run on crop protection (for example, with the development of resistance against insect pests and tolerance of certain herbicides). The exclusive use of herbicide-tolerant GM crops would also make the farmer dependent on these chemicals. These groups fear a dominant position of the chemical industry in agricultural development, a trend which they do not consider to be sustainable.

Q.19. What further developments can be expected in the area of GMOs?

Ans. Future GM organisms are likely to include plants with improved disease or drought resistance, crops with increased nutrient levels, fish species with enhanced growth characteristics and plants or animals producing pharmaceutically important proteins such as vaccines. At the international level, the response to new developments can be found in the expert consultations organized by FAO and WHO in 2000 and 2001, and the subsequent work of the Codex ad hoc Task Force on Foods Derived from Biotechnology. This work has resulted in an improved and harmonized framework for the risk assessment of GM foods in general. Specific questions, such as the evaluation of allergenicity of GM foods or the safety of foods derived from GM microorganisms, have been covered and an expert consultation organized by FAO and WHO will focus on foods derived from GM animals in 2003.

Q.20. What is WHO doing to improve the evaluation of GM foods?

Ans. WHO will take an active role in relation to GM foods, primarily for two reasons:

(1) On the grounds that public health could benefit enormously from the potential of biotechnology, for example, from an increase in the nutrient content of foods, decreased allergenicity and more efficient food production; and

(2) Based on the need to examine the potential negative effects on human health of the consumption of food produced through genetic modification, also at the global level. It is clear that modern technologies must be thoroughly evaluated if they are to constitute a true improvement in the way food is produced. Such evaluations must be holistic and all-inclusive, and cannot stop at the previously separated, non-coherent systems of evaluation focusing solely on human health or environmental effects in isolation.

Work is therefore under way in WHO to present a broader view of the evaluation of GM foods in order to enable the consideration of other important factors. This more holistic evaluation of GM organisms and GM products will consider not only safety but also food security, social and ethical aspects, access and capacity building. International work in this new direction presupposes the involvement of other key international organizations in this area. As a first step, the WHO Executive Board will discuss the content of a WHO report covering this subject in January 2003. The report is being developed in collaboration with other key organizations, notably FAO and the United Nations Environment Programme (UNEP). It is hoped that this report could form the basis for a future initiative towards a more systematic, coordinated, multi-organizational and international evaluation of certain GM foods.

9

Microbial Toxins in Food

Microbial toxins are toxins produced by micro-organisms. Microbial toxins promote infection and disease by directly damaging host tissues and by disabling the immune system. Ingestion of water and wide variety of food contaminated with pathogenic microorganisms (bacteria, viruses, protozoa, and fungi), their toxins and chemicals results in diseases commonly categorized as microbial food borne diseases. Pathogenic bacteria, fungi, parasites, viruses, marine phytoplankton, and cyanobacteria are the known causes of microbial food-borne diseases. These microorganisms can use our food as a source of nutrients for their own growth. By growing in the food, metabolizing them and producing by-products, they not only render the food inedible but also pose health problems upon consumption. Many of our foods will support the growth of pathogenic microorganisms or at least serve as a vector for their transmission. Food can get contaminated from plant surfaces, animals, water, sewage, air, soil, or from food handlers during handling and processing.

Microbial food-borne illnesses are among the most widespread diseases of the modern day world. Several factors have contributed to the rapid increase in the number of reported cases of the Microbial food borne illnesses. Despite the increasing awareness among the consumers and also the focus of the law enacting and enforcing agencies only a small proportion of cases of microbial food borne illnesses reach the notice of health agencies and even fewer are investigated. It is believed that in industrialized countries less than 10% of the cases are reported, and in developing countries reported cases probably account for less than 1% of the total. In India the occurrence of such cases is very common and needs to be dealt with utmost competence to avoid these diseases and also save the economic damages incurred by them.

The pathogenic microbes themselves are a major cause of food borne diseases. Their presence even in small numbers is sufficient for the symptoms to appear but the actual clinical presentation depends on the virulence of the pathogen dose and resistance/susceptibility of the host. The pathogenic microbes may result in food borne illnesses by below mentioned three means:

1. Infection: *Ingestion of a harmful microorganism within a food.*

2. Toxicoinfection : *Ingestion of a harmful microorganism within a food that produces a toxin in the human body.*

3. Intoxication: *Ingestion of a harmful toxin produced within a food.*

The food borne illnesses including toxicoinfections and intoxication are the direct result of the toxins produced by the microbes.

The microbial toxins produced by the microbes ingested in the human host's body along with the food sources leads to the conditions of toxicoinfection. These toxin or toxins damage the tissues or interfere with normal organ or tissue function. Examples of microbes capable of causing toxicoinfections include bacteria like *Vibrio cholerae, Bacillus cereus, Clostridium perfringens, C. botulinum* (infant botulism), and enterotoxigenic *Escherichia coli.* The predominant clinical manifestation of food-borne toxicoinfections is diarrhea. Some organisms, such as enterotoxigenic *Escherichia coli,* may produce hemorrhagic colitis, hemolytic uremic syndrome (HUS), and other debilitating sequelae. The onset times for toxicoinfections are frequently, but not necessarily, longer than those for intoxications but shorter than those for infections.

 Food borne intoxication is caused when during the microbial growth; specific pathogenic bacteria release toxins into food that subsequently is consumed. Intoxications can be differentiated from food borne infections and toxicoinfections based on the time duration in which symptoms develop after consumption of foods containing microbial toxins. Generally, intoxications are manifested more rapidly after consumption of contaminated food than are infections or toxicoinfections because time for growth and invasion or elaboration of the toxin *in vivo* is not required. Bacteria capable of causing food-borne intoxications include *Staphylococcus aureus, Bacillus cereus,* and *Clostridium botulinum.*

The microbial toxins may be categorized on the basis of either the type of organism producing it or on the basis of the clinical manifestation of the toxin on the host.

In order of economic and public health significance, bacterial toxins are the most important, followed by mycotoxins and algal biotoxins. Although mycotoxins have been responsible for individual acute poisoning outbreaks, primary concerns regarding mycotoxin contamination in foods and feeds are related to both human illnesses due to long-term, low level exposure and animal health. On the other hand, although there is a paucity of information on aquatic biotoxins, contamination of seafoods with these toxins has the highest potential human health risks because of the widespread distribution of susceptible seafoods and the etiology of toxin production and subsequent accumulation.

A. Bacterial Toxins

Bacterial toxins have been defined as soluble substances that alter the normal metabolism of host cells with deleterious effects on the host. Bacterial toxins were recognized by the 1890s as the potent substances responsible for such infectious diseases as diphtheria, tetanus, and btulinum. The pathogenic bacteris found in human food may be categorized into three groups as follows:

I. **Group I** includes Infectious bacteria associated with food poisoning like *Brucella*, *Campylobacter jejuni*, enteroinvasive *Escherichia coli*, enterohemorrhagic *E. coli*, *Listeria monocytogenes*, *Salmonella*, *Shigella*, *Vibrio parahaemolyticus*, *V. vulnificus*, and *Yersinia enterocolitica*. These organisms must be ingested for poisoning to occur, and in many instances only a few cells need be consumed to initiate a gastrointestinal infection. *Salmonella* and *C. jejuni* are the most prevalent causes of food-borne bacterial infections. They produce molecules that provide a defense against host immune system and transmission within the invaded organism. When the bacteria reach intestinal epithelium, they penetrate tissues by the outgrowth in cell cytosol or vacuoles. The condition resulting from this kind of food poisoning is also called as Food borne infections.

II. **Group II** includes food-poisoning bacteria that produce toxin in the gastrointestinal tract following their ingestion and lead to the conditions of toxicoinfections. These include *Bacillus cereus*, *Clostridium perfringens*, enterotoxigenic *E. coli*, and *V. cholerae*. *Bacillus cereus* and *C. perfringens* are spore-forming bacteria that often survive cooking and grow to large numbers in improperly refrigerated foods. Following ingestion, their cells release enterotoxins in the intestinal tract. Enterotoxigenic *E. coli* is a leading cause of travelers' diarrhea.

III. **Group III** *includes* bacteria responsible for food poisonings resulting from ingestion of preformed toxin leading to food intoxication. *Staphylococcus aureus* and *Clostridium botulinum* are included in this group. *Staphylococcus aureus* produces heat-stable toxins that remain active in foods after cooking. *Clostridium botulinum* produces one of the most potent toxins known. Botulinal toxin causes neuromuscular paralysis, often resulting in respiratory failure and death.

As far as toxins produced by bacteria are concerned the organisms belonging to Group II and Group III are very important. To keep the focus of the chapter in view the bacteria belonging to the Group II and Group III shall be the topics of discussion in this section.

Toxicoinfections causing bacteria

Bacillus cereus is a Gram-positive, facultatively anaerobic, endospore forming, beta hemolytic large rod. *B. cereus* is widespread in the environment and often is isolated from soil and vegetation. The optimal growth temperature is 28 C to 35 C, with a minimum growth temperature of 4 C and a maximum of 48 C. Growth can occur in pH ranges from 4.9 to 9.3, and the organism tolerates 7.5% salt concentration.

B. Cereus food poisoning is the general description of illness associated with this organism, although two recognized types of illness are caused by two distinct metabolites (toxins):

a) The *diarrheal type* of illness is caused by a large-molecular-weight protein.

b) The *vomiting (emetic) type* of illness is associated with cereulide, an ionophoric low molecular-weight dodecadepsipeptide that is pH-stable and heat- and protease- resistant. The non-antigenic peptide is stable after heating at 121 C for 30 minutes, cooling at 4 C for 60 days, and at a pH range of 2 to 11.

Mortality

The emetic enterotoxin of *B. cereus* foodborne illness has been implicated in liver failure and death in otherwise healthy individuals. Similarly, a newly identified cytotoxin has been isolated from a *B. cereus* strain that caused a severe outbreak and three deaths. But generally speaking mortality due to *B. cereus* toxicoinfections is very rare.

Infective dose

The presence of large numbers of *B. cereus* (greater than 10^6 organisms/g) in a food is indicative of active growth and proliferation of the organism and is consistent with a potential human health hazard. The number of organisms most often associated with human illness is 10 to 10^5; however, the pathogenicity arises from preformed toxin.

Disease Complications

Toxicoinfections associated with the diarrheal and emetic toxins produced by *B. cereus* are generally mild and self-limiting. In some cases more severe and fatal forms of the illness have been reported. Other clinical manifestations of *B. cereus* invasion and infection include severe systemic and pyogenic infections, gangrene, septic meningitis, cellulitis, panophthalmitis, lung abscesses, infant death, and endocarditis.

Bacillus cereus might cause many more cases of foodborne illness than is known. Most people have fairly mild, brief symptoms, which is one of the major reasons it is under reported. But it can cause serious illness in some people, such as those with compromised and weak immune system, elderly and very young subjects. This bacterium can cause two different types of sickness.

1. In the first type, after contaminated food is eaten the bacteria make a toxic substance in the small intestine. This can lead to diarrhea, cramps, and, sometimes, nausea (but usually not vomiting). Many kinds of contaminated foods have been linked to this illness. Symptoms start in about 6 to 15 hours and usually clear up within a day or so.

2. The second type occurs if *B. cereus* makes a different kind of toxin in contaminated food. It most often affects rice and other starchy foods. It causes nausea and vomiting in a half hour to 6 hours and usually clears up in about a day.

Both kinds of illness generally go away by themselves, but can cause serious complications, although rarely in otherwise healthy people.

One of the most important things to avoid infection with *B. cereus* is to keep the food refrigerated at 40 F or lower. The reason is that, at higher temperatures, *B. cereus* can form spores – a survival mode in which they make an inactive form that can exist without nutrition and that develops very tough protection against the outside world – that grow and turn into more *B. cereus* bacteria. The more bacteria, the more toxin, and the greater the chances of infection. Cooking may kill the bacteria, but it might not disable the toxin that causes the vomiting type of illness.

Sources

1. A wide variety of foods, including meats, milk, vegetables, and fish, have been associated with the diarrheal-type food poisoning. The vomiting-type outbreaks generally have been associated with rice products; however, other starchy foods, such as potato, pasta, and cheese products, also have been implicated. Food mixtures, such as sauces, puddings, soups, casseroles, pastries, and salads, frequently have been linked with food-poisoning outbreaks (FDA, 2012)

2. *Clostridium perfringens* was first described in 1892 by William Welch and George Nutall. *C. perfringens* is gram-positive, rod-shaped, spore-forming bacteria and is present almost everywhere in nature especially in soil. *C. perfringens* is very durable due to its ability to produce spores. The spores allow *C. perfringens* to be dormant during periods that are not environmentally friendly and make it very easy for these bacteria to cause contamination in foods because during the dormant stage *C. perfringens* is resistant to disinfectants, temperature, starvation and many other extreme conditions.

TOXINS

Strains of *C. perfringens* are classified as 5 biotypes A – E depending on the differential production of four major (i.e. lethal) exotoxins (alpha, beta, epsilon and iota). In addition, strains of *C. perfringens* may also produce a number of other toxins, including: neuraminidase and enterotoxin on account of the presence of the *cpe* gene.

FOOD POISONING

In the United Kingdom and United States *C. perfringens* is the third most common cause of food poisoning, with poorly prepared meat and poultry the main culprits. Spores survive cooking and, during slow cooling and unrefrigerated storage, germinate to form large numbers of cells which are then ingested.

Incubation time is between 8 and 16 hours after ingestion of contaminated food. The bacterial enterotoxins cause intense abdominal cramps and diarrhoea which last about 24 hours. It is likely that many cases of *C. perfringens* food poisoning remain sub clinical, as antibodies to the toxin are common amongst the population. This has led to the conclusion that most, if not all, of the population has experienced food poisoning due to *C. perfringens*. Foodborne illness caused by *C. perfringens* can take two forms.

1) The **gastroenteritis form** is very common and often is mild and self-limiting. Depending on the strain, it may also develop as more severe gastroenteritis that leads to damage of the small intestine and, potentially, but rarely, fatality. It is mostly caused due to the production of a enterotoxin called CPE protein (encoded by *cpe* gene) which is usually is released into the intestines when the vegetative cells lyse on completion of sporulation. This enterotoxin is responsible for the clinical symptoms in humans. The enterotoxin induces fluid and electrolyte losses from the GI tract. The principal target organ for CPE is believed to be the small intestine.

2) The other form, **enteritis necroticans or "pig-bel disease"** (a name reportedly derived from pidgin English, referring to the characteristic swollen bellies and other severe symptoms that resulted from feasts on contaminated pork in New Guinea), is rare in the United States, more severe than the other form of the illness, and often fatal (FDA, 2012). Pig-bel disease involves production of beta toxin, which is highly trypsin-sensitive and leads to necrotic enteritis.

Both forms of the disease result from ingestion of large numbers of *C. perfringens*, which have very high ability of replication in the host as compared to other pathogenic bacteria.

Symptoms

Like other food-borne illnesses, the symptoms of *Clostridium perfringens* infection mainly involve the gut. These symptoms can include:

- abdominal bloating, pain and cramps
- increased gas
- diarrhea (profuse and watery)
- nausea
- loss of appetite and weight loss
- muscle aches
- fatigue

Infection with *Clostridium perfringens* does not generally cause vomiting or fever.

Mortality: In 1999, the Centers for Disease Control and Prevention (CDC) estimated that, overall, *C. perfringens* annually accounts for 26 deaths in the U.S.

- **Common gastroenteritis form**: A few deaths resulting from diarrhea-induced dehydration and other complications have been reported, and usually were among debilitated or elderly people.

- **Pig-bel form (enteritis necroticans)**: This disease is often fatal. As noted, it is extremely rare in the U.S.

Infective dose

Symptoms are caused by ingestion of large numbers (> 10^6) vegetative cells or >10^6 spores/g of food. Toxin production in the digestive tract (or in vitro) is associated with sporulation. This disease is characterized as a food infection; only one episode has ever implied the possibility of intoxication (i.e., disease from preformed toxin).

Sources of infection

Eating food that has been slowly cooked or improperly cooled, stored or reheated increases the risk of infection. Foods high in protein or starch pose greater risk. Foods associated with *Clostridium perfringens* infection, include:

- thick soups
- stews
- raw meat, poultry and beef
- meat products
- gravies
- dried or pre-cooked foods
- cooked beans
- meat pies

Normal cooking temperatures do not kill *Clostridium perfringens* spores, which is why it is so important that foods are properly stored, cooled and reheated.

Complications

Complications are rare in the typical, mild gastroenteritis form of the disease, particularly among people under 30 years old. Elderly people are more likely to have prolonged or severe symptoms, as are immunocompromised people. The more severe form of the disease may cause necrosis of the small intestine, peritonitis, and septicemia.

GAS GANGRENE

This condition caused by *C. perfringens* is not associated with food intake. Gas gangrene is a deep wound infection most often associated with the alpha-toxin (exotoxin) of *C. perfringens* type A. It is also known as Clostridial myonecrosis. It is characterised by rapid inflammation at the site of infection, extreme swelling, acute pain, and, eventually, necrosis of the infected tissue. In addition to the damaging toxins, the bacteria also generate a gas: a composition of 5.9% hydrogen, 3.4% carbon dioxide, 74.5% nitrogen and 16.1% oxygen was reported in one clinical case. The alpha-toxin enters into the plasma membrane of the cells. The alpha-toxin produces holes in the plasma membrane with disrupts normal cell function and the tissue will begin to decompose from the inside out. Treatment usually involves excision/amputation, and antibiotics. Hyperbaric oxygen therapy (HBOT) may also be used to inhibit the growth of and kill the anaerobic *C. perfringens*.

Escherichia coli is a Gram-negative, rod-shaped bacterium that is commonly found in the lower intestine of warm-blooded organisms (endotherms). It was discovered by German paediatrician and bacteriologist Theodor Escherich in 1885. Most *E. coli* strains are harmless. *Escherichia coli* typically colonizes the gastrointestinal tract of human infants within a few hours after birth. Usually, *E. coli* and its human host coexist in good health and with mutual benefit for decades. They colonize the gut of the host and can benefit them by producing Vitamin K_2 and preventing the establishment of the harmful bacteria to the intestinal wall. Among the intestinal pathogens there are six well-described categories: enteropathogenic *E. coli* (EPEC), enterohaemorrhagic *E. coli* (EHEC), enterotoxigenic *E. coli* (ETEC), enteroinvasive *E. coli* (EIEC), enteroaggregative *E. coli* (EAEC) and diffusely adherent *E. coli* (DAEC). Of these, the first four groups are well known to be transmitted via contaminated food or water; EHEC, especially, are often implicated in major foodborne outbreaks worldwide.

Pathogenic *E. coli* are generally grouped based on their virulence properties or factors that they carry and which elicits an immune response in animals, namely:

1. O antigen: part of lipopolysaccharide layer

2. K antigen: capsule

3. H antigen: flagellin

For example *E.coli* strain EDL933 is of the O157:H7 group.

O antigen

The outer membrane of an *E. coli* cell contains millions of lipopolysaccharide (LPS) molecules, which consists of:

1. O antigen, a polymer of immunogenic repeating oligosaccharides (1–40 units)

2. Core region of phosphorylated nonrepeating oligosaccharides

3. Lipid A (endotoxin)

The O antigen is used for serotyping *E.coli* and these O group designations go from O1 to O181, with the exception of some groups which have been historically removed, namely O31, O47, O67, O72, O93 (now K84), O94, and O122; groups 174 to 181 are provisional (O174=OX3 and O175=OX7) or are under investigation (176 to 181 are STEC/VTEC). Additionally subtypes exist for many O groups (*e.g.* O128ab and O128ac). It should be noted though that antibodies towards several O antigens cross-react with other O antigens and partially to K antigens not only from *E. coli*, but also from other *Escherichia* species and Enterobacteriaceae species.

The O antigen is encoded by the rfb gene cluster. rol (cld) gene encodes the regulator of lipopolysaccharide O-chain length.

K antigen

The acidic capsular polysaccharide (CPS) is a thick, mucous-like, layer of polysaccharide that surrounds some pathogen *E. coli*. There are two separate groups of K-antigen groups, named group I and group II (while a small in-between subset (K3, K10, and K54/K96) has been classified as group III). The former (I) consist of 100 kDa (large) capsular polysaccharides, while the latter (II), associated with extraintestinal diseases, are under 50 kDa in size.

Group I K antigens are only found with certain O-antigens (O8, O9, O20, and O101 groups), they are further subdivided on the basis of absence (IA, similar to that of *Klebsiella* species in structure) or presence (IB) of amino sugars and some group I K-antigens are attached to the lipid A-core of the lipopolysaccharide (K_{LPS}), in a similar way to O antigens (and being structurally identical to O antigens in some instances are only considered as K antigens when co-expressed with another authentic O antigen).

Group II K antigens closely resemble those in **Gram-positive** bacteria and greatly differ in composition and are further subdivided according to their acidic components, generally 20–50% of the CPS chains are bound to phospholipids. In total there are 60 different K antigens that have been.

H antigen

The flagella allows *E. coli* to move. H antigens groups go from H1 to H56 with some exceptions (H13 and H22 were not *E. coli* antigens but from *Citrobacter freundii*, also a coliform, and H50 being the same as H10). These are encoded by the fliC gene.

The descriptions of pathogenic *E. coli* that are most often transmitted via contaminated food or water is given below.

i. Enterotoxigenic *Escherichia coli* (ETEC)

Enterotoxigenic *Escherichia coli* (ETEC) are highly motile, Gram-negative, rod-shaped bacteria. They are characterized by production of several virulence factors, including both heat-labile (LT) toxin and heat-stable (ST) toxins, as well as several colonization-factor antigens. ETEC uses fimbrial adhesins (projections from the bacterial cell surface) to bind enterocyte cells in the small intestine. ETEC can produce two proteinaceous enterotoxins:

- The larger of the two proteins, **LT enterotoxin**, is similar to cholera toxin in structure and function.

- The smaller protein, **ST enterotoxin** causes cGMP accumulation in the target cells and a subsequent secretion of fluid and electrolytes into the intestinal lumen.

Mortality

ETEC strains are noninvasive, and they do not leave the intestinal lumen. ETEC is the leading bacterial cause of diarrhea in children in the developing world, as well as the most common cause of traveler's diarrhea. Each year, ETEC causes more than 200 million cases of diarrhea and 380,000 deaths, mostly in children in developing countries.

Infective dose

Volunteer feeding studies showed that a high dose, ranging from 10 million to 10 billion ETEC cells, may be needed to cause an infection in adults. Children may be affected by a smaller dose. Onset of the symptoms is usually 26 hours after ingestion of contaminant, but can range from 8 to 44 hours.

Symptoms

Infection is characterized by sudden onset of diarrhea that is watery and without blood or mucus, rarely accompanied by high fever or vomiting. Other symptoms include abdominal cramps, low-grade fever, nausea, and malaise.

Sources

Contaminated food or water is the most common cause ETEC outbreaks. ETEC is often found in feces of asymptomatic carriers, and humans appear to be the most likely source of ETEC. In 1975, a large outbreak affecting 2,000 people was traced to sewage-contaminated water at a national park. Contaminated well water in Japan and water supplies aboard cruise ships also have been implicated in ETEC outbreaks. Foodborne outbreaks of ETEC have occurred in restaurants and at various catered functions (FDA, 2012).

Examples of implicated foods include Brie cheese, curried turkey, mayonnaise, crabmeat, deli food, and salads. In most of these cases, foods became contaminated with ETEC via infected food handlers or through the use of contaminated water during preparation. ETEC infection does not appear to be transmitted by person-to-person contact, but some hospital infections have occurred and probably were caused by unsanitary conditions.

Disease / complications

Illness from ETEC is usually self-limiting, mild, and brief. However, some severe forms last longer and resemble cholera, with up to five or more daily passages of rice-water-like stools that result in severe dehydration. Antibiotic treatment usually is not required in ETEC infections, but seems to be effective in reducing the duration and severity of illness. In infants and elderly and debilitated patients, particularly, appropriate electrolyte replacement therapy may be necessary.

ii. Enteropathogenic *Escherichia coli* (EPEC)

EPEC are Gram-negative, rod-shaped bacteria. EPEC was the first pathotype of *E. coli* to be described. Large outbreaks of infant diarrhoea in the United Kingdom led Bray, in 1945, to describe a group of serologically distinct *E. coli* strains that were isolated from children with diarrhea but not from healthy children. Although large outbreaks of infant diarrhoea due to EPEC have largely disappeared from industrialized countries, EPEC remains an important cause of potentially fatal infant diarrhoea in developing countries (Natro and Kaper, 1998). For decades, the mechanisms by which EPEC caused diarrhoea were unknown and this pathotype could only be identified on the basis of O:H serotyping. However, since 1979, numerous advances in our understanding of the pathogenesis of EPEC diarrhoea have been made, such that EPEC is now among the best understood of all the pathogenic *E. coli*.

This virotype has an array of virulence factors that are similar to those found in *Shigella*, and may possess a shiga toxin. They are characterized by the presence of the locus for enterocyte effacement (LEE) pathogenicity island, which carries multiple virulence factors, including the *eae* gene that encodes for intimin and, together with the *tir* gene (intimin receptor), allows intimate adherence of EPEC to intestinal epithelial cells. Adherence to the intestinal mucosa causes a rearrangement of actin in the host cell, causing significant deformation. EPEC cells are moderately invasive (i.e. they enter host cells) and elicit an inflammatory response. The changes caused in intestinal cell ultrastructure due to "attachment and effacement", is likely the prime cause of diarrhea in those afflicted with EPEC. This adherence of the bacteria to the intestinal mucosa causes extensive disarrangement of the digestive-absorptive enzyme system, resulting in nutrient malabsorption. The disease usually associated with EPEC is infantile diarrhea.

Mortality

Mortality rates from 25% to 50% have been reported in the past. In developed countries, better treatment and medical facilities have greatly reduced mortality, but some deaths still occur.

Infective dose

EPEC is highly infective in infants, and the dose is presumably very low. EPEC infections most often occur in infants, especially those who are being bottle fed. Poor-quality water used to rehydrate infant formulae in underdeveloped countries may be the source of EPEC in bottle-fed infants. Adults, however, are not as susceptible. Volunteer feeding studies showed that 10 million to 10 billion cells are needed to cause diarrhea in adults, provided that gastric acid first has been neutralized by bicarbonate. Onset of diarrhea is often rapid, occurring as soon as 4 hours post ingestion of the bacteria. The most common symptoms include profuse, watery diarrhea; vomiting; and low-grade fever. Diarrhea occasionally is protracted, lasting from 21 to 120 days.

Complications

The diarrhea can be mild; however, the infection sometimes can be severe. Fluid and electrolyte imbalance may need to be corrected, to prevent dehydration.

Sources

Source(s) and prevalence of EPEC are controversial, because foodborne outbreaks are sporadic. Foods implicated in past EPEC outbreaks have included raw beef and chicken, but any food exposed to fecal contamination is strongly suspect. In the mid 1990s, an EPEC outbreak in Minnesota was traced to a buffet, but no specific food item was identified. In 1995, two outbreaks in France affected 59 people and were traced to mayonnaise, lettuce, and pickles.

iii. Enterohemorrhagic *Escherichia coli* (EHEC)

First recognized as a cause of human disease in 1982, EHEC causes bloody diarrhoea (haemorrhagic colitis), non-bloody diarrhea and haemolytic uremic syndrome (HUS). They are gram-negative rod shaped bacteria characterized by the ability to produce shiga toxin (*stx*). They are known by a number of names, including enterohemorrhagic *E. coli* (EHEC), shiga-like toxin-producing *E. coli* (STEC or SLTEC), hemolytic uremic syndrome–associated enterohemorrhagic *E. coli* (HUSEC) and verocytotoxin- or verotoxin-producing *E. coli* (VTEC). The key virulence factor for EHEC is Stx, which is also known as verocytotoxin (VT). Stx consists of five identical B subunits that are responsible for binding the holotoxin to the glycolipid globotriaosylceramide (Gb3) on the target cell surface, and a single A subunit that cleaves ribosomal RNA, causing protein synthesis to cease. The Stx family contains two subgroups — Stx1 and Stx2 — that share approximately 55% amino acid homology. Stx is produced in the colon and travels by the bloodstream to the kidney, where it damages renal endothelial cells and occludes the microvasculature through a combination of direct toxicity and induction of local cytokine and chemokine production, resulting in renal inflammation (Andreoli et al., 2002). This damage can lead to HUS, which is characterized by haemolytic anaemia, thrombocytopoenia and potentially fatal acute renal failure. Stx also induces apoptosis in intestinal epithelial cells — a process that is regulated by the Bcl-2 family. Stx was first purified from *Shigella dysenteriae*, and HUS can also result from infection with this species, although not with other *Shigella* species or EIEC,which do not produce Stx. Stx also mediates local damage in the colon, which results in bloody diarrhoea, haemorrhagic colitis, necrosis and intestinal perforation.

In addition to Stx, most EHEC strains also contain the LEE pathogenicity island that encodes a type III secretion system and effector proteins that are homologous to those that are produced by EPEC. Animal models have shown the importance of the intimin adhesin in intestinal colonization, and HUS patients develop a strong antibody response to intimin and other LEEencoded proteins. EHEC O157:H7 is believed to have evolved from LEE-containing O55 EPEC strains that acquired bacteriophage encoding Stx (Reid et al., 2000).Although more than 200 serotypes of *E. coli* can produce Stx, most of these serotypes do not contain the LEE pathogenicity island and are not associated with human disease. This has led to the use of Shiga toxin-producing *E. coli* (STEC) or verotoxin-producing *E. coli* (VTEC) as general terms for any *E. coli* strain that produces Stx, and the term EHEC is used to denote only the subset of Stx positive strains that also contain the LEE.

Although O157:H7 is currently the predominant strain and accounts for ~75% of the EHEC infections worldwide, other non-O157 EHEC serotypes are emerging as a cause of foodborne illnesses. In the United States a group often referred to as the "big 6" (O111, O26, O121, O103, O145, and O45) accounts for the majority of the non-O157:H7 serotypes isolated from clinical infections and, therefore, is currently a focus of concern. However, other EHEC serotypes, such as O113, O91, and others, also can cause severe illness. As a result, the non-O157 EHEC serotypes of public health concern can change quickly, depending on outbreak incidents, and can vary with countries and geographic regions.

Mortality: Patients whose illness progresses to HUS have a mortality rate of 3% to 5%.

Infective dose: The infective dose of EHEC O157:H7 is estimated to be very low, in the range of 10 to 100 cells. The infective dose of other EHEC serotypes is suspected to be slightly higher. Symptoms usually begin 3 to 4 days after exposure, but the time may range from 1 to 9 days.

Disease / complications

Infections from EHEC may range from asymptomatic-to-mild diarrhea to severe complications. The acute symptoms are called hemorrhagic colitis (HC), characterized by severe abdominal cramps and bloody diarrhea, which may progress to such life-threatening complications as HUS or thrombotic thrombocytopenia purpura (TTP) – conditions that are most often associated with O157:H7, but that also can occur with other EHEC serotypes. About 3% to 7% of HC cases progress to HUS or TTP. Some evidence suggests that Stx2 and intimin are associated with progression to severe disease, such as HUS. Kidney cells have a high concentration of Stx receptors; hence, the kidney is a common site of damage. Some survivors may have permanent disabilities, such as renal insufficiency and neurological deficits.

Symptoms

Hemorrhagic colitis is characterized by severe cramping (abdominal pain), nausea or vomiting, and diarrhea that initially is watery, but becomes grossly bloody. In some cases, the diarrhea may be extreme, appearing to consist entirely of blood and occurring every 15 to 30 minutes. Fever typically is low-grade or absent. In uncomplicated cases, duration of symptoms is 2 to 9 days, with an average of 8 days.

Sources

Raw or undercooked ground beef and beef products are the vehicles most often implicated in O157:H7 outbreaks. Earlier outbreaks also implicated consumption of raw milk. O157:H7 can develop acid tolerance, as evidenced by infections in which acid foods (<pH4.6) were implicated, such as yogurt, mayonnaise, fermented sausages, cheeses, and unpasteurized fruit juices. Various water sources, including potable, well, and recreational water, also have caused EHEC infections, as has contact with animals at farms or petting zoos. Products like, bagged lettuce, spinach, and alfalfa sprouts, increasingly is being implicated in O157:H7 infections. Person-to-person transmission of infection is well documented.

iv. Enteroinvasive *Escherichia coli* (EIEC)

EIEC is a Gram-negative, rod-shaped, enterotoxin-producing bacterium that closely resembles *Shigella*. Both are characterized by their ability to invade colonic epithelial cells. The genetic information required for the invasion phenotype is encoded within a 37 kilobase region on a virulence plasmid, which can vary in size from 180 kb in *S. sonnei* to 220 kb in *S. flexneri* and EIEC. EIEC might cause an invasive inflammatory colitis, and occasionally dysentery, but in most cases EIEC elicits watery diarrhea that is indistinguishable from that due to infection by other *E. coli* pathogens.

The early phase of EIEC/*Shigella* pathogenesis comprises epithelial cell penetration, followed by lysis of the endocytic vacuole, intracellular multiplication, directional movement through the cytoplasm and extension into adjacent epithelial cells. Movement within the cytoplasm is mediated by nucleation of cellular actin into a 'tail' that extends from one pole of the bacterium. In addition to invasion into and dissemination within epithelial cells, *Shigella* (and presumably EIEC) also induces apoptosis in infected macrophages. Genes that are required to effect this complex pathogenetic scheme are present on a large virulence plasmid that is found in EIEC and all *Shigella* species. The illness caused by EIEC is a mild form of bacillary dysentery, similar to that caused by *Shigella* spp.

Mortality

A recent estimate of domestically acquired foodborne illness in the United States, by the Centers for Disease Control and Prevention (CDC), lists a death rate of zero for diarrheagenic *E. coli* other than Shiga-toxigenic and enterotoxigenic *E. coli*.

Infective dose

The infective dose of EIEC is thought to be in the range of 200 to 5,000 cells, somewhat higher than that of *Shigella*. The difference in the dose may depend on which virulence plasmid these pathogens harbor. The symptoms usually occur within 12 to 72 hrs after ingestion of contaminated food.

Complications: The illness generally is self-limiting, with no known complications.

Symptoms: Mild dysentery; abdominal cramps, diarrhea, vomiting, fever, chills, and generalized malaise. Stools often contain blood and mucus.

Sources

No specific foods are frequently associated with EIEC infections. Infected humans are the only known reservoirs of EIEC; hence, any food contaminated with human feces from an ill individual, either directly or via contaminated water, can be infectious (FDA, 2012).

1. *Aeromonas* spp.

   A. hydrophila are Gram-negative, rod-shaped facultative anaerobes, ranging in size from 0.3-1.0 µm wide by 1.0-3.5 µm long. They are motile by a single polar flagellum. The bacteria can produce heat-labile enterotoxins, which can be associated with haemolysin and cytotoxin production. Infection with *Aeromonas hydrophila* can result in gastrointestinal or non-gastrointestinal complications. Symptoms of gastrointestinal infection range from watery diarrhea to dysenteric or bloody diarrhea. Chronic infection is also possible. Non-gastrointestinal complications that may arise subsequent to *A. hydrophila* infection include hemolytic syndrome and kidney disease, cellulitis, wound and soft-tissue infection, meningitis, bacteremia and septicemia, ocular infections, pneumonia and respiratory tract infections, urinary tract infection in neonates, osteomyelitis, peritonitis and acute cholecystitis. Severe infection can result from non resolved intermittent diarrhea, which can occur months after the initial infection. *A. hydrophila* can cause disease in aquatic animals, such as red leg disease in frogs which is caused by endotoxin and haemolysin produced by the bacteria and can be fatal. The entire genome of *A. hydrophila* has been sequenced and was reported in 2006. Symptoms of *Aeromonas* infection range from mild diarrhea to dysentery-like symptoms, including blood and mucus in the stool, to symptoms of septicemia.

Mortality

For gastroenteritis, the mortality rate is not known. The mortality rate for septicemia caused by *Aeromonas* may be 33% or higher. (Infections that were not foodborne – skin or soft tissue infections caused by *Aeromonas*, particularly in immunocompromised people with conditions such as liver disease or malignancy – can result in mortality rates of 60% to 75%.)

Infective dose

The infective dose of this organism is unknown, but SCUBA divers who have ingested small amounts of water have become ill, and *A. hydrophila* has been isolated from their stools. Although the organism possesses several virulence factors that could cause human illness, volunteer feeding studies using healthy adults and high concentrations of organism (10^4 to 10^{10} cells) have failed to elicit human illness. However, an outbreak associated with shrimp salad contaminated with *A. hydrophila*, at approximately 10^9 cfu/gm of food, has been reported. The incubation period associated with gastroenteritis is unknown (as strong challenge studies of volunteers and an animal model are lacking), although the onset of diarrhea appears to be greater than 24 hours.

Complications

The link between *A. hydrophila* and human gastroenteritis has not yet been firmly established. The link between the pathogen and disease in humans is based mostly on epidemiologic data. Clinically, different types of gastroenteritis are associated with *A. hydrophila,* including mild diarrhea to a *Shigella*-like dysenteric illness characterized by loose stools containing blood and mucus, and colitis. In people with weak or impaired immune systems, diarrhea can be chronic and severe. Rarely, the dysentery-like syndrome is severe. In people with impaired immune systems, *A. hydrophila* may spread throughout the body and cause systemic infections. Examples of those at risk include people with cirrhosis or various kinds of cancer and those treated with immunosuppressive drugs or who are undergoing cancer chemotherapy. *A. caviae* and *A. veronii* biovar *sobria* also may cause enteritis and, in immunocompromised people or those with malignancies, septicemia. Along with *hydrophila,* these bacteria account for the majority of human clinical isolates of *Aeromonas*. Aside from foodborne infections, *Aeromonas* spp. are well documented as causative agents of wound infection, usually linked to water-related injuries or aquatic recreational activities.

Sources

A. hydrophila frequently has been found in fish and shellfish. It has also been found in market samples of meats (beef, pork, lamb, and poultry) and produce.

2. Vibrio cholerae

Vibrio cholerae, a member of the family Vibrionaceae, is a facultatively anaerobic, Gram-negative, non-spore-forming curved rod, about 1.4–2.6mm long. Differences in the sugar composition of the heat-stable surface somatic "O" antigen are the basis of the serological classification of *V. cholerae*; currently the organism is classified into 206 "O" serogroups. Until recently, epidemic cholera was exclusively associated with *V. cholerae* strains of the O1 serogroup. All strains that were identified as *V. cholerae* on the basis of biochemical tests but that did not agglutinate with "O" antiserum were collectively referred to as non-O1 *V. cholerae*. The non-O1 strains are occasionally isolated from cases of diarrhoea and from a variety of extraintestinal infections, from wounds, and from the ear, sputum, urine, and cerebrospinal fluid.

The simple distinction between *V. cholerae* O1 and *V. cholerae* non-O1 became obsolete in early 1993 with the first reports of a new epidemic of severe, cholera-like disease in Bangladesh (Albert et al., 1993) and India. At first, the responsible organism was referred to as non-O1 *V. cholerae* because it did not agglutinate with O1 antiserum. However, further investigations revealed that the organism did not belong to any of the O serogroups previously described for *V. cholerae* but to a new serogroup, which was given the designation O139 Bengal after the area where the strains were first isolated (Shimada et al., 1993). Since recognition of the O139 serogroup, the designation non-O1 non-O139 *V. cholerae* has been used to include all the other recognized serogroups of *V. cholerae* except O1 and O139.

The emergence of *V. cholerae* O139 as the new serogroup associated with cholera, and its probable evolution as a result of horizontal gene transfer between O1 and non-O1 strains (Bik et al., 1995), has led to a heightened interest in the *V. cholerae* non-O1 non-O139 serogroups. There is evidence for horizontal transfer of O antigen among *V. cholerae* serogroups; it is reported that isolates of nearly identical *asd* gene (chromosomal housekeeping gene, which encodes aspartate semialdehyde dehydrogenase) sequences had different O antigens and that isolates with the O1 antigen did not cluster together but were found in different lineages.

Vibrio cholerae serogroups O1 and O139 are responsible for epidemics and pandemic cholera outbreaks. Virulence of *V. cholerae* serogroups O1 and O139 is predicted by the production of an enterotoxin called cholerae toxin (CT) and the toxin co-regulated pilus (TCP). *V. cholerae* O1 and O139 are the most hardy of the pathogenic *Vibrio* spp. and have the ability to survive in freshwater and in water composed of up to ~3% salt. However, these organisms are very susceptible to disinfectants, cold temperatures (especially freezing), and acidic environments. They are readily inactivated at temperatures >45 C, and cooking food is lethal to *V. cholerae* O1 and O139. *V. cholerae* O139 is unique among *V. cholerae* strains, in that it is encapsulated. However, this does not appear to provide greater pathogenicity or resistance to common disinfectants, such as ethanol and bleach (FDA, 2012).

V. cholerae causes cholera, a gastrointestinal illness. After passage through the acid barrier of the stomach, the organism colonizes the epithelium of the small intestine by means of the toxin-coregulated pili and possibly other colonization factors such as the different haemagglutinins, accessory colonization factor, and core-encoded pilus, all of which are thought to play a role. Cholera enterotoxin produced by the adherent vibrios is secreted across the bacterial outer membrane into the extracellular environment and disrupts ion transport by intestinal epithelial cells. The subsequent loss of water and electrolytes leads to the severe diarrhoea characteristic of cholera. It is known that CT is a multi-subunit toxin encoded by the *ctx*AB operon. Additionally, genes responsible for formation of the TCP (toxin coregulated pilus) are essential for infection.

Mortality

Cholera is usually transmitted by the faecal–oral route, with the infecting dose being around 10^8. Individuals with reduced gastric acidity and blood group O are more susceptible to infection. Without rehydration therapy, this disease has a 30% to 50% mortality rate; however, with timely treatment, the fatality rate is less than 1%. The Symptoms of the infection usually appear within a few hours to 3 days of ingestion. The illness generally presents with abdominal discomfort and diarrhea that may vary from mild and watery to acute, with rice-water stools. Vomiting also occurs in some cases.

Complications

Infection with *V. cholerae* serogroups O1 or O139 causes mild to severe diarrhea. Approximately 20% of those infected have watery diarrhea, and 10% to 20% of those develop severe watery diarrhea (characteristic rice-water stools) and vomiting. Cholera gravis, the most severe form of cholera infection, is characterized by severe fluid and electrolyte loss from vomiting and profuse, watery diarrhea. Complications include tachycardia, hypotension, and dehydration. *V. cholerae* O1 and O139 infections can be treated with antibiotics, though rehydration therapy is generally sufficient. Doxycycline and/or tetracycline are the antibiotics of choice; however, some resistance to tetracycline has been reported.

Sources

In the U.S., infections with these organisms have been associated with a variety of seafoods, including molluscan shellfish (oysters, mussels, and clams), crab, lobster, shrimp, squid, and finfish. Illness generally results from consumption of these seafoods raw, improperly cooked, or cross contaminated by a raw product. Although cooking kills these bacteria, serogroups O1 and O139 can grow, in shellfish that have been contaminated *after* cooking, and prompt refrigeration of food remnants is important for prevention of this illness. In areas where *V. cholerae* serogroup O1 and/or O139 is endemic, infections can occur from ingestion of water; ice; unwashed, contaminated food; and seafood.

Food Intoxication Causing Bacteria

This group includes bacteria responsible for food poisonings resulting from ingestion of preformed toxin leading to food intoxication. *Clostridium botulinum* and *Staphylococcus aureus* are included in this group.

Clostriddium botulinum is an anaerobic, Gram-positive, spore-forming rod that produces a potent neurotoxin. The spores are heat-resistant and can survive in foods that are incorrectly or minimally processed.

Based on the antigenic specificity of toxins (neurotoxins) produced by various strains of *C. botulinum*, the following serovars are identified: A, B, C1, C2, D, E, F, G. Types A, B, E and F cause human botulism. Types C and D cause botulism in animals. Types C and E also cause botulism in birds. No outbreaks of type G have been reported. Most strains produce only one type of toxin, but strains producing dual toxin types are known.

C. botulinum strains are divided into four types:

- Type I (so-called 'proteolytic'): produces A, B, and F neurotoxins; harmful for humans; minimum temperature for growth is 12⁰C.

- Type II (so-called 'non-proteolytic'): produces B, E, and F neurotoxins; harmful for humans; the minimum temperature for growth is 3.3⁰C.

- Type III: produces C and D toxins; dangerous for birds, minks, and calves; do not affect humans; the minimum temperature for growth is 15⁰C.

- Type IV: produces G toxin; harmful for humans; the minimum temperature for growth is 12⁰C.

The bacterium causes an illness known as "Botulism". Botulism is characterised by symmetrical, descending, flaccid paralysis of motor and autonomic nerves usually beginning with cranial nerves. It occurs when neuromuscular transmission is interrupted by a protein neurotoxin produced by the bacterium. Paralysis begins with the cranial nerves, then affects the upper extremities, the respiratory muscles, and, finally, the lower extremities in a proximal-to-distal pattern. In severe cases, extensive respiratory muscle paralysis leads to ventilatory failure and death unless supportive care is provided. There are five clinical categories of botulism:

1. **Foodborne botulism**

   Onset generally occurs 18 to 36 hours after exposure (range, 6 hours to 8 days). Initial symptoms can include nausea, vomiting, abdominal cramps or diarrhoea. After the onset of neurologic symptoms, constipation is typical. Dry mouth, blurred vision, and diplopia are usually the earliest neurologic symptoms. They are followed by dysphonia, dysarthria, dysphagia, and peripheral muscle weakness. Symmetric descending paralysis is characteristic of botulism.

2. **Wound botulism**

This can be defined as clinical evidence of botulism following lesions, with a resultant infected wound and no history suggestive of foodborne illness. Except for the gastrointestinal symptoms, the clinical manifestations are similar to those seen in foodborne botulism. However, the incubation period is much longer as time is required for the incubation of spores, growth of clostridium and release of toxins (4 to 14 days).

3. **Infant botulism**

This is caused by the absorption of toxin produced by *Clostridium botulinum* that colonize the intestinal tracts of infants under one year of age. It is often associated with ingestion of honey and the first clinical sign is usually constipation. After a few weeks, progressive weakness and poor feeding are observed. The weakness is symmetrical and descending. It evolves over hours or several days. The infant is afebrile and has a weak cry, has either absent or diminished spontaneous movements, decreased sucking, floppy head and decreased motor response to stimuli. The autonomic nervous system manifestations include dry mucous membranes, urinary retention, diminished gastro-intestinal motility, fluctuation of heart rate, and changes in skin colour. Duration of hospitalisation may last from a few days to six months.

4. **Adult infectious botulism**

It occurs as a result of intestinal colonization with C. *botulinum* and in vivo toxin production in a manner similar to that of infant botulism. These patients often have a history of abdominal surgery, achlorhydria, Crohn's disease or recent antibiotic treatment. The disease may simulate a Guillain- Barré Syndrome.

5. **Inadvertent botulism**

This has been reported in patients who have been treated with intramuscular injections of botulinum toxin. Marked clinical weakness is observed as well as electrophysiologic abnormalities.

Mode of action of Botulinum toxin

Botulinum neurotoxin reaches nerve terminals at the neuromuscular junction, where it binds to the neuronal membrane, moves into the cytoplasm of the axon terminal, and acts to block excitatory synaptic transmission, leading to flaccid paralysis. There are three steps involved in toxin mediated paralysis:

1) internalisation
2) disulphide reduction and translocation
3) inhibition of the neurotransmitter release.

The toxin must enter the nerve ending to exert its effect. Binding of toxin to both peripheral and central nerves is selective and saturable. The C-terminal half of the heavy chain determines cholinergic specificity and is responsible for binding, while the light chain is the intracellular toxic moiety. If the disulphide bond that links the two chains is broken before the toxin is internalised by the cell, the light chain cannot enter and there is virtually complete loss of toxicity. The toxin blocks the release of acetylcholine but not its synthesis or storage. Botulinum toxin is a zinc endopeptidase specific for protein components of the neuroexocytosis apparatus. It cleaves synaptobrevin, a membrane protein of synaptic vesicles. The types A, C and E act on proteins of the presynaptic membrane. Types A and E cleave SNAP-25 while serotype C cleaves syntaxin.

Characteristics of the botulinum toxin

All clostridial neurotoxins are synthesized as a single inactive polypeptide chain of 150 kDa without a leader sequence and hence are presumably released from the cell by bacterial lysis. Bacterial or tissue protease cleaves these toxins within an exposed highly protease-sensitive loop and generates the active di-chain neurotoxins composed of a heavy chain (H, 100 kDa) and a light chain (L, 50 kDa) joined by disulphide bonds, that is associated with one atom of zinc. This interchain S-S bond plays a critical role in cell penetration, and its cleavage by reduction abolishes toxicity.

The heavy chain can be divided functionally into an amino terminal domain (Hn) and a carboxyl terminal domain (Hc). The light chain (amino acids 1-448) acts as a zinc endopeptidase, with proteolytic activity concentrated at the N-terminal end. The heavy chain (amino acids 449-1280) provides cholinergic specificity and promotes light chain translocation across the endosomal membrane of the neurotransmitter. If the disulphide bond that links the two chains is broken before the toxin is internalised in the cell, the light chain cannot enter the axon terminal membrane, and there is a virtually complete loss of toxicity.

The toxin in the complex is rather stable, especially under acidic conditions (pH 3,5 to 6,5), but the complex dissociates under slightly alkaline conditions and the biological activity is readily inactivated in this state. The neurotoxin can be separated from the nontoxic components and purified by ion-exchange chromatography. Although botulinum spores are relatively heat resistant the toxin itself is heat sensitive. Heating it at 80^0C for 30 minutes or 100^0C for 10 minutes destroys the active toxin.

Mortality: The mortality rate is high if treatment is not immediately administered. The disease is generally fatal in 5% to 10% of cases. An extremely small amount of infective dose – a few nanograms – of the toxin can cause illness.

The symptoms of the illness in adult and infant are as follows:

Adult: Initial symptoms may include double vision, blurred vision, drooping eyelids, slurred speech, difficulty swallowing, dry mouth, and muscle weakness. If the disease is not treated, symptoms may progress to paralysis of the arms, legs, trunk, and respiratory muscles. Early signs of intoxication consist of marked lassitude, weakness and vertigo, usually followed by double vision and progressive difficulty in speaking and swallowing. Difficulty in breathing, weakness of other muscles, abdominal distention, and constipation may also be common symptoms

Infant: Constipation after a period of normal development is often the first sign of infant botulism. This is followed by flat facial expression; poor feeding (weak sucking); weak cry; decreased movement; trouble swallowing, with excessive drooling; muscle weakness; and breathing problems.

Sources

The types of foods involved in botulism vary according to food preservation and cooking practices. Any food conducive to outgrowth and toxin production can be associated with botulism. This can occur when food processing allows spore survival and the food is not subsequently heated before consumption, to eliminate any live cells.

Almost any type of food that is not very acidic (pH above 4.6) can support growth and toxin production by *C. botulinum*. Salt concentration from 4% to 5% is needed for inhibition of its spores (especially regarding type E), with a 5% concentration completely inhibiting their growth. Salt concentrations slightly lower than those providing inhibition tend to extend spore outgrowth time at low temperatures.

A variety of foods, such as canned corn, peppers, green beans, soups, beets, asparagus, mushrooms, ripe olives, spinach, tuna fish, chicken and chicken livers, liver pate, luncheon meats, ham, sausage, stuffed eggplant, lobster, and smoked and salted fish have been associated with botulinum toxin.

Infant botulism: Of the various potential environmental sources, such as soil, cistern water, dust, and foods, honey is the one dietary reservoir of *C. botulinum* spores linked to infant botulism by both laboratory and epidemiologic studies. *Honey should not be fed to infants under 12 months of age.*

Staphylococcus aureus

S. aureus is a Gram-positive, spherical bacterium (coccus) with a diameter of 1 – 1.3 µm. When viewed microscopically, *S. aureus* appears in clusters, like bunches of grapes (*staphyle* is Greek for "bunch of grapes," and *coccus* means "grain" or "berry") and hence has been named so. Growing in food, some strains can produce toxins which cause acute gastro-intestinal diseases if ingested. S. aureus are non-motile, catalase-positive, non spore forming, ubiquitous and impossible to eradicate from the environment. Many of the 32 species and subspecies in the genus *Staphylococcus* are potentially found in foods due to environmental, human, and animal contamination. Several staphylococcal species have the ability to produce highly heat-stable enterotoxins that cause gastroenteritis in humans. S. aureus is the etiologic agent predominantly associated with staphylococcal food poisoning.

S. aureus is a versatile human pathogen capable of causing staphylococcal food poisoning, toxic shock syndrome, pneumonia, postoperative wound infection, and nosocomial bacteremia. *S. aureus* produces a variety of extracellular products, many of which act as virulence factors. Staphylococcal enterotoxins can act as superantigens capable of stimulating an elevated percentage of T-cells.

Staphylococci are mesophilic. *S. aureus* growth, in general, ranges from 7 C to 47.8 C, with 35 C being the optimum temperature for growth. The growth pH range is between 4.5 and 9.3, with an optimum between 7.0 and 7.5. *S. aureus* are highly tolerant to salts and sugars.

Staphylococcal food poisoning (SFP) is an intoxication that results from the consumption of foods containing sufficient amounts of one (or more) preformed enterotoxin. Symptoms of SFP have a rapid onset (2–8 h), and include nausea, violent vomiting, abdominal cramping, with or without diarrhea. The disease is usually self-limiting and typically resolves within 24–48 h after onset. Occasionally it can be severe enough to warrant hospitalization, particularly when infants, elderly or debilitated people are concerned.

S. aureus Enterotoxins

Staphylococcal enterotoxins (SEs) are single-chain proteins with molecular weights of 26,000 to 29,000. The SEs are short proteins (from 194 to 245 aa) which are soluble in water. They are potent gastrointestinal exotoxins synthesized by the bacteria and are known to be highly stable, having the ability to resist most proteolytic enzymes, such as pepsin or trypsin, and thus keep their activity intact in the digestive tract after ingestion. They are also highly resistant to heat and can servive temperatures upto 100⁰C for 30 minutes.

Till to date 22 SEs have been described, with some of them proven to be emetic. There are five classical enterotoxin serotypes: SEA, SEB, SEC1,2,3, SED, and SEE and the more recently described SEG, SEH, and SEI; all exhibit emetic activity. There are also SE-like enterotoxin serotypes, SElJ-SElU; these SE-like designations have not been confirmed to exhibit emetic activity. The different SE serotypes are similar in composition and biological activity, but are different in antigenicity and are identified serologically as separate proteins.

Staphylococcal food poisoning (staphyloenterotoxicosis; staphyloenterotoxemia) is the name of the condition caused by the enterotoxins. The main symptoms of SFP are nausea, vomiting, retching, abdominal cramping and prostration, often accompanied by diarrhoea and sometimes fever. In severe cases, patients may suffer from headache, muscle cramping, severe fluid and electrolytes loss with weakness and low blood pressure or shock. Patients usually recover within two days, but can take longer in severe cases that may require hospitalization. Death following a case of staphylococcal food poisoning is very rare and may occur among the elderly, infants, and severely debilitated persons.

Mortality: Death from staphylococcal food poisoning is uncommon, although it has occurred among the elderly, infants, and severely debilitated people.

Infective dose: The intoxication dose of SE is less than 1.0 microgram. This toxin level is reached when *S. aureus* populations exceed 100,000 organisms/g in food. This level is indicative of unsanitary conditions in which the product can be rendered injurious to health. In highly sensitive people, ingestion of 100 to 200 ng of enterotoxin can cause symptoms. The population of *S. aureus* at the time of analysis may be significantly different, and not representative of, the highest population that occurred in the product. This should be taken into consideration when examining foods.

Onset: The onset of symptoms usually is rapid (1 to 7 hours) and in many cases acute, depending on individual susceptibility to the toxin, amount of toxin ingested, and general health.

Complications: Staphylococcal food poisoning generally causes self-limiting, acutely intense illness in most people. Not all people demonstrate all symptoms associated with the illness. The most common complication is dehydration caused by diarrhea and vomiting.

Source

Foods that are commonly regarded as the cause of staphylococcal intoxication include meat and meat products, poultry and egg products, milk and dairy products, salads, bakery products, particularly cream-filled pastries and cakes, and sandwich fillings. Salted food products, such as ham, have also been implicated.

Food handlers carrying enterotoxin-producing *S. aureus* in their noses or on their hands are regarded as the main source of food contamination, via manual contact or through respiratory secretions. In fact, *S. aureus* is a common commensal colonizer of the skin and mucosal membranes of humans, with estimates of 20–30% for persistent and 60% for intermittent colonization. *S. aureus* does not compete well with indigenous microbiota in raw foods, therefore contamination is mainly associated with improper handling of cooked or processed foods, followed by storage under conditions which allow growth of *S. aureus* and enterotoxin(s) production. However, *S. aureus* is also present in food animals, and dairy cattle, sheep and goats, particularly if affected by subclinical mastitis, are likely contaminants of milk. Air, dust, and food contact surfaces can also serve as vehicles in the transfer of *S. aureus* to foods.

Fungal Toxins

The secondary metabolites toxic to humans produced by fungi are called mycotoxins. Mycotoxins are a group of chemically diverse naturally occurring substances produced by a range of filamentous fungi or moulds. They have toxic effects on both humans and animals ranging from acute toxicity and death, through reduced egg and milk production, lack of weight gain, impairment or suppression of immune function to tumour formation, cancers and other chronic diseases. The mycotoxins of greatest concern are produced by mould species from three main genera - *Aspergillus*, *Penicillium* and *Fusarium*. These are mainly storage moulds affecting commodities such as nuts, dried fruits and cereals. The moulds grow and produce toxins when commodities are stored incorrectly - usually at too high moisture levels. Specific mycotoxins of greatest concern are detailed below:

A. Aflatoxins

Aflatoxins (AF) are produced mainly by some strains of *Aspergillus flavus* and most, if not all, strains of *A. parasiticus*. There are four main aflatoxins, B1, B2, G1 and G2, plus two additional ones that are significant, M1 and M2. The aflatoxin M1, is produced by mammals after consumption of feed (or food) contaminated by aflatoxin B1. Cows are able to convert B1 into M1 and transmit it through their milk. Although M1 in milk is, by far, not as hazardous as the parent compound, a limit of 0.5 parts per billion is applied, largely because milk tends to constitute a large part of the diet of infants and children. The aflatoxins are potent liver toxins in most animals and carcinogens in some, with aflatoxin B1 being the most toxic and carcinogenic. There is sufficient evidence that AFB1 can interact with DNA, producing damage. If the DNA is not repaired, a mutation can occur that may initiate the cascade of events required to produce cancer. This condition may develop due to following biochemical events.

After activation by cytochrome P450 monooxygenases, AFB1 is metabolized to form a highly reactive metabolite, AFB1-exo-8,9-epoxide. The exo-epoxide binds to the guanine moiety of DNA at the N7 position, forming trans-8,9-dihydro-8-(N7-guanyl)-9hydoxyAFB1 adducts, which can rearrange and form a stable adduct. This can be measured in tumor tissues. AFB1-DNA adducts can result in GC-to-AT transversions. This specific mutation at codon 249 of the p53 tumor suppressor gene may be important in the development of HCC. Studies of liver-cancer patients in Southeast Asia and sub-Saharan Africa, where AF contamination in foods was high, have shown that a mutation in the p53 at codon 249 is associated with a G-to-T transversion.

Mould growth and aflatoxin production are greatest in warm temperatures and high humidity, particularly in tropical and sub-tropical regions, mainly on corn (maize), peanuts, cottonseed and tree nuts.

Mortality: The mortality rates due to aflatoxin food poisoning is very high as indicated by following outbreaks in various parts of the world:

1. In northwest India, in 1974, there were 108 fatalities from 397 illnesses. AF levels of 0.25 to 15 mg/kg were found in corn.

2. In 1982, in Kenya, there were 20 hospital admissions, with a 60% mortality rate, with AF intake at 38 µg/kg of body weight.

3. In 1988, in Malaysia, 13 Chinese children died of acute hepatic encephalopathy after eating Chinese noodles. Aflatoxins were confirmed in postmortem samples from the patients.

4. In 2004 and 2005, one of the largest aflatoxicosis outbreaks on record occurred in rural Kenya, resulting in illness in 317 people, 125 of whom died. AF-contaminated homegrown maize with an average concentration of 354 ng/g was the source of the outbreak.

Toxic dose: The toxic level of aflatoxin (AF) in humans is largely unknown. In one example, a laboratory worker who intentionally ingested B1 at 12 µg/kg body weight for 2 days developed a rash, nausea, and headache, but recovered without ill effect. In a 14-year follow-up of the worker, a physical examination and blood chemistry, including tests for liver function, were normal.

Complications

From acute exposure: Acute exposure to high doses of AFs can result in aflatoxicosis, with the target organ being the liver, leading to serious liver damage. AFs inhibit the normal functions of the liver, including carbohydrate and lipid metabolism and protein synthesis.

From chronic exposure at sublethal doses: cancer, impaired protein formation, impaired blood coagulation, toxic hepatitis, and probable immunosuppression. In animals, AFs may cause, in addition, reduced weight gain and reduced feed-conversion efficiency.

B1 is the most potent known natural carcinogen and is the most abundant of the AFs. The International Agency for Research on Cancer has classified AFB1 as a group 1 carcinogen and M1as a group 2b carcinogen (carcinogenic to laboratory animals and possibly carcinogenic to humans, respectively). Combined exposure to aflatoxin and hepatitis B increases the risk for development of human hepatocellular carcinoma (HCC).

Other significant health effects of AF exposure follow from the finding that they are probably immunosuppressive in humans. AFs have been shown primarily to affect the cellular immune processes in most of the laboratory animal species studied. Some animals exhibit a decrease in antibody formation, and there is evidence of transplacental movement of AFs, allowing embryonic exposure and reducing immune responses in offspring.

Symptoms: The disruption and inhibition of carbohydrate and lipid metabolism and protein synthesis associated with aflatoxicosis can lead to hemorrhaging, jaundice, premature cell death, and tissue necrosis in liver and, possibly, other organs. Other general symptoms include edema of the lower extremities, abdominal pain, and vomiting.

Sources

In the U.S., AFs are commonly found in corn (maize), sorghum, rice, cottonseed, peanuts, tree nuts, copra, cocoa beans, figs, ginger, and nutmeg. AFM1 may be found in milk and dairy products. Aflatoxin M1 also may be found in human breast milk, as has been the case in Ghana, Kenya, Nigeria, Sudan, Thailand, and other countries, from a mother's chronic exposure to dietary AFs. The maximum acceptable limit of the aflatoxin in select countries is depicted in Table 9.1:

Table 9.1 : Maximum acceptable levels for aflatoxin for select countries (AFB, unless otherwise stated)

Country	Limit ($\mu g kg^{-1}$)	Foods
United	2	Nuts, dried figs and their products
Kingdom	5	As above but intended for further processing
United	20	Total aflatoxins in all foods
States	0.5	Aflatoxins M1 in whole milk, low
		fat milk and skim milk

Contd...

Table 9.1 Contd...

Country	Limit (µgkg⁻¹)	Foods
Australia	5	All foods except peanut products
	15	Peanut products
India	30	All foods
Japan	10	All foods
China	50	Rice, peanuts, maize, sorghum, beans, wheat, barley, oats

Source: WHO, Basic Food Safety, 2000.

B. Ochratoxins

The family of ochratoxins consists of three members, A, B, and C which are produced by *Aspergillus ochraceus* and related species, as well as *Penicillium verrucosum*. Ochratoxin A (OTA), the major and the most abundant compound, has been found in more than 10 countries in Europe and the USA. It was first isolated from *Aspergillus ochraceus* in 1965 by a research group in South Africa. Ochratoxin A is a neurotoxic, immunosuppressive, genotoxic, carcinogenic and teratogenic mycotoxins present in human food, mainly cereals and cereals products, alcoholic beverages and mill products (coffee, cocoa). Ochratoxin A causes liver damage in rats, dogs and pigs. Ochratoxins are also teratogenic to mice, rats and chicken embryos, and are now thought to be a potent nephrotoxin and carcinogen in humans. The carcinogenic potential of Ochratoxin A is recognized by the International Agency for Research on Cancer which classifies it as a group 2b potential human carcinogen. Ochratoxin A is structurally similar to phenylalanine. Due to this similarity OTA has shown to inhibit protein synthesis both *in vitro* and *in vivo*, by competition with phenylalanine. OTA might act on other enzymes that use phenylalanine as a substrate, such as phenylalanine hydroxylase, and lower the levels of phosphoenolpyruvate carboxykinase, a key enzyme in gluconeogenesis. Inhibition of protein and RNA synthesis is also considered another toxic effect of OTA.

OTA has been implicated in the aetiology of Balkan Endemic Nephropathy (BEN) and Urinary Tract Tumours (UTT). Endemic nephropathy is a fatal human renal disease, affecting predominantly rural populations in the central Balkan Peninsula. The disease has been reported in Bosnia and Herzegovina, Bulgaria, Croatia, Romania, and Serbia (Krogh, 1976). The Joint Food and Agriculture Organization/World Health Organization Expert Committee on Food Additives (JECFA) have established a provisional tolerable weekly intake (PTWI) of 0.1µg/kg body weight per week for ochratoxin A.

OTA, $C_{20} H_{18} ClNO_6$ (molecular weight: 403.82 daltons), is a phenylalanyl derivative of a substituted isocoumarin. It is listed in Chemical Abstracts' index as L-phenylalanine N-[5-chloro-3,4-dihydro-8-hydroxy-3-methyl-1-oxo-1 H2-benzopyran-7-yl]carbonyl-(R)-(C.A. No. 303-47-9). OTA is structurally similar to the amino acid phenylalanine (Phe). For this reason, it has an inhibitory effect on a number of enzymes that use Phe as a substrate, in particular, Phe-tRNA synthetase, which can result in inhibition of protein synthesis. For the same reason, OTA may also stimulate lipid peroxidation. OTA is a colourless crystalline compound soluble in organic solvents and in alkaline water. It crystallises from benzene to give a product melting at 90 °C containing one molecule of benzene. This can be removed under vacuum at 120 °C to give a substance melting at 168 °C. It crystallises in a pure form from xylene. OTA is optically active and exhibits blue fluorescence under UV light, but the ultraviolet spectrum varies with pH and with the solvent polarity. Fluorescence emission is maximum at 467 nm in 96 % ethanol and 428 nm in absolute ethanol (Scott, 1994).

Ochratoxin A is found mainly in cereal and cereal products. This group of commodities has been reported to be the main contributors to ochratoxin A exposure in exposure assessments carried out by the European Commission (EC, 1997, 2002), accounting for 50% of total dietary exposure of ochratoxin A in European countries. Besides cereals and cereal products, ochratoxin A is also found in a range of other food commodities, including coffee, cocoa, wine, beer, pulses, spices, dried fruits, grape juice, pig kidney and other meat and meat products of non-ruminant animals exposed to feedstuffs contaminated with this mycotoxin. The legal limits of ochratoxin A (OTA) in various food sources as set by European Commission is depicted in Table 9.2.

Table 9.2 : Legal limits for ochratoxin A in different food products set by the European Commission

	Products	Maximum levels (µg/kg)
1.	Raw cereal grains (including raw rice and buckwheat)	5.0
2.	All products derived from cereals (including processed cereal products and cereal grains intended for direct human consumption)	3.0
3.	Dried vine fruits (currants, raisins and sultanas)	10.0
4.	Roasted coffee beans and ground roasted coffee with the exception of soluble coffee	5.0
5.	Soluble coffee (instant coffee)	10.0

Contd...

Table 9.2 Contd....

Products	Maximum levels (µg/kg)
6. Wine (red, white and rose) and other wine and/ or grape must based drinks	2.0
7. Grape juice, grape juice ingredients in other beverages, including grape nectar and concentrated grape juice as reconstituted	2.0
8. Grape must and concentrated grape must as reconstituted, intended for direct human consumption	2.0
9. Baby foods and processed cereal-based foods for infants and young children	0.50
10. Dietary foods for special medical purposes intended specifically for infants	0.50

Source: EC Regulation No. 123/2005 of 26 January 2005.

C. Patulin

Patulin is a polyketide lactone, produced by certain fungal species of *Penicillium*, *Aspergillus* and *Byssochlamys* growing on fruit, including apples, pears, grapes and other fruit. However, the most common producer of patulin is *Penicillium expansum*, which occurs commonly in rotting apples, as a result of which patulin has frequently been found in commercial apple juice. Patulin is toxic to many biological systems, including bacteria, mammalian cell cultures, higher plants and animals. Its role in causing animal and human disease is unclear, but it is believed to be carcinogenic and has been found to cause intestinal injury, ulceration and oxidative damage to DNA.

The International Agency for Research on Cancer has evaluated the toxicity data and in 1986 classified patulin a Group 3 carcinogen or "a compound for which there is not enough data to allow its classification". Several European countries have established regulatory limits for patulin in apples and apple products. Switzerland, Sweden, Belgium, Russia, and Norway, have set maximum permitted concentrations of 50ppb. In addition, the World Health Organization has established a maximum recommended concentration of 50 µg/L (50 ppb) in apple juice. Patulin possesses wide-spectrum antibiotic properties and has been tested in humans to evaluate its ability to treat common colds. However, its effectiveness has never been proven and, in the light of its toxicity, use for treatment of medical conditions has not been pursued because of its being irritant to the stomach and causing nausea and vomiting. In acute and short-term studies, patulin causes gastrointestinal hyperaemia, distension haemorrhage and ulceration.

For patulin, the LD_{50} for the rat has been reported as 15 mg kg^{-1} body and 25 mg kg-1after sub-cutaneous injection. Death was usually caused by pulmonary oedema. Lungs were oedematous, with the alveoli filled with protein-rich fluid and many leucocytes. The pulmonary vessels were congested but haemorrhages were few. Hepatic and intestinal blood vessels were congested and in sections of the kidneys there was slight congestion, mild degeneration of the tubular epithelium, and a few loci of haemorrhages. Patulin injected in large amounts over a 2-month period was carcinogenic, resulting in induction of sarcomas at the injection site. In long-term studies at lower dose levels, these effects were not observed. It has also been shown to be immunotoxic, and neurotoxic.

Source

By far the most important source of patulin for humans is apples and apple juice, particularly that produced by direct pressing of apples. Other products containing apples, such as pies and jam, may contain smaller amounts. Pears, grapes, bilberries and other fruit may also be affected. Sweet cider may also be affected but only if additional apple juice is added to the fermented cider. Patulin has also been reported in vegetables, cereal grains and animal silage. Patulin is reported to be formed when silage spoils and is sometimes suspected of causing haemorrhagic symptoms in cattle, although when these incidents are investigated patulin is rarely proven to be the cause.

Up to the present, patulin has not been subject to statutory regulation in most countries. However, the quality of fruit juice is controlled in some countries by the setting of a 'guideline' or a 'recommended' maximum concentration agreed with the apple processing industry. This is commonly set at 50 µg/litre. In the UK regular monitoring of apple juice has been carried out since 1992, and this has reduced the concentrations and incidence of patulin in juices to a very low level, chiefly through better storage of apples, the avoidance of damaged or poor-quality fruit, and better production protocols.

At the 32nd session of the Codex Committee on Food Additives and Contaminants, held in March 2000, discussions took place and a limit of 50 mg/kg for patulin in apple juice and apple juice ingredients in other beverages was proposed for adoption at Step 8 to the Codex Alimentarius Commission. In this latter meeting, a consensus could not be reached and the Commission returned the draft maximum level to Step 6 for further consideration.

Although various exposure assessments indicate that the average lifetime exposure of patulin is well below the provisional maximum tolerable daily intake (PMTDI), recent assessments indicate that the exposure of children to patulin through the consumption of apple juice is in the range of, or even exceeds, the PMDTI during a considerable period of the childhood. The Committee was of the opinion that this aspect needed a closer examination with regard to the potential health risks for children and that it was premature to adopt the level of 50 mg/kg as a maximum level for patulin in apple juice.

D. Cyclopiazonic acid (CPA)

Cyclopiazonic acid is a toxic indole tetramic acid, first isolated from *Penicillium cyclopium* and subsequently from other *Penicillium* species (e.g. *P. commune* and *P. camembertii*), *Aspergillus flavus and A. versicolor*. It is thus an interesting mycotoxin because it is produced by a number of different fungi that infect different foodstuffs. Because it can be formed by *A. flavus*, a species that is a major producer of aflatoxins, it has the potential to co-occur with these mycotoxins in a range of commodities. Cyclopiazonic acid (CPA) is produced by several moulds which occur on agricultural products or are used in some food fermentations. It also occurs naturally in infected corn (maize) and peanuts. It affects rats, dogs, pigs and chickens, where it may cause anorexia, weight loss, diarrhoea, pyrexia, dehydration and other symptoms. Organs affected include liver, spleen, kidneys, and pancreas. It has the ability to chelate metal ions such as calcium, magnesium and iron, which may be an important mechanism of toxicity.

Cyclopiazonic acid (molecular weight 336.39) occurs as an optically active colourless crystalline compound or an off-white hygroscopic powder with a melting point of 245⁰C, soluble in chloroform, dichloromethane, methanol and acetonitrile, and sodium bicarbonate. It is stable in dry state if stored at +4⁰ C. It reacts with 0.1N H_2SO_4 in methanol, gives a blue-violet Ehrlich colour reaction and an orange-red reaction with ferric chloride.

Toxicity

Cyclopiazonic acid only appears to be toxic when present in high concentrations. It has been found to be a neurotoxin when injected intraperitoneally into rats and the LD50 in male rats was 2.3 mg/kg. Oral administration produced no convulsions and LD50 values found in rats for administration by this route were 36 mg/kg and 63 mg/kg for males and females respectively. In addition, lesions in the liver, kidney, spleen and other organs were observed. The effects reported include decreased weight gain, diarrhoea, dehydration, depression hyperaesthesia, hypokinesis, convulsion and death. It is reported that some of its effects in the body are due to its interference with the uptake and release of Ca^{2+} so it could pose a particular risk to humans taking drugs such as calcium antagonists designed to carefully control calcium homeostasis.

Studies of the effect of cyclopiazonic acid are also reported on broiler chicks although its importance for the poultry industry is unclear. Toxicity observed may be masked or caused by other co-occurring mycotoxins of which aflatoxins and T2-toxin have been cited.

It has been found mutagenic for *Salmonella typhimurium* TA98 and TA100 in the Ames assay. It can co-occur with aflatoxins and may enhance the overall toxic effect when this happens. There is a dearth of human exposure data and this precludes an assessment of possible health effects. However, 'Kodua' poisoning in India resulting from ingestion of contaminated millet seeds has been linked to this toxin. It has similar pharmacological properties to the anti-psychotic drugs, chlorpromazine and reserpine, in mice and rabbits. Near lethal doses of 11 to 14 mg/kg body weight induce continuous involuntary tremors and convulsions. It may be able to produce similar effects in humans.

Source

It has been detected at levels up to 10 mg/kg or higher in maize, millet, peanuts, pulses, cheese, ham, sausage, frankfurters, mixed feeds, hay, tomato, milk and other foods and feeds. Some cheeses are surface ripened with the species *P. camembertii* that can produce cyclopiazonic acid, so there is intensive scrutiny of the strains used to ensure that they are non-toxin producers. The co-occurrence of aflatoxins with cyclopiazonic acid has been reported recently in 2 out of 50 samples of peanuts grown in Argentina. To date no regulatory standards have been set for cyclopiazonic acid because its natural occurrence in human food appears to be very low so human exposure would be very limited. It may be that its occurrence in some products susceptible to aflatoxin contamination is indirectly controlled by regulations in place for the aflatoxins. An attempt to estimate an acceptable daily intake has been reported, based on a no observed effect level (NOEL) of 1 mg/kg/day, which takes into account data for several animal species and species variation. This indicates that an appropriate acceptable daily intake (ADI) would be approximately 10 micro g/kg/day or 700 micro g/day. In the context of human exposure, if the uppermost limit of CPA found in cheese is 4 microgrammes/g and the average individual consumes 50 g of cheese daily, this allows an intake of 200 µg, less than one third of a traditionally established ADI.

E. Zearalenone

Zearalenone (also known as F-2 toxin) is described chemically as a phenolic resorcyclic acid lactone and can be produced by a number of species of *Fusarium* including *F. culmorum*, *F. graminearum* and *F. crookwellense*. These species are known to colonise cereals and tend to develop particularly during cool, wet growing and harvest seasons. It occurs naturally in high moisture corn (maize) in late autumn and winter, mainly from the growth of *F. culmorum* in Northern Europe and *F. graminearum* in North America. Production of this and other *Fusarium* toxins is favoured by high humidity and low temperatures, conditions which often occur in temperate regions during autumn harvest. It has been found in mouldy hay, high-moisture corn (maize), corn infected before harvest and pelleted feed rations, so it is an important contaminant of animal feed. The involvement of zearalenone in human disease is unconfirmed, but it is regarded as an endocrine disruptor having estrogenic properties and hence a potential hazard. It has the ability to bind to estrogenic receptors and may lead to infertility in both the sexes in mammals and humans.

Zearalenone is a white crystalline compound, which exhibits blue-green fluorescence when excited by long wavelength UV light (360) and a more intense green fluorescence when excited with short wavelength UV light (260 nm). In methanol, UV absorption maxima occur at 236 (e =29,700), 274 (e =13,909) and 316 (e =6,020). Maximum fluorescence in ethanol occurs with irradiation at 314nm and with emission at 450nm. Solubility in water is about 0.002g/100ml. It is slightly soluble in hexane and progressively more so in benzene, acetonitrile, methylene chloride, methanol, ethanol and acetone. It is also soluble in aqueous alkali. In fungal cultures a number of closely related metabolites are formed, but there is only limited evidence that these occur in foodstuffs, although there is experimental evidence for some transmission of zearalenone and α - and β -zearalenols into the milk of sheep, cows and pigs fed high concentrations.

Toxicity

The most important effect of zearalenone is on the reproductive system. In New Zealand, zearalenone in pasture is a recognised cause of infertility in sheep although its acute toxicity is low. Animal studies show that zearalenone is fairly rapidly absorbed following oral administration and can be metabolised by intestinal tissue in pigs and possibly also in humans with the formation of a - and b -zearalenols, which are subsequently conjugated with glucuronic acid. The proportions of these various products have been shown to vary considerably between species.

The ability of zearalenone to cause hyperestrogenism, particularly in swine has been known for many years. Several of a number of closely related metabolites of zearalenone produced by *Fusarium* spp also possess similar properties, although few have been proven to occur naturally. It is reported that swine fed a diet containing 50 mg/kg of pure zearalenone suffered abortion and stillbirths, while levels above 10 mg/kg reduced the litter size and reduced the weight of piglets. Trial feeding of female pigs demonstrated that a concentration of 0.25 mg/kg or less, produced distinct redness and swelling of the vulva, slight swelling of the mammae with numerous vesicular follicles and some cystic follicles on the ovaria. It was also found that lower levels of zearalenone in swine fed naturally contaminated feed could produce these effects. Although swine have been found to be the most sensitive domestic animal to zearalenone, calves have been reported to show earlier sexual maturity, dairy cows have been reported to have vaginitis, prolonged oestrus and infertility and sheep are reported to become sterile. The effective dose for sheep may be approximately 1 mg/kg.

Sub-acute and sub-chronic toxicity studies, of up to 14 weeks duration have been completed using several species and results showed that most effects were due to the oestrogenic effects of zearalenone. The oestrogenic potency of zearalenone has been compared the with other plant derived oestrogens in MCF-7 or T-47D breast cancer cells and this suggested that in comparison with 17-b -oestradiol, it is one of the most potent natural xenoestrogens.

It has been concluded that there is limited evidence in experimental animals for the carcinogenicity of zearalenone while the evidence for genotoxicity has been contradictory although it has suggested that zearalenone is genotoxic in mice. However, these effects may be species dependant and further studies are required to confirm whether zearalenone should be considered as a potential human mutagen or carcinogen. Although the association between zearalenone exposure and human diseases remains speculative at present, it was considered as a possible causative agent in the outbreaks of precocious pubertal changes in thousands of young children in Puerto Rico and has been suggested to have a possible involvement in human cervical cancer.

A risk assessment of the mycotoxin was carried out some time ago and the authors concluded that no adverse human health effects would be anticipated from zearalenone contamination of corn in Canada, but expressed concern that other unidentified sources might add to the oestrogenic burden. Since the publication of that work, there has been increasing awareness of the potential effects of such natural compounds and more recently zearalenone was evaluated in 2000 by JECFA.

Source

Zearalenone may be produced in wheat, barley, rice, maize, and other cereals and in some other food crops and can survive into consumer products. In cereals and animal feeds, closely related compounds or conjugated products are known to also occur. Zearalenone has been shown to occur in almost every agricultural products and a variety of food-grade grains and foods have been found to contain this mycotoxin including corn and corn products, breakfast cereals, corn beer, wheat flour, bread and walnuts and in animal feed products. As zearalenone is metabolised by yeasts during brewing, mainly to b -zearalenol, this metabolite should be looked for in beer. The presence of zearalenone in whole plants and parts of maize used for silage making was investigated in Germany during 1989-1990 and zearalenone was detected at concentrations up to 300 µg/kg mainly accumulating at the end of the ripening process, with subsequent contamination of the silage. Because zearalenone and its metabolites are produced by the same fungi that give rise to deoxynivalenol and nivalenol it is not surprising that mixtures of all these mycotoxins can occur in the same sample.

Zearalenone was evaluated by JECFA in June 2000 and the Committee concluded that its safety could be evaluated on the basis of the dose that had no hormonal effect in pigs, the most sensitive species. It established a temporary TDI of 0.2 µg/kg of body weight per day. This decision was based on the NOEL of 40 µg/kg of body weight obtained in a 15 day study with pigs and the lowest observed effect level of 200 µg/kg of body weight per day in this study. A safety factor of 200 was also applied. Estimates of average dietary intakes for some 'European' consumers were of the order of 0.02 µg/kg of body weight per day suggesting a significant margin of safety based on current knowledge. However further Research is required on hormonal effects in pigs, potential genotoxicity, long term carcinogenicity tests and blood levels in humans. Maximum levels for zearalenone in cereals have not yet been set by the EC although in a review published in 1997, nine countries had set guidelines or maximum tolerable levels in food (mainly cereals) ranging from non detectable to 1000 µg/kg.

F. Tricothecenes

The trichothecenes are a large group of chemicals characterised by a double bond between C9 and C10 and an epoxy ring at the C12- C13 position in the chemical structure. The '12,13-epoxytrichothecenes' are a group of related and biologically active mycotoxins often wrongly referred to as the *Fusarium* toxins as several other fungal genera including *Trichoderma, Stachybotrys, Verticimonosporium, Cephalosporium* and *Myrothecium* can also produce them. Although the number of compounds of this type runs into the hundreds, only a few have been shown to be agriculturally important. However the fusaria are by far the most important mycotoxin-producing species occurring widely in field crops with more than 20 species of *Fusarium*, including *F. poae, F. sporotrichioides, F. moniliforme, F. culmorum*, and *F. graminearum* among the most important trichothecene producers. They are often classified as Group A and Group B compounds depending on whether they have a side chain on the C7 atom. The most commonly reported Group A trichothecenes include, T-2 toxin, HT-2 toxin, neosolaniol, monoacetoxy scirpenol and diacetoxyscirpenol. Common group B trichothecenes are deoxynivalenol, nivalenol, 3- and 15- acetoxynivalenol and fusarenon X (a separate fact sheet is devoted to deoxynivalenol). In addition to producing mycotoxins these fungi include important plant pathogens that cause a number of serious diseases in growing crops.

Another group of trichothecenes which are generally more acutely toxic than T-2 toxin are known as the macrocyclic trichothecenes produced by mould species such as *Stachybotrys atra*. These include the satratoxins, verrucarins and roridins.

All trichothecenes containing an ester group are hydrolysed to their respective parent alcohols when treated with alkali. A dilute solution of potassium carbonate, sodium hydroxide or ammonium hydroxide hydrolyses T-2 toxin and neosolaniol to T-2 tetraol and diacetoxy- and monoacetoxy- scirpenol to scirpentriol. Many of the alcohols are unaffected, even by hot dilute alkali. Trichothecenes are thus chemically stable and can persist for long periods once formed. Prolonged boiling in water or under highly acidic conditions causes a skeletal rearrangement due to opening of the epoxide ring. Owing to the hindered nature of the epoxide and stability of the ring system, reactions of the trichothecenes usually proceed in a manner predictable from sound chemical principles, e.g. primary and secondary hydroxyl groups are easily oxidised to the aldehyde and ketone derivatives by reagents such as CrO_3-H_2SO_4 in acetone, CrO_3-pyridine and CrO_3-acetic acid.

Group A trichothecenes, T-2 toxin, HT-2 toxin, neosolaniol, monoacetoxy scirpenol and diacetoxyscirpenol are highly soluble in ethyl acetate, acetone, chloroform, methylene chloride and diethyl ether. The Group B trichothecenes, deoxynivalenol (commonly called 'DON' or 'vomitoxin'), nivalenol, 3-acetyldeoxynivalenol, 15-acetyldeoxynivalenol, fusarenone-X, scirpentriol and T-2 tetraol are highly hydroxylated and relatively polar being soluble in methanol, acetonitrile and ethanol.

Toxicity

When given orally or by intraperitoneal injection, the trichothecenes are acutely toxic at low concentrations although the acute toxicity varies considerably as shown. T-2 toxin and the macrocyclic mycotoxins are far more toxic than deoxynivalenol, but occur less commonly in agricultural products. Acute trichothecene toxicity is characterised by gastrointestinal disturbances, such as vomiting, diarrhoea and inflammation, dermal irritation, feed refusal, abortion, anaemia and leukopenia. This group of toxins are acutely cytotoxic and strongly immunosuppresive.

LD$_{50}$ values for mice (intraperitoneal route) for some trichothecenes

Dosed animals become listless or inactive and develop diarrhoea and rectal haemorrhaging. Necrotic lesions may develop in the mouth parts. The mucosal epithelium of the stomach and small intestine erodes, accompanied by haemorrhage, which may develop, into severe gastroenteritis, followed by death. In larger animals, massive haemorrhages develop in the small intestine. The cells of the bone marrow, lymph nodes and intestines undergo a pathological degeneration. The trichothecenes have not been shown to be mutagenic or carcinogenic, but do inhibit DNA and protein synthesis.

Trichothecene	LD$_{50}$ (mg/kg bw)
deoxynivalenol	70
diacetoxyscirpenol	23
neosolaniol	14.5
HT-2 toxin	9.0
T-2 toxin	5.2
nivalenol	4.1
verrucarin A	0.5

A characteristic of a number of the trichothecenes is to cause vomiting and this may limit the amount of food ingested by livestock. For example, pigs are very sensitive to the presence of deoxynivalenol and will reject contaminated feed effectively limiting any further toxic effects. However, many compounds of this group are immunosuppresive in low concentrations and this may be more important than their acute toxicities. Because of the number of closely related metabolites likely to occur in combination in foods or animal feeds, the toxicology is complex with both synergistic and antagonistic effects observed.

Alimentary toxic aleukia (ATA) is the most well recognised human trichothecene mycotoxicosis. T-2 toxin is thought to have contributed to the epidemiology of alimentary toxic aleukia in Russia last century, which was responsible for widespread disease and many deaths. Continuous exposure to trichothecenes results in skin rashes, which may proceed to necrotic lesions. Many outbreaks of acute human diseases involving nausea, vomiting, gastrointestinal upset, dizziness, diarrhoea and headache have occurred particularly in Asia and these outbreaks have been attributed to the consumption of *Fusarium*-contaminated grain. High concentrations of deoxynivalenol have been detected in some samples from such outbreaks.

Source

Surveys have shown that trichothecenes occur in cereal grains such as wheat, barley, maize, oats, rice, soya beans and in derived products such as breakfast cereals and beer. There are also reports of occurrences in other food commodities including sorghum, potatoes, bananas, mustard seed, groundnuts, mangoes, sunflower seeds and cassava. Past surveillance of cereals commonly targeted deoxynivalenol only although other trichothecenes are highly likely to be present and the recent trend is to screen for the range of related compounds that may be expected to occur.

Satratoxins, verrucarins and roridins and may be produced in hay and straw stored under unsatisfactory conditions and may cause symptoms including decreased performance in race horses, haemorrhaging and death, particularly in equines. However, there is little evidence that these compounds occur in human food although the presence of macrocyclic trichothecenes in air-borne fungal spores may contribute to some forms of 'sick building' syndrome.

Legislation for selected trichothecenes has existed in only a few countries. Recently, high levels of deoxynivalenol were found in infant/foods in the Netherlands and this mycotoxin and related trichothecenes have since come under close scrutiny within the EC. One difficulty in considering possible legislation is how to deal with mixtures of toxins of different toxicity that can occur together but often in widely varying proportions. However in 2000 the EC proposed action levels for deoxynivalenol of 500ppb for cereal products as consumed, and for other cereal products at the retail stage, 750 ppb for flour used as raw material in food products and 750 ppb as a monitoring level for raw cereals. At the time, The Commission indicated that these levels were unlikely to be published but asked Member States to consider the practicalities of advising on and using the levels. Trichothecenes were evaluated by JECFA in February 2001 and among the recommendations was the need to obtain much more information on many aspects related to the toxicity and occurrence of these mycotoxins.

G.   Fumonisins

The fumonisins are a group of at least 15 closely related mycotoxins that frequently occur in maize, the most important being fumonisin B_1. Fumonisins were only identified during the mid-1980' s, although their effects on horses had been recognised for at least 150 years before. They are polar metabolites produced by several species of *Fusarium*, including *F. moniliforme, F. proliferatum, F. nygamai, F. anthophilum, F. dlamini* and *F. napiforme*. Their structures are based on a long hydroxylated hydrocarbon chain containing methyl and amino groups. Two hydroxyl groups are esterified to two propane-1, 2, 3-tricarboxylic acids. Fumonisin B_1 differs from fumonisin B_2 in that it has an extra hydroxyl group at the 10 position. Fumonisins often occur together with other mycotoxins, which can include, for example, aflatoxins, deoxynivalenol and zearalenone. Fumonisin B_1 (FB_1) has the empirical formula $C_{34}H_{59}NO_{15}$ (relative molecular mass: 721). The pure substance is a white hydroscopic powder that is soluble in water, acetonitrile-water or methanol. Fumonisins are soluble in polar solvents because of the 4 free carboxyl groups, the hydroxyl groups and the amino group. Their insolubility in many organic solvents such as chloroform and hexane commonly used in mycotoxin analysis partly explains the difficulty in their original identification.

Toxicity

They have been linked to several diseases, including liver cancer and oesophagal cancer in humans. The effects of fumonisins have been observed in a sporadic fatal disease in horses and related species called equine leucoencephalomalacia (ELEM) for many years. On a weight for weight basis, fumonisins are far less acutely toxic than the aflatoxins. However, fumonisins commonly occur in concentrations of parts per million in maize; up to 300 mg/kg has been reported. This contrasts with aflatoxins, which are usually measured in the low parts per billion concentrations in foods.

Fumonisins are considered to be toxic principally because of their effects on sphingolipid synthesis. Alteration in sphingolipid base ratios occurs almost immediately after exposure because fumonisin inhibits ceramide sythetase an enzyme involved in sphingolipid synthesis. The disruption to sphingolipid metabolism increases the ratio of two sphingoid precursors, sphinganine and sphingosine. This property is indicative of fumonisin exposure in a number of species, including horses and pigs. Animal studies with ^{14}C-labelled fumonisin B$_1$ generally show the uptake to be poor and elimination rapid. The range of effects that fumonisins cause in mammals appears to be species-related. ELEM was firstly linked to the presence of *Fusarium moniliforme* in feed and more recently to the presence of fumonisins. In equines, affected animals commonly lose appetite, become lethargic and develop neurotoxic effects after a period of ingesting contaminated feed. Autopsy shows oedema in the brain and liquefaction of areas within the cerebral hemispheres. The liver is also generally affected and, in severe cases, gross liver lesions may be seen with fibrosis of the centrilobular areas. In pigs, fumonisins induce pulmonary oedema and hydrothorax, with thoracic cavities filled with a yellow liquid. There may also be respiratory problems and foetal mortality.

Rats fed culture material from *F. moniliforme* develop primary hepatocellular carcinomas. Similar effects were reproduced using purified fumonisins B$_1$, B$_2$ and B$_3$ although experimental carcinogenicity studies have been hampered by lack of pure standards. Fumonisin B$_1$ has also been shown to affect the foetus in pregnant rats, causing low litter weights and foetal bone development when compared with controls.

In humans, there appears to be a link between the high maize consumption in some areas of the world and the occurrence of oesophageal cancer. Further epidemiological studies are required to more precisely define the role of *F. moniliforme* and its metabolites in oesophageal cancer in the Transkei, China and Northern Italy, where incidence is high. Many studies of the toxicology of fumonisins are in progress. The full significance of fumonisins in maize for humans and animal health still remains to be determined.

Effects have been demonstrated on other organisms and fumonisin B_1 has shown to inhibit cell growth and cause accumulation of free sphingoid bases and alteration of lipid metabolism in *Saccharomyces cerevisiae*. It is phytotoxic, damages cell membranes and reduces chlorophyll synthesis. It also disrupts the biosynthesis of sphingolipids in plants and may play a role in the pathogenicity of maize by fumonisin-producing *Fusarium* species.

Source

When the fumonisins were first identified, it was considered that their occurrence was confined to maize. Subsequently, their presence is being noted in a range of products, which include rice, sorghum and navy beans, but so far in much lower concentrations than are common in maize. Significant accumulation of FB_1 in maize occurs when weather conditions favour *Fusarium* kernel rot.

Surveillance has shown that fumonisins may be present in a number of finished foods, such as polenta, maize-based breakfast cereals and beer and snack products. They have not been detected in milk, meat or eggs.

Human exposure to fumonisins is common worldwide, but there are considerable differences in the extent of human exposure between different maize-growing regions. This is most evident when comparing fully developed and developing countries. For example, although fumonisins can occur in maize products in the USA, Canada and Western Europe, human consumption of those products is modest. In parts of Africa, South-Central America and Asia, some populations consume a high percentage of their calories as maize meal and this often coincides with the growing areas where contamination may be the highest.

To date there has been no wide-scale introduction of limits for fumonisins. Limits have been set in some countries to protect susceptible animals such as horses (5 mg/kg) and pigs (50 mg/kg), and temporary guidelines have been introduced in a few countries to limit the exposure for humans; for example, Switzerland has set a limit for the sum of fumonisin B_1 and B_2 at 1,000 µg/kg in maize intended for human consumption. Fumonisins were considered by the Joint FAO/WHO Committee on Food Additives at a meeting in February 2001 and this body allocated a group provisional maximum tolerable intake (PMTDI) for fumonisins B_1, B_2 and B_3 of 2 µg/kg of body weight per day on the basis of the no observed effect level (NOEL) and a safety factor of 100. All estimates of fumonisins B_1 based on data available from national consumption were well below the group PMTDI, even if an allowance was included for fumonisins B_2 and B_3.

H.   Moniliformin

Moniliformin is formed in cereals by a number of *Fusarium* species that include *F. avenaceum. F. subglutinans,* and *F. proliferatum* and occurs as the sodium or potassium salt of 1-hydroxycyclobut-1-ene-3,4-dione. Studies that ascribe moniliformin production to *F. moniliforme,* which is now called *F. verticillioides* and does not produce moniliformin, actually tested an aggregate consisting of more than one species. These fungi also commonly produce other important mycotoxins so that moniliformin is frequently present in a mixture of mycotoxins.

This mycotoxin has not yet received much attention because it does not appear to be carcinogenic and relatively high amounts appear to be necessary to cause significant toxicological effects. These have been demonstrated in a limited number of animal species. Its stability and fate during processing is also poorly studied so that the degree of consumer exposure is uncertain.

Toxicity

There is a limited amount of data on the effects of moniliformin on mammalian species. The oral LD50 in rodents is approximately 25-50 mg/kg and for day old cockerels 4 mg/kg. The ip. LD50 was 21 and 29 mg/kg respectively for female and male mice. In acute studies, the main lesion appears to be intestinal haemorrhage, but in sub-acute and chronic studies in a variety of avian species and laboratory rodents, the principal target is the heart. It is a potent inhibitor of mitochondrial pyruvate and ketoglutarate oxidation. Data on the effects of moniliformin on reproduction and the foetus and its mutagenic and carcinogenic potential are negative but extremely limited. In a few studies it was found that moniliformin caused chromosomal aberrations. It is cytotoxic for mammalian cells at higher concentrations. In studies in which broiler chicks were fed diets containing 50 mg/kg moniliformin, the birds consumed more feed but put on less weight. They had increased heart and proventriculus (the thin-walled part of the stomach) weights, and decreased mean cell volumes, and the results showed that diets containing moniliformin at this concentration were toxic to chicks fed to market age. Phytotoxic effects have also been observed. In humans, moniliformin has casually been linked with Keshan disease, endemic to certain areas of China.

Some of the published data in which maize containing moniliformin has been fed to animals may need re-evaluation on the basis that contaminated maize may contain a cocktail of toxic *Fusarium*-derived residues such as fumonisins, zearalenone and trichothecenes.

Source

Data on the occurrence of moniliformin in food is scarce. Concentrations up to 12 mg/kg occurred in maize in the Transkei intended for human consumption. More recently, analysis of imported milled maize products, destined for incorporation into animal feed stuffs in the UK, showed 60% of samples contaminated with concentrations up to 4.6 mg/kg moniliformin. It has also been shown to occur in other cereals including wheat, rye and rice. Samples with similar maximum concentrations have been reported in maize from Gambia and South Africa while field samples of maize, oats, wheat, rye and triticale showing visible fungal damage in Poland contained levels ranging from 0.5 to nearly 400 mg/kg. In consumer products, moniliformin has been found in 12 out of 14 corn tortillas examined at levels of 0.022 to 0.1 mg/kg.

I. Other mycotoxins

There may exist several hundred fungal metabolites that could be classed as mycotoxins, but many of these are poorly studied, or information about their toxicity is lacking. A few of these fungal metabolites that have been considered to be mycotoxins are as follows:

1. *Aspergillus clavatus* toxins

The mould *A. clavatus* is a soil fungus that is particularly well adapted to growing in malting barley and has the potential to produce a range of toxic products that include agroclavine (one of the ergot alkaloids), cytochalasin E and K, and several compounds of the tryptoquivaline structure (these have tremorgenic properties). It is the causative agent in 'malt workers' lung. While the fungus can produce many of these compounds in culture, they have not been found to any significant extent in barley. The fungus has been implicated in the intoxication of cattle consuming infected grain in a number of countries, although the toxin(s) responsible have not been identified.

2. *Aspergillus fumigatus* toxins

The *A. fumigatus* group of moulds occurs widely, and they are pathogens that can cause fatal diseases in birds and animals. They can also produce a range of toxic compounds that include some of the tryptoquivalines, fumigaclavines and gliotoxin. *A. fumigatus* is often associated with heating in mouldy grain and this can be associated with a range of different symptoms including haemorrhagic and neurological problems. The occurrence of these compounds is only likely in spoiled cereals and is thus only likely to affect animal feed.

3. Citreoviridin

Citreoviridin is produced by *P. citreonigrum* (synonyms *P. citreoviride* and *P. toxicarium*), particularly in rice after harvest. It can cause cardiac beriberi in man. Acute cardiac beriberi in Japan is now only of historical interest although *P. citreonigrum* and citreoviridin are still reported in other parts of Asia. The fungus is said to be favoured by the lower temperatures and shorter hours of daylight occurring in the more temperate rice growing areas. The toxin is also produced by *P. ochrosalmoneum*. Citreoviridin has been found in un-harvested corn in the USA. Citreoviridin is an unusual molecule consisting of a lactone ring conjugated to a furan ring, with a molecular weight of 402. It is a neurotoxin.

4. Lesser known *Fusarium* toxins

The genus *Fusarium* is responsible for the formation of many toxic metabolites and a number of the most important mycotoxins have been described in separate fact sheets. Those less studied ones that may be of importance for human or animal health include beauvericin, enniatin and fusaproliferin.

5. Gliotoxin

This toxin may be produced by *Aspergillus fumigatus* and limited number of other *Aspergillus* and *Penicillium* species. It is a potent immunosuppressive metabolite and brings about apoptosis in cells. Because of its effects on the immune system it may have a place in transplant surgery. There is limited evidence for its occurrence in moulded cereals. *A. fumigatus* is a potent pathogen which can colonise the lungs and other body tissues after ingestion of spores. There is some limited evidence that gliotoxin may be formed *in situ* in such circumstances.

6. Griseofulvin

A number of *Penicillium* species particularly *P. griseofulvum* produce griseofulvin, which has been detected in mouldy cereals, although its survival into food products does not appear to have been studied. It is strongly fungistatic and has been used for treating many fungal infections. As it stops fungal cells dividing without killing them outright, therapeutic use needs to be continued for several weeks or months. However newer drugs work better than griseofulvin.

7. Mycophenolic acid

This compound is produced by several species of *Penicillium*. It has been detected in cheese as it can be produced by some species of *P. roqueforti*. It has antibiotic activity against bacteria. LD_{50} in rodents is between 500 and 2500 mg/kg bodyweight per day. Monkeys fed 150 mg/kg daily for 2 weeks developed abdominal pain, and diarrhoea with bleeding and anaemia. Mutagenic activity has been reported.

8. β-Nitropropionic acid

Oryzae is used for the production of soy and other sauces. However, along with other food-borne moulds, it can produce b-nitropropionic acid. Its mode of action is apparently irreversible succinate dehydrogenase inhibition that can cause a variety of symptoms, often neurological in nature. Reports of livestock poisoning via ingestion in feed showed that ingestion of b-nitropropionic acid could produce significant toxic effects up to and including death. *A. oryzae* has been shown *to* produce this toxin in cooked sweet potato, potato and ripe banana. Ames type assays for mutagenicity showed positive responses on some strains of *Salmonella*. It has been implicated in food poisonings in China.

9. Kojic acid

Kojic acid is produced by koji, a solid culture of the koji mould fungal starter, used for centuries in oriental food fermentations. It is a commonly produced metabolite that possesses antibacterial and anti fungal activity. Few oral studies exist although toxic effects have been shown in chickens consuming 4-8 mg/kg in feed. Kojic acid is also reported to have moderate cardio toxic and cardio tonic activity. 19 of 47 *A. oryzae* strains tested in one study produced kojic acid. Even though it is apparent that the koji moulds, including *A. oryzae*, can produce kojic acid, this toxin may not be present in the fermented foods. It has been reported to occur in dried fruit such as figs.

10. Penicillic acid

This is a toxic antibiotic produced by several species of *Penicillium* and *Aspergillus*. It has been reported in corn and dried beans and in commercial tobacco. Penicillic acid is a hepatocarcinogen in some animal species, and has also been reported to affect the heart.

11. PR-toxin

A metabolite formed by *P. roqueforti* with an LD50 of 5.8 mg/kg (i.p.) in mice and 11 mg/kg in rats. Symptoms reported include congestion and oedema of lung, kidney and brain and degeneration and haemorrhaging in the liver and kidney. It has been reported in cheese, mouldy grains and silage.

12. Penitrem A

The occurrence of serious outbreaks of tremorgenic and other types of neurotoxicity in domestic animals was originally linked to a number of different *Penicillium* species. The toxin responsible is now considered to be penitrem A, and its major source has been shown to be *P. crustosum*. This fungus is now recognised as a very common species in foods and feeds. *P. crustosum* has also been reliably reported to produce cyclopiazonic acid and roquefortine. Penitrem A is a potent neurotoxin and death or severe brain damage has been reported in field outbreaks involving sheep, cows, horses and dogs. The symptoms of penitrem A are essentially the same as those of a range of other fungal tremorgens. The potential hazard of penitrem A to man remains unknown, while the role of penitrem A and perhaps other fungal neurotoxins in human illness or neurological disorders still awaits elucidation. *P. crustosum* is a ubiquitous spoilage fungus and has often been isolated from cereal and animal feed samples. It can cause spoilage of corn, processed meats, nuts, cheese and fruit. The occurrence of penitrem A in animal feeds is well documented although its occurrence in human foods remains to be assessed.

13. Roquefortines A, B and C

Roquefortines are produces by several moulds included some used to produce mould-ripened cheeses. *P. roqueforti* is an essential internal component in such cheeses such as Roquefort and Gammelost (France), Gorgonzola (Italy), Stilton (UK), Tulum (Turkey), Danish blue (Denmark) and Blauschimmelkase (Switzerland). There is no evidence that roquefortines are formed in significant levels in cheese. They occur in infected feed grain, wilted grasses or whole-crop maize silages.

14. Stachybotryotoxin toxins, satratoxins G and H

Effects of stachybotryotoxin/satratoxins G and H are usually seen in horses but have also been suspected in small animals, including dogs. Symptoms induced by feeding fungal cultures of *Stachybotrys atra* are anorexia, depression, and death.

15. Viomellein, vioxanthin and xanthomegnin

These compounds are produced in cereals by some *Penicillium* and *Aspergillus* species. They have been shown to co-occur with ochratoxin A and citrinin and because they can affect the kidneys, they may contribute to the overall nephrotoxic effect caused by ochratoxin A, particularly in pigs. Current analytical methods are insensitive and there is no evidence for or against their survival into human food products

16. Walleminols

Wallemia sebi is an interesting xerophilic mould that occurs widely in dry products including cereals, dried fish and hay. It is easily missed on standard culture medium. Fungal cultures of this fungus can be very toxic probably due to the presence of metabolites called walleminols and other compounds. The occurrence of these metabolites in materials used to produce human food is poorly studied and the possibility of significant amounts reaching the consumer has not been investigated.

10
Chemopreventives in Food

Many dietary compounds have been identified as potential chemopreventive agents. These include vitamins, minerals, carotenoids, and the large class of phytochemicals (polyphenols, isothiocyanates, organosulfur compounds). These compounds can be divided into two main groups on the basis of the mechanism of action against cancer: cancer-blocking and cancer-suppressing agents. The former prevents carcinogens to hit their cellular targets by several mechanisms including enhancing carcinogen detoxification, modifying carcinogen uptake and metabolism, scavenging ROS (reactive oxygen species) and other oxidative species, enhancing DNA repair. The latter inhibits cancer promotion and progression after formation of preneoplastic cells occurred.

Apart from their role in preventing cancer food sources or their parts have been associated with prevention of several diseases in humans. The regular use of adequate quantity of vegetables in diet has a positive impact on the health of the consumer and prevents him from several pathological events ranging from hepatocellular diseases, DNA damage or oxidative stress to other chronic diseases such as cancer, diabetes, high blood pressure, cataract, macular degeneration, osteoporosis, arthritis and even wrinkles resulting from aging. Studies have indicated that food sources particularly fruits, vegetables, spices etc are rich sources of phytonutrients which have limitless health benefits in terms of their role as chemopreventive agents.

The term "chemoprevention" was coined by Dr. Michael Sporn referring to the possibility that natural forms of vitamin A could prevent the development and progression of epithelial cancer. Dr. Sporn recently pointed out, a more modern and complete definition of chemoprevention includes the use of natural or pharmacological agents to suppress arrest or reverse carcinogenesis at its early stages (Sporn, 2002). This new approach of chemoprevention using dietary sources to prevent various diseases such as cancer, hypertension, diabetes, and aging process has attracted the attention of leading researchers around the world. Chemoprevention of cancer using dietary sources has been a thrust area of research recently. Chemoprevention of cancer can be divided into three main areas:

1. primary prevention in high-risk healthy individuals;
2. cancer prevention in individuals that already had developed pre-malignant lesions;

3. prevention of secondary forms of cancers in patients already treated for a primary cancer.

Consuming a diet rich in plant foods provides a milieu of phytochemicals, nonnutritive substances in plants that possess health-protective benefits. Nuts, whole grains, fruits, and vegetables contain an abundance of phenolic compounds, terpenoids, pigments, and other natural antioxidants that have been associated with protection from and/or treatment of chronic disease such as heart disease, cancer, diabetes, and hypertension as well as other medical conditions. The foods and herbs with the highest anticancer activity include garlic, soybeans, cabbage, ginger, licorice, citrus fruits and the umbelliferous vegetables. The phytochemicals in grains reduce the risk of cardiovascular disease and cancer. A significant finding that has been observed repeatedly is that individuals who consume relatively large amounts of vegetables, fruits, grains and herbs, are at decreased risk of cancer of many organs. A report of 24 epidemiological investigations showed that consumption of relatively large amount of vegetables and fruits were associated with decreased incidence of lung cancer. Multiple mechanisms are undoubtedly involved in the protective effect of diets rich in fruits and vegetables. However, it is difficult to identify the relative contribution of various components of a plant-based food to overall cancer risk reduction. The issue is further complicated by the recent demonstration of synergism among protectors. Attention has recently been focused on intercellular-signaling as common molecular target for various chemopreventive phytochemicals.

The chemopreventive phytochemicals found in food sources may be classified on the basis of their role in the body.

The focus of this chapter shall be the non nutrient phytochemicals/chemopreventives found in food. Many chemopreventives/phytochemicals have been identified in our food sources. Some of the promising chemopreventives having disease prevention capability are as follows:

A. Non-nutrients

I. Alkaloids

1. Caffeine

Caffeine is a water-soluble alkaloid. Pure caffeine is a white odourless crystalline powder with a very bitter taste. Caffeine is closely related to other alkaloids such as theophylline (mainly found in tea) and theobromine (mainly found in cacao beans). Caffeine is found in many everyday products, including tea, cola nuts, coffee, chocolate, mate and guarana. It is also found in some softdrinks (mainly colas and energy drinks) where it is artificially added. Caffeine acts on the nervous system by blocking adenosine receptor thereby slowing down nerve cell activity. Caffeine stimulates the central nervous system, respiration and blood circulation. Caffeine also acts as a diuretic. Caffeine increases the circulation and oxidation of fatty acids. This is why caffeine is used by sportsmen to increase fatty acid metabolism. Caffeine is often used in combination with aspirin to treat headaches. Caffeine can also have negative impact on health, especially if overdosed.

Coffee consumption is associated with a lower overall risk of cancer. This is primarily due to a decrease in the risks of hepatocellular and endometrial cancer, but it may also have a modest effect on colorectal cancer. There does not appear to be a significant protective effect against other types of cancers, and heavy coffee consumption may increase the risk of bladder cancer. On the other hand, caffeine has been shown to inhibit cellular DNA repair mechanisms, but only at extreme high concentrations (which would be lethal in humans). There is little or no evidence that caffeine consumption increases the risk of cardiovascular disease, and it may somewhat reduce the risk of type 2 diabetes. Drinking four or more cups of coffee per day does not affect the risk of hypertension compared to drinking little or no coffee. However those who drink 1–3 cups per day may be at a slightly increased risk. Caffeine increases intraocular pressure in those with glaucoma but does not appear to affect normal individuals (Li et al., 2011). It may protect people from liver cirrhosis (Muriel and Arauz, 2010). There is no evidence that coffee stunts a child's growth. Caffeine may increase the effectiveness of some medications including ones used to treat headaches. Similarly, intravenous caffeine is often used in hospitals to provide temporary pain relief for headaches associated caused by low cerebrospinal fluid pressure.

Inside the body caffeine acts through several mechanisms, but its most important effect is to counteract a substance called adenosine that naturally circulates at high levels throughout the body, and especially in the nervous system. In the brain, adenosine plays a generally protective role, part of which is to reduce neural activity levels. Consumption of caffeine antagonizes adenosine and increases activity in neurotransmission including acetylcholine, epinephrine, dopamine, serotonin, glutamate, norepinephrine, cortisol, and in higher doses, endorphins which explains the analgesic and stimulant effect to some users. At very high doses (exceeding 500 milligrams) caffeine inhibits GABA neurotransmission. Caffeine is both water-soluble and lipid-soluble, and therefore it readily crosses the blood–brain barrier that separates the bloodstream from the interior of the brain. Once in the brain, the principal mode of action is as a nonselective antagonist of adenosine receptors (in other words, an agent that reduces the effects of adenosine). The caffeine molecule is structurally similar to adenosine, and is capable of binding to adenosine receptors on the surface of cells without activating them, thereby acting as a competitive inhibitor.

The long term effects of moderate caffeine consumption can be a reduced risk of developing Parkinson's disease. Parkinson's disease (PD) is the degeneration of dopamine producing neurons. Dopamine producing neurons stimulate the motor cortex effecting motor control. Loss of dopamine produces loss of motor control skills, cognitive function, and autonomic nervous system. Epidemiological studies have shown that the risk of developing PD decreases with increasing levels of caffeine intake. Caffeine binds to the adenosine receptor (A2aR) and indirectly prevents MPTP (1-methyl-4-phenyl-1,2,3,6-tetrahydropyridine, an experimental neurotoxin known to cause PD) from destroying dopamine producing neural cells thus preventing neural degeneration and loss of motor control.

Despite the studies indicating some beneficial effects of caffeine on our body many of the ill effects it has cannot be overlooked. Excessive dependency on caffeine has been associated with increased risks of cardiovascular diseases, anxiety, few forms of cancer (like colon cancer), withdrawal symptoms and many other critical conditions including addiction to caffeine in extreme cases.

2. Theophylline

Theophylline is naturally found in cocoa beans and is also known as dimethylxanthine. Amounts as high as 3.7 mg/g have been reported in Criollo cocoa beans. Trace amounts of theophylline are also found in brewed tea. Theophylline is a bronchodilator. It works by relaxing muscles in the lungs and chest, making the lungs less sensitive to allergens and other causes of bronchospasm. Theophylline is used to treat symptoms such as wheezing or shortness of breath caused by asthma, bronchitis, emphysema, and other breathing problems. Theophylline is known to inhibit the enzyme cAMP phosphodiesterase, which results in release of hormones that cause stimulatory effect. The main actions of theophylline involve:

- relaxing bronchial smooth muscle
- increasing heart muscle contractility and efficiency; as a positive inotropic
- increasing heart rate: (positive chronotropic)
- increasing blood pressure
- increasing renal blood flow
- anti-inflammatory effects
- central nervous system stimulatory effect mainly on the medullary respiratory center.

The main therapeutic uses of theophylline are aimed at:

- chronic obstructive pulmonary disease (COPD)
- asthma
- infant apnea
- Blocks the action of adenosine, an inhibitor neurotransmitter that induces sleep, contracts the smooth muscles and relaxes the cardiac muscle.

II. Monoterpenes (Limonene)

Monoterpenes are nonnutritive dietary components found in the essential oils of citrus fruits, cherry, mint and herbs. Limonene is a colourless liquid hydrocarbon classified as a cyclic terpene. The more common D isomer possesses a strong smell of oranges. A number of dietary monoterpenes have antitumor activity, exhibiting not only the ability to prevent the formation or progression of cancer, but to regress existing malignant tumors. Limonene has well established chemopreventive activity against many cancer types. Limonene has been shown to inhibit the development of spontaneous neoplasms in mice receiving 1200 mg/kg orally; dietary limonene also reduces the incidence of spontaneous lymphomas in p532/2 mice (Hursting et al. 1995). Furthermore, when administered either in pure form or as orange peel oil (95% *d*-limonene), limonene inhibits the development of chemically induced rodent mammary, skin cancers. In rat mammary carcinogenesis models, the chemopreventive effects of limonene are evident during the initiation phase of 7-12-dimethylbenz[*a*]anthracene (DMBA)2-induced cancer and during the promotion phase of both DMBA- and nitrosomethylurea (NMU)-induced cancers. Dietary limonene also inhibits the development of *ras* oncogene–induced mammary carcinomas in rats. It is reported that the development of azoxymethane-induced aberrant crypt foci in the colon of rats was significantly reduced when they were given 0.5% limonene in the drinking water. Limonene has promising chemotherapeutic activity against established rodent pancreatic and mammary tumors.

Mode of action of Limonene

Chemopreventive agents may have cancer blocking and/or suppressing activity. Blocking chemopreventive agents act during the initiation phase of carcinogenesis to prevent the interaction of chemical carcinogens with DNA, e.g., by modulating carcinogen metabolism to less toxic forms. Suppressing chemopreventive agents, on the other hand, act during the promotion phase of carcinogenesis to prevent the outgrowth of initiated cells. The blocking chemopreventive effects of limonene and other monoterpenes during the initiation phase of mammary carcinogenesis are likely due to the induction of Phase I and Phase II carcinogen-metabolizing enzymes, resulting in carcinogen detoxification. Chemopreventive doses of dietary limonene induce total cytochrome P450. The specific cytochrome P450 isozymes induced by limonene include CYP 2B1 and CYP2C. Both limonene and sobrerol, another chemopreventive monoterpene, induce epoxide hydratase as well. Limonene induces glutathione-S-transferase and UDP-glucuronyl transferase resulting in formation of fewer "DMBA-DNA" adducts in monoterpene-treated rats than in controls, and more DMBA is excreted in the urine. These results correlate well with the reduction in tumor incidence and multiplicity observed in rats treated with dietary limonene or other monoterpenes like sobrerol during the initiation phase of DMBA-induced mammary cancer.

The cancer suppressing chemopreventive activity of monoterpenes during the promotion phase of mammary and liver carcinogenesis may be due to inhibition of tumor cell proliferation, acceleration of the rate of tumor cell death and/or induction of tumor cell differentiation. Monoterpenes have multiple pharmacologic effects on mevalonate metabolism; some of these effects may account for their tumor suppressive activity. Some monoterpenes, including limonene and menthol, inhibit hepatic 3-hydroxy- 3-methylglutaryl (HMG) CoA-reductase activity and reduce serum cholesterol.

Many monoterpenes, including limonene, perillyl alcohol and their active serum metabolites inhibit protein isoprenylation. Protein isoprenylation involves the post-translational modification of a protein by the covalent attachment of a lipophilic farnesyl or geranylgeranyl isoprenoid group to a Cys residue at or near the carboxyl terminus. Isoprenoid substrates for prenyl:protein transferase enzymes include farnesylpyrophosphate and geranylgeranylpyrophosphate, two intermediates in the mevalonate pathway. Monoterpenes can directly inhibit prenyl-protein transferases in vitro at doses that are attainable in vivo, suggesting that the inhibition of protein prenylation by monoterpenes occurs at the level of prenyl-protein transferase enzymes. Known mammalian prenylated proteins include Ras-related small GTP-binding proteins, heterotrimeric G proteins and nuclear lamins. Prenylation of Ras enables it to associate with the plasma membrane, which is required for its oncogenic activity. Many prenylated proteins regulate cell growth and/or transformation, and impairment of the prenylation of one or more of these proteins might account for the antitumor activity of monoterpenes. It is reported that limonene prevented the formation of mammary tumors expressing normal or oncogenic *ras* genes with equal efficiency. Together, these data suggest that either the antitumor activity of monoterpenes is due to prenylation-independent mechanisms or, alternatively, that prenylation of proteins other than Ras may be affected by monoterpenes.

III. Organosulfides

1. Allicin

Allicin is an organosulfur compound obtained from garlic, a species in the family Alliaceae. Allicin is the major biologically active component of garlic. First reported that allicin is the key ingredient responsible for the broad-spectrum of anti-bacterial activity in garlic. Research also showed that allicin is responsible for lipid-lowering, anti-blood coagulation, anti-hypertension, anti-cancer, antioxidant and anti-microbial effects.

Medicinal Activity in Garlic is best measured by its Allicin content. Nonetheless, allicin is not found in fresh garlic. The chemistry of garlic is extremely complex. Fresh garlic contains an enzyme called "allinase" and "alliin", which are contained in different parts of the garlic plant. This unique structure is designed as a defense mechanism against microbial pathogens of the soil. When fungi or other soil pathogens attack the cloves, the membrane of those compartments is destroyed, and within 10 seconds, all the alliin is converted into a new compound called allicin. The allicin produced has a very short half-life (the time needed for one-half of a given amount of the component to deteriorate) and has a typical odour of freshly crushed garlic. This is a very efficient weapon because the clove's defense systems only comes to life (activated) in a very small location and for a short period of time, whereas the rest of the allinase and alliin remain preserved in their respective compartments and are available for subsequent microbial attacks. More importantly, as a large amount of allicin generated could also be harmful for the plant tissues and enzymes, this very limited short-lived production that is confined to the area where the microbial attack takes place, minimizes self-damage to the plant.

Animal studies published between 1995 and 2005 indicate that allicin may reduce atherosclerosis and fat deposition, normalize the lipoprotein balance, decrease blood pressure have anti-thrombotic and anti-inflammatory activities, and function as an antioxidant to some extent. A randomized clinical trial funded by the National Institutes of Health (NIH) in the United States and published in the *Archives of Internal Medicine* in 2007 found that the consumption of garlic in any form did not reduce blood cholesterol levels in patients with moderately high baseline cholesterol levels. The fresh garlic used in this study contained substantial levels of allicin, so the study casts doubt on the ability of allicin when taken orally to reduce blood cholesterol levels in human subjects.

In 2009, Vaidya, Ingold and Pratt clarified the mechanism of the antioxidant activity of garlic, such as trapping damaging free radicals. When allicin decomposes, it forms 2-propenesulfenic acid, and this compound is what binds to the free-radicals.

Allicin has been found to have numerous antimicrobial properties, and has been studied in relation to both its effects and its biochemical interactions. One potential application is in the treatment of methicillin-resistant Staphylococcus aureus (MRSA), an increasingly prevalent concern in hospitals. A screening of allicin against 30 strains of MRSA found high level of antimicrobial activity, including against strains that are resistant to other chemical agents. Of the strains tested, 88% had minimum inhibitory concentrations for allicin liquids of 16 mg/L, and all strains were inhibited at 32 mg/L. Furthermore, 88% of clinical isolates had minimum bactericidal concentrations of 128 mg/L, and all were killed at 256 mg/L. Of these strains, 82% showed intermediate or full resistance to mupirocin. This same study examined use of an aqueous cream of allicin, and found it somewhat less effective than allicin liquid. At 500 mg/L, however, the cream was still active against all the organisms tested—which compares well with the 20 g/L mupirocin currently used for topical application.

A water-based formulation of purified allicin was found to be more chemically stable than other preparations of garlic extracts. They proposed that the stability may be due to the hydrogen bonding of water to the reactive oxygen atom in allicin and also to the absence of other components in crushed garlic that destabilize the molecule.

Allicin has in few cases and research studies demonstrated antiviral properties. A small (146 healthy adults) double-blind, placebo-controlled study found that a daily supplement containing purified allicin, had dramatic results by reducing the risk of catching a cold by 64%, the symptom duration was reduced by 70% and those in the treatment group were much less likely to develop more than 1 cold. In contrast to these claims concerning the cold-preventing properties of garlic (or its active ingredient, allicin), a 2012 report in the Cochrane Database of Systematic Reviews concludes that "there is insufficient clinical trial evidence regarding the effects of garlic in preventing or treating the common cold. A single trial suggested that garlic may prevent occurrences of the common cold but more studies are needed to validate this finding. Claims of effectiveness appear to rely largely on poor-quality evidence. Similar concerns are voiced in a 2013 report, which states "Garlic as a preventative or treatment option for the common cold could not be recommended, as only one relatively small trial evaluated the effects separately.

2. Indole-3-carbinol

Indole-3-Carbinol, also known as I3C, is found in cruciferous vegetables such as collards, mustard greens, turnips, cabbage, broccoli, kale, cabbage, cauliflower and Brussels sprouts. Cruciferous vegetables are recognized as being one of world's healthiest food sources, providing multiple nutrients and anti-cancer properties. Research has shown that Indole-3-Carbinol supports a hormonal balance as it prevents cellular damage thus also benefiting the body's immune system. Indole-3-Carbinol is produced by the breakdown of glucosinolate glucobrassicin (found in cruciferous vegetables) and is then transformed to diindolylmethane in the stomach. The substance that is found in the bloodstream after ingestion is not Indole-3-Carbinol, but is actually diindolymethane. Trials are being conducted to determine the authenticity of consuming Indole-3-Carbinol supplements to prevent illnesses, particularly cancer. Although it does not provide an active cure to cancer, Indole-3-Carbinol is scientifically proven to support the health of reproductive organs and cellular reproduction for both men and women. It also assists in detoxifying the intestines and liver. As an antioxidant, it stimulates the production of enzymes that detoxify toxins and protects cell structures including DNA.

Indole-3-carbinol is the subject of on-going Biomedical research into its possible anticarcinogenic, antioxidant, and anti-atherogenic effects. Research on indole-3-carbinol has been conducted primarily using laboratory animals and cultured cells. Limited and inconclusive human studies have been reported. A recent review of the biomedical research literature found that "evidence of an inverse association between cruciferous vegetable intake and breast or prostate cancer in humans is limited and inconsistent" and "larger randomized controlled trials are needed" to determine if supplemental indole-3-carbinol has health benefits.

Investigation of mechanisms by which consumption of indole-3-carbinol might influence cancer incidence focuses on its ability to alter estrogen metabolism and other cellular effects. Controlled studies have been performed on such animals as rats, mice, and rainbow trout, introducing various controlled levels of carcinogens, and levels of Indole-3-carbinol into their daily diet. Results showed dose-related decreases in tumor susceptibility due to Indole-3-carbinol (inferred by decreases in aflatoxin-DNA binding). The first direct evidence of pure anti-initiating activity by a natural anticarcinogen (indole-3-carbinol) found in human diet. Indole-3-Carbinol was found to impede estrogen receptors in breast membranes, reducing the risk of breast cancer. There is a repair protein known as BRCA (Breast Cancer Type 1 Suceptibility Protein) that prevents damaged genetic DNA being passed to the next generation. These proteins are coded by the BRCA genes which are also called as the caretaker gene as the protein coded by this gene is responsible for repairing the damaged DNA in the breast cells and other tissues in the body. If the DNA is not in a repairable condition BRCA destroys the cell thereby preventing any risks of cancer. Faulty BRCA genes increase the risk of developing cancers. As low amounts of BRCA are seen in cancer cells, it is suggested that higher levels of BRCA will prevent further growth. It is proposed that Indole-3-Carbinol assists in boosting this repair protein.

In 2006, Hsu et al. proved that indole-3-carbinol induces a G1 growth arrest of human reproductive cancer cells. This is significant in the prevention and treatment of cancer, as the G1 phase of cell growth occurs early in the cell lifecycle, and, for most cells, is the major period of cell cycle during its lifespan. The G1 phase is marked by synthesis of various enzymes that are required in the next ("S") phase, including those needed for DNA replication.

Indole-3-carbinol can shift estrogen metabolism towards less estrogenic metabolites. SLE (or Systemic lupus erythematosus), a currently incurable autoimmune disease, is associated with estrogen. In a study using mice bred to develop lupus, I3C was fed to one group while another group was fed a standard mouse diet; the group fed the I3C diet lived longer and had fewer signs of disease. Women with lupus can manifest a metabolic response to I3C and might also benefit from its antiestrogenic effects. Clinical trials are currently underway to determine the efficacy of treating human patients suffering from lupus with I3C.

Another study of lupus prone mice with I3C defined the mechanism for the improvement of their disease to be due to sequential blocks in the development of B and T cells of these mice. The maturation arrests resulted in a fall in autoantibody production, thought to be a crucial component of lupus causation. In addition, I3C supplementation of the disease prone mice led to a normalization of their T cell function.

Research studies have provided evidence suggesting that indole-3-carbinol has an effect on human papilloma virus infected cells in both pediatrics and adult patients.

3. Isothiocyanates

Isothiocyanates are abundant in cruciferous vegetables such as broccoli, watercress, Brussels sprouts, cabbage, Japanese radish and cauliflower. Vegetables of the Cruciferae family are in the botanical order Capparales, which includes the *Brassicas* genus (common crops like rape, black and brown mustard, and root crops such as turnips and rutabagas, kale, kohlrabi etc). Cruciferous vegetables have been widely accepted as potential diet components that may reduce the risk of cancer. The chemopreventative effect of cruciferous vegetables is thought to be partially due to their relatively high content of glucosinolates (β-thioglucoside N-hydroxysulfates) which degrades enzymatically by the action of myrosinase to form isothiocyanates.

Over 100 different glucosinolates have been identified, and they are classified into 4 groups: saturated aliphatic, unsaturated aliphatic, aromatic and indolyl. The identities and amount of glucosinolate in plants vary with species, variety and growing conditions. In *Brassica* vegetables, there are typically 0.5–28 µmol aliphatic/aromatic glucosinolates per gram dry weight and 0.7–8 µmol indolyl glucosinolates per gram dry weight. Glucosinolates are normally localized to the cytoplasm of plant tissue. Myrosinase is expressed on the external surface of the plant cell wall, so it cannot access the glucosinolates. When the tissue is ruptured by chewing, preparation for cooking, heating, or insect attack, myrosinase interacts with the released glucosinolates and hydrolysis products are formed. The myrosinase acting on the glucosinolates may also originate from other species. Most of the dietary isothiocyanate absorbed by mammals from ingested plant material is formed by the action of myrosinase originating from the gastrointestinal tract bacteria.

The capacity of organic isothiocyanates to block chemical carcinogenesis was first recognized more than 30 years ago with α-naphthyl isothiocyanate. The anticarcinogenic activities of isothiocyanates have been demonstrated in rodent models using a wide variety of chemical carcinogens, including polycyclic aromatic hydrocarbons, azo dyes, ethionine, fluorenyl acetamide and several nitrosamines. Protection is conferred to a variety of target organs including the lungs, liver, forestomach, mammary gland, esophagus, small intestine, colon and bladder.. Isothiocyanates inhibited 7,12-dimethylbenz[a]-anthracene (DMBA)-induced mammary tumor formation in female Sprague-Dawley rats when administered 4 h prior to DMBA administration. Addition of BITC to the diet containing benz(a)pyrene prevented carcinogenesis in mouse forestomach. PEITC, BITC and phenyl isothiocyanate (PITC) were tested for their abilities to inhibit lung tumorigenesis and O^6-methylguanine formation (DNA-adduct formation in the 4-(methylnitrosamino)-1-(3-pyridyl)-1-butanone (NNK)-induced tumors) in the DNA of lung cells from A/J mice treated with NNK. PEITC also inhibited N-nitrosomethylbenzylamine (NMBA)-induced esophageal tumorigenesis and DNA methylation in rats.

The length of the alkyl chain of the phenylalkyl moiety of isothiocyanate affected the inhibitory potency: the inhibition of tumorigenesis increased as the alkyl chain was increased from 1 to 6 methylene groups. Phenylhexyl isothiocyanate (PHITC) was approximately 50 100 times more potent than PEITC. At longer alkyl chain lengths (C_8–C_{10}), the inhibitory potency declined.

Mechanism of anticarcinogenic activity

Depression of activation of carcinogens

Cytochrome P-450 (CYP) enzymes (phase I enzymes) are important for normal metabolic processing of numerous endogenous and exogenous compounds, but they may also activate certain carcinogens. Isothiocyanates are direct and very potent inhibitors (both competitively and irreversibly, depending on conditions) of members of the cytochrome P-450 family. In a detailed correlative comparison of the arylalkyl isothiocyanates and some alkyl isothiocyanates, Jiao and co-workers found that:

(a) increased alkyl chain length (Ph-$[CH_2]_n$-NCS, n=0–6, 8, 10) enhanced the inhibitory activity of arylalkyl isothiocyanates against NNK lung tumorigenesis;

(b) the phenyl moiety was not essential for the inhibitory activity, because long-chain alkyl isothiocyanates (eg CH_3-$[CH_2]_{11}$-NCS) also exhibited strong inhibitory effects in the same model. The ability of isothiocyanate to inhibit or enhance tumorigenesis depended on the structure of the isothiocyanates, the animal species, target tissue, and the specific carcinogen employed.

Acceleration of carcinogen disposal

The phase 2 enzymes are a diverse family of enzymes that metabolize a variety of reactive carcinogens, mutagens, and other toxins. The phase II genes that are induced contain antioxidant (or electrophile) response elements (AREs) in their promoters and include genes encoding NAD(P)H: quinone oxidoreductase (NQO1), GSTs, uridine 5-diphosphate-glucuronosyl transferase (UGT), epoxide hydrolase, ferritin, γ-glutamate-cysteine ligase, and catalase.

Isothiocyanates are inducers of phase 2 enzymes. The induction of quinone reductase (QR) and GST activity in various rodent tissues is a characteristic property of isothiocyanates. Aromatic isothiocyanates, α- or β-naphthyl isothiocyanate, allyl isothiocyanate (AITC), SFN, and *exo-2-acetyl-exo-6-isothiocyanato-norbornane* were shown to be inducers of QR and GST in several bowel, colon, kidney, stomach, lung and nasal mucosa. These compounds were administered either in the diet (3–4 μmol/g of diet) for 5–28 days or by intragastric administration (5–100 μmol in single or several daily doses), and the specific activities of GST and QR in the cytosol of these organ were increased by 1.2- to 9.4-fold over those of control animals (Zhang et al., 1994). The coordinated nature of induction of phase 2 enzymes was studied in detailed in Wistar rats with BITC. BITC (0.5% (*w/w*) in the diet for 2 weeks) increased liver and small intestinal GST, QR and UDP-glucuronyl transferase activities by 1.7- to 11-fold. BITC also increased GSH levels in the esophagus and small bowel of ICR/Ha mice by 63%–75% (Talalay and Zhang. 1996). Thus, similar to many chemically unrelated inducers, administration of isothiocyanate to rodents evoked the 'electrophile counter-attack' response. Molecular studies have shown that isothiocyanates can induce phase 2 enzymes by stimulating transcription of phase II genes *via* a common antioxidant/electrophile enhancer element (ARE/EpRE) present in the upstream regions of several phase 2 enzyme genes.

Aralkyl isothiocyanates have been recently, implicated in mediating antitumor activities. These compounds have inhibitory effects on the growth of several types of cultured cancer cells, including leukemia, prostate cancer, breast cancer, lung cancer, cervical cancer, and colorectal cancer.

Mechanism of antitumor activity

The mechanism for the antitumor activity of isothiocyanates has not been fully elucidated; however, studies have implicated numerous pathways

Induction of apoptosis

The induction of apoptosis by isothiocyanates study showed that PEITC and other structurally related isothiocyanates, phenylmethyl isothiocyanate, phenylbutyl isothiocyanate, and phenylhexyl isothiocyanate, but not phenyl isothiocyanate, induced apoptosis in HeLa cells in a time- and dose-dependent manner. In addition, treatment with apoptosis-inducing concentrations of isothiocyanates caused rapid and transient induction of caspase-3/CPP32-

like activity. Furthermore, these isothiocyanates, except phenyl isothiocyanate, stimulated proteolytic cleavage of poly-(ADP-ribose) polymerase, which followed the caspase activation and preceded DNA fragmentation. Pretreatment with a potent caspase-3 inhibitor AC-DEVD-CHO inhibited isothiocyanate-induced caspase-3 activation and apoptosis. These results suggest that isothiocyanates induce apoptosis through a caspase-3-dependent mechanism.

PEITC and AITC inhibit leukemia cell growth by inducing apoptosis. Activities of caspase-3 and caspase-8 were increased during isothiocyanate-induced apoptosis, but caspase-1 activity was not. The general caspase inhibitor Z-VAD-fmk and the specific caspase-8 inhibitor Z-IETD-fmk inhibited apoptosis, but specific caspase-1 and caspase-3 inhibitors did not. This suggests that caspase-8 is critical and caspase-3 may exert a supporting role during apoptosis in leukemia cells. Apoptosis was associated with cleavage of p22 BID protein to p15, p13, and p11 fragments, activation of JNK, and tyrosine phosphorylation. This suggests that during isothiocyanate-induced human leukemia, cell apoptosis depends on the caspase pathway, and the JNK pathway may play a supporting role.

The mitochondria are involved in the apoptosis induced by isothiocyanates. PEITC induced apoptosis in HT-29 human colorectal carcinoma cells. Both caspase-3 and -9 activities were stimulated by PEITC. The release of cytochrome c from the mitochondrial inter-space was time- and dose-dependent, with a maximal release at 50 µmol/L after 10 h of treatment.

MAPK (Mitogen Activated Protein Kinase) pathway

Three MAPKs [JNK (c-Jun N-terminal kinase), extracellular signal-regulated protein kinase (ERK) and p38 kinase] were activated shortly after PEITC treatment in HT-29 cells. The JNK inhibitor SP600125, but not the ERK and p38 inhibitors, suppressed PEITC-induced apoptosis. Similarly, this JNK inhibitor attenuated both cytochrome c release and caspase-3 activation induced by PEITC, suggesting that activation of JNK is critical for the initiation of apoptosis.

In ovarian cancer OVCAR-3 cells, PEITC suppressed the activation of Akt and ERK1/2 while simultaneously activating pro-apoptotic p38 and JNK1/2. Specific inhibitors of JNK1/2 and p38 reversed the cytotoxic effect of PEITC. These findings suggest that PEITC inhibits Akt- and ERK1/2-mediated survival signaling while simultaneously activating pro-apoptotic p38 and JNK1/2 signaling.

SFN, PEITC, and AITC each potently induced AP-1 activity and caused a significant elevation in the phosphorylation of ERK1/2, JNK1/2, Elk-1, and c-Jun. Transfection with ERK2 and the upstream kinase DNEE-MEK1 activated AP-1 activity, and transfection with the dominant-negative mutant ERK2 (dnERK2) potently decreased AP-1 activation induced by SFN, PEITC and AITC. Transfection with JNK1 and upstream kinase MKK7 activated AP-1 activity, and transfection with dominant-negative mutant JNK1-APF significantly attenuated AP-1 activation induced by SFN, PEITC, and AITC. Pretreatment with the MEK1-ERK inhibitor U0126 and the JNK inhibitor SP600125 substantially attenuated the decrease in cell viability induced by SFN, PEITC, and AITC. Transfection with dnERK2 and JNK1-APF significantly reversed the decrease in Bcl-2 expression elicited by these isothiocyanates. Furthermore, transfection with dnERK2 and JNK1-APF blocked the apoptosis induced by these isothiocyanates in PC-3 cells. Taken together, these results indicate that the activation of the ERK and JNK signaling pathways is important for AP-1 transcriptional activity and is involved in the regulation of cell death elicited by isothiocyanates in PC-3 cells.

Oxidative stress

Reactive oxygen species (ROS) stimulate cell proliferation and induce genetic instability, and their increased level in cancer cells is often viewed as an adverse event. Abnormal increases in ROS can be exploited to selectively kill cancer cells. Oncogenic transformation of ovarian epithelial cells with *H-Ras* or expression of *Bcr-Abl* in hematopoietic cells caused elevated ROS generation and rendered the malignant cells highly sensitive to PEITC. PEITC effectively disables the glutathione (GSH) antioxidant system and causes ROS accumulation preferentially in the transformed cells due to their active ROS output. Excessive ROS cause oxidative mitochondrial damage, cytochrome *c* release, inactivation of redox-sensitive molecules (GXP), and massive cell death.

Oxidative stress caused by isothiocyanates can be used to treat drug-resistant cancer cells. Chronic lymphocytic leukemia (CLL) is the most common adult leukemia, and resistance to fludarabine-based therapies is a major challenge in CLL treatment. Because CLL cells have elevated levels of reactive oxygen species (ROS), Trachootham *et al* tested a novel ROS-mediated strategy to eliminate fludarabine-resistant CLL cells based on this redox alteration. Using primary CLL cells and normal lymphocytes from patients and healthy individuals, they found that both fludarabine-resistant and -sensitive CLL cells were highly sensitive to PEITC, exhibiting mean IC_{50} values of 5.4 and 5.1 µmol/L, respectively. Normal lymphocytes were significantly less sensitive to PEITC (IC_{50}=27 µmol/L, $P<0.0001$). CLL cells exhibited intrinsically higher ROS levels and lower cellular GSH, which were shown to be the critical determinants of CLL sensitivity to PEITC. Exposure of CLL cells to PEITC induced severe GSH depletion, ROS accumulation, and oxidation of mitochondrial cardiolipin leading to massive cell death. Such ROS stress also caused deglutathionylation and rapid degradation of the cell survival molecule MCL1. This study demonstrated that PEITC was effective in eliminating fludarabine-resistant CLL cells through a redox-mediated mechanism with low toxicity to normal lymphocytes.

Isothiocyanates induce cellular oxidative stress by rapidly conjugating and thus depleting cells of GSH in leukemia cells (Xu and Thornalley, 2001). PEITC induced apoptosis of human leukemia HL-60 and myeloblastic leukemia ML-1 cells, which was associated with an initial decrease in GSH and GSSG (oxidized GSH) and concomitant formation of the GSH adduct *S*-(*N*-phenethylthiocarbamoyl) glutathione inside cells. This adduct was then exported from cells.

Inhibition of cell cycle progression

The induction of cell cycle arrest by isothiocyanates was first reported by Hasegawa and coworkers in 1993. The accumulation of cells at G_2/M phase was observed 16 h after treatment with 10 µmol/L AITC, 2.5 µmol/L BITC or PEITC, the concentrations at which cell growth was inhibited by 41% 79% compared with the control. These results suggest that isothiocyanates delay the cell cycle progression of HeLa cells, resulting in the inhibition of cell growth.

Isothiocyanates may induce cell cycle arrest in different phases in a cell line dependent manner. AITC arrested HL-60 cells at the G_1 phase, whereas BITC arrested the cells at both the G_1 and the G_2/M phases. When AITC induced prostate cancer PC-3 cell arrest at G_2/M phase, cyclin B1 levels were dramatically decreased, as well as cdk1, cdc25B, and cdc25C. This suggested that cyclin B1, cdk1, cdc25B, and cdc25C may be targeted by AITC. In HL-60 cells, BITC significantly up-regulated expression of G_2/M cell cycle arrest-regulating genes including p21, GADD45, and 14-3-3 sigma. A similar result was observed in human Capan-2 pancreatic cancer cells. BITC-mediated G_2/M arrest was associated with the up-regulation of p21 and the activation of checkpoint kinase 2 (Chk2), whereas the expression of other G_2/M regulatory proteins, including CyclinB1, Cdc2, and Cdc25C, was down-regulated.

Inhibition of angiogenesis

Inhibition of angiogenesis may be an important mechanism employed by PEITC to prevent cancer. PEITC treatment decreased the survival of human umbilical vein endothelial cells (HUVEC) in a concentration- and time-dependent manner. The formation of a capillary-like tube structure (*in vitro* neovascularization) by HUVECs and their migration (invasion potential) were also inhibited significantly in the presence of PEITC at pharmacologically relevant concentrations (<1 μmol/L). The PEITC-mediated inhibition of angiogenic features of HUVEC *in vitro* was associated with suppression of vascular endothelial growth factor (VEGF) secretion, down-regulation of VEGF receptor 2 protein levels, and inactivation of Akt. PEITC treatment reduced the migration of PC-3 human prostate cancer cells, which correlated with inactivation of Akt, suppression of VEGF and epidermal growth factor (EGF) expression, and granulocyte colony-stimulating factor (G-CSF) secretion. The PEITC-mediated inhibition of PC-3 cell migration was significantly attenuated by ectopic expression of constitutively active Akt. More importantly, PEITC treatment inhibited *ex vivo* angiogenesis as assessed using a chicken egg chorioallantoic membrane assay.

Inhibition of histone deacetylation

Isothiocyanates are histone deacetylase inhibitors (Dashwood and Ho, 2008). SFN was first reported to inhibit HDAC activity in human colon cancer cells. In human embryonic kidney 293 cells and human colorectal cancer HCT116 cells, SFN dose-dependently increased the activity of a beta-catenin-responsive reporter (TOPflash) without altering beta-catenin or HDAC protein levels. Cytoplasmic and nuclear extracts from these cells had diminished HDAC activity, and global and localized histone acetylation was increased in both cell lines.

PHITC inhibits the growth of human leukemia HL-60 cells *via* chromatin remodeling. PHITC reduced the expression of HDAC and increased the levels of acetyl transferase p300, in favor of accumulation of acetylated histones. The global acetylation of histones was enhanced within hours.

Regulation of translation initiation

Hu *et al* reported a novel response of PEITC at pharmacologically relevant concentrations on the regulation of translation initiation. Treatment of human colorectal cancer HCT-116 cells and human prostate cancer PC-3 cells, but not a normal prostate epithelial cell line (PrEC), with PEITC caused an increase in expression of the eukaryotic translation initiation factor 4E (eIF4E) binding protein (4E-BP1) and inhibition of 4E-BP1 phosphorylation. Results from pull-down assays indicated that PEITC treatment reduced cap-bound eIF4E, confirming that increased 4E-BP1 expression and inhibition of 4E-BP1 phosphorylation reduced the availability of eIF4E for translation initiation. Accordingly, results from *in vivo* translation experiments using a luciferase reporter assay indicated that PEITC treatment inhibited cap-dependent translation, particularly the translation of mRNA with secondary structure (stem-loop structure). Ectopic expression of eIF4E prevented PEITC-induced translation inhibition and conferred significant protection against PEITC-induced apoptosis. These results indicate that PEITC modulates the availability of eIF4E for translation initiation leading to inhibition of cap-dependent translation. This suggests that inhibition of cap-dependent translation may be an important mechanism for PEITC-induced apoptosis.

4. Sulforaphane

Sulforaphane (SFN), one of naturally occurring isothiocyanates (ITCs), has huge cancer chemopreventive potential. Sulforaphane is a molecule within the isothiocyanate group of organosulfur compounds. It exhibits anti-cancer and antimicrobial properties in experimental models. It is obtained from cruciferous vegetables such as broccoli, Brussels sprouts or cabbages. It is produced when the enzyme myrosinase transforms glucoraphanin, a glucosinolate, into sulforaphane upon damage to the plant (such as from chewing) which allows the two compounds to mix and react. Young sprouts of broccoli and cauliflower are particularly rich in glucoraphanin. Sulforaphane is an effective cancer protective substance in cell culture and carcinogen-induced and genetic animal cancer models. Early research focused on its "blocking activity" via Phase 2 enzyme induction, as well as inhibition of enzymes involved in carcinogen activation, but there has been growing interest in other mechanisms of action. Sulforaphane protects against tumor development during the "post-initiation" phase, including cell cycle arrest and apoptosis induction. Sulforaphane can stimulate cellular adaptation to redox stressors through transcription factor Nrf2. it is an indirect antioxidant that protects animal tissues from chemical or biological insults by stimulating the expression of several NF-E2-related factor-2 regulated phase 2 enzymes involved in xenobiotic transformation (such as quinone reductase and glutathione S-transferase).

SFN induced prostate cancer cell apoptosis, by activation of caspases, ERK1/2, and Akt, and increasing p53 and bax protein levels. Apoptosis induction was also observed in medulloblastoma and human pancreatic cancer cells. Recent results demonstrated the ability of SFN to induce apoptosis in glioblastoma cell lines through the activation of multiple molecular mechanisms.

The histone deacetylase inhibitory activity was also studied in other cells. SFN treatment significantly inhibited HDAC activity in four breast cancer cell lines: MDA-MB-231, MDA-MB-468, MCF-7, and T47, particularly in the ER-negative cell lines, MDA-MB-231, and MDA-MB-468 cells. Despite this significant inhibition in global HDAC activity, no significant changes were observed in the acetylation of H3 or H4 in any cell line following 48 h of exposure to 15 μmol/L sulforaphane.

Sulforaphane (SFN) has been shown to inhibit the catalytic activity of a number of Cytochrome P-450 (CYP) enzymes, including CYP1A1, 1A2, 2B1/2, 2E1, and 3A4. SFN (20 μmol/L) completely inhibited the growth of LM8 cells and caused G_2/M-phase arrest. SFN induced the expression of p21(WAF1/CIP1) protein, which caused cell cycle arrest in a dose-dependent manner. An additional study showed that SFN inhibited human lung adenocarcinoma LTEP-A2 cell growth by causing G_2/M-phase arrest .

IV. Carotenoids

1. β-Carotene

Beta-Carotene is one of 30-50 carotenoids found in plant foods that can be converted by the body into Vitamin A. Beta-Carotene is a fat-soluble compound that is absorbed intact in the presence of bile salts from the intestine. Beta-Carotene is made up of two Vitamin A molecules (attached together). Within intestinal cells they are split to yield retinol (preformed Vitamin A). Approximately one third of all the carotene in food can be converted into Vitamin A. It performs following functions in the body:

    i.   **Vitamin A Precursor** Beta-Carotene can be converted into Vitamin A, and it supports Vitamin A nutritional status and all vitamin A-related functions.

    ii.   **Antioxidant**: Beta-Carotene is an antioxidant and does not need to be converted into Vitamin A to perform antioxidant functions.

    iii. **Immune System**: Beta-Carotene appears to enhance thymus gland function and increases interferon's stimulatory action on the immune systema.

    iv. **Other Functions**: Beta-Carotene exhibits a number of immune-enhancing and anti-cancer properties, and has therefore, been tested in patients with immune-compromised states, precancerous, and cancerous conditions, as well as in patients at high risk in developing certain cancers.

Compromised Immune Function

A number of studies reveal that older subjects can enhance various aspects of immune function through the supplementation of at least 15 mg of Beta-Carotene (25,000 I.U.) per day (Santos et al., 1998; 1996). The immune system tends to weaken as humans age, thus researchers have examined various nutrients that may prevent or reverse age-related decline in immune function. High doses of Beta-Carotene have been used in the treatment of immune compromised states and studies on normal human volunteers indicate that supplementation with 180 mg (300,000 I.U.) of Beta-Carotene per day, significantly increased in the number of T-helper cells by approximately 30% after seven days of supplementation, with a 30% increase in a total T-cell count after 14 days. This may be of great significance in HIV/AIDS patients, who have low T-helper cell counts and other parameters of immune function compromise.

Beta-Carotene supplementation at 50,000 I.U., twice per day administered to AIDS patients has resulted in a 66% rise in total lymphocyte count and a small rise in T-helper cell levels. With discontinuation of Beta-Carotene supplementation, lymphocyte and T-helper cell counts returned to base line levels within six weeks. In a second study, 60 mg (100,000 I.U.) administered to seven AIDS patients resulted in a rise of T-helper cells over the four-week trial period. This is important as it is the T-helper cell (CD$) count that is adversely affected by the HIV virus and largely accounts for the dramatic reduction in immune function seen in HIV and AIDS patients. Not all Beta-Carotene studies with AIDS patients have shown these benefits, but the lack of adverse side effects with Beta-Carotene suggests that it can be used safely as a complementary therapy in these cases. Moderate dosages of Beta-Carotene supplementation may help to slow down or halt the age-related decline in immune function that increases susceptibility to infection and possibly cancer associated with aging.

Cancer Prevention

At this time it is inadvisable to give high dose Beta-Carotene supplementation (50,000 I.U. or greater) to patients who smoke one pack of cigarettes per day or more. The Alpha-Tocopherol, Beta-Carotene study and the CARET study suggested that Beta-Carotene, in these cases, may slightly increase the risk of lung cancer, although this needs confirmation. However, Beta-Carotene does demonstrate a number of anti-cancer properties and has been shown to reverse leukoplakia – a pre-cancerous condition of the oral cavity, as well as early-stage cervical dysplasia, a pre-cancerous condition of the uterine cervix. In the Linxian China study, the combination of modest dosages of Beta-Carotene, Vitamin E, and selenium significantly reduced stomach and esophageal cancers, as well as total cancer incidence in high-rish individuals, compared to other vitamin and mineral combinations. Beta-Carotene is an antioxidant, an immune system modulator and enahances cellular differentiation of epithelial cells. All of these effects are associates with the prevention of cancer and the reversal of some early stage cancers and states of dysplasia (pre-cancerous states).

Cervical dysplasia

Beta-Carotene has been shown to influence cellular differentiation of surface lining cells (epithelial cells) and enhances immune-system function. Beta-Carotene has been shown to halt the progression of cervical dysplasia and cause a reversal in some cases involving early and moderate stages of this condition, which is known to be a pre-cancerous condition.

Cardiovascular Disease

Beta-Carotene supplementation has been shown to decrease oxidation of LDL-cholesterol, but to a lesser degree than Vitamin E. In this regard, it may help to reduce the risk of cardiovascular disease, as oxidized LDL-cholesterol appears to be more inclined to narrow arteries as part of the atherosclerotic process that leads to heart disease and ischemic stroke. However, evidence is stronger for Vitamin E. Both Vitamin E and Beta-Carotene are transported through the bloodstream within VLDL and LDL lipoproteins, where they are able to act as antioxidants in regards to reducing the oxidation of fatty acids and cholesterol within these lipoproteins (VLDL and LDL). The Physicians Health Study failed, to show a benefit in cardiovascular disease reduction with Beta-Carotene supplementation of 50 mg (83,333 I.U.), taken every other day for 12 years. However, a subgroup analysis of about 22,000 subjects with prior history of heart disease, Beta-Carotene supplementation produced a small reduction in risk of fatal and non-fatal heart attack. A number of prospective studies have suggested that higher intakes of Beta-Carotene is associated with a significant reduction in heart attack and stroke, as highlighted in the Western Electric Study in Chicago.

2. **Lycopene**

Lycopene (derived from *Lycopersicum* or tomato species) is a bright red carotene and carotenoid pigment found in tomatoes and other red fruits and vegetables, such as red carrots, red bell peppers, watermelons, gac, and papayas. Lycopene is a natural pigment synthesized by plants and microorganisms but not by animals. It is a carotenoid, an acyclic isomer of -carotene, and has no vitamin A activity. Lycopene may be obtained from vegetables and fruits such as the tomato, but another source of lycopene is the fungus *Blakeslea trispora*. In plants, algae, and other photosynthetic organisms, lycopene is an important intermediate in the biosynthesis of many carotenoids, including beta carotene, responsible for yellow, orange or red pigmentation, photosynthesis, and photo-protection. Like all carotenoids, lycopene is a polyunsaturated hydrocarbon (an unsubstituted alkene). Structurally, it is a tetraterpene assembled from eight isoprene units, composed entirely of carbon and hydrogen, and is insoluble in water. Lycopene's eleven conjugated double bonds and two non conjugated double bonds give it its deep red color and are responsible for its antioxidant activity. Due to its strong color and non-toxicity, lycopene is a useful food coloring (registered as **E160d**) and is approved for usage in the USA, Australia and New Zealand (registered as **160d**) and the EU. Lycopene is not an essential nutrient for humans, but is commonly found in the diet, mainly from dishes prepared from tomatoes. When absorbed from the stomach, lycopene is transported in the blood by various lipoproteins and accumulates in the liver, adrenal glands, and testes.

As a polyene it undergoes *cis-trans* isomerization induced by light, thermal energy or chemical reactions. Lycopene from natural plant sources exists predominantly in *trans* configuration the most thermodynamically stable form. Lycopene, ingested in its natural *trans* form found in tomatoes, is poorly absorbed. Recent studies have shown that heat processing of tomatoes and tomato products induces isomerization of lycopene to the *cis* form which in turn increases its bioavailability.

It is demonstrated that serum and prostate levels of lycopene in prostate cancer patients were significantly lower than their age matched controls. They hypothesized that prostate cancer patients perhaps lack the ability to isomerize dietary lycopene and therefore do not absorb it efficiently. Because preliminary research has shown an inverse correlation between consumption of tomatoes and cancer risk, lycopene has been considered a potential agent for prevention of some types of cancers, particularly prostate cancer.

After ingestion, lycopene is incorporated into lipid micelles in the small intestine. These micelles are formed from dietary fats and bile acids, and help to solubilize the hydrophobic lycopene and allow it to permeate the intestinal mucosal cells by a passive transport mechanism. Little is known about the liver metabolism of lycopene, but like other carotenoids, lycopene is incorporated into chylomicrons and released into the lymphatic system. In blood plasma, lycopene is eventually distributed into the very low and low density lipoprotein fractions. Lycopene is mainly distributed to fatty tissues and organs such as the adrenal glands, liver, prostate and testes.

Lycopene is one of the most potent antioxidants and has been suggested to prevent carcinogenesis and atherogenesis by protecting critical biomolecules including lipids, low-density lipoproteins (LDL), proteins and DNA. Several studies have indicated that lycopene is an effective antioxidant and free radical scavenger. Lycopene, because of its high number of conjugated double bonds, exhibits higher singlet oxygen quenching ability compared to β-carotene or α-tocopherol. In *in vitro* systems, lycopene was found to inactivate hydrogen peroxide and nitrogen dioxide.

Oxidative modification of LDL is hypothesized to be the key step in the atherogenic process, and LDL associated antioxidants provide protection against this oxidation. *In vitro* lycopene and other carotenoids are able to inhibit oxidation of LDL.

Levy *et al.* showed that lycopene inhibited the growth of human endometrial, mammary and lung cancer cells grown in cultures and was more effective than α- or β-carotene. Lycopene along with vitamin D3 synergistically inhibited cell cycle progression and induced differentiation of the HL60 promyelocytic leukemia cell line. In mouse embryo fibroblast cells, lycopene enrichment upregulated gap-junction-communication by enhancing the expression of the connexin43 gene, which encodes a major gap junction protein, and thereby acted as an anticarcinogenic agent. Lycopene was also shown to protect against microcystinCR-induced mouse hepatocarcinoma by suppressing the phosphorylation of regulatory proteins and arresting cells in the G0/G1 phase of the cell cycle. Preliminary *in vitro* evidence indicates that lycopene reduces cellular proliferation induced by IGF-1 in various cancer cell lines. In a recent investigation, lycopene, together with α-tocopherol at physiological concentrations, synergistically inhibited cell proliferation of an androgen insensitive prostate carcinoma cell line. In the J774A.1 macrophage cell line, lycopene was shown to act as a hypocholesterolemic agent by inhibiting the HMG-CoA reductase pathway.

Lycopene may play an important protective role in several human cancers. Animal models have been used to measure lycopene's absorption and tissue distribution. It is recently demonstrated that 10 ppm dietary lycopene in rat diet was absorbed and distributed to various tissues. Liver, spleen and prostate showed the highest levels of lycopene, whereas brain had the lowest level. The varying levels of lycopene in different tissues suggest its selective uptake involving tissue-specific mechanism(s). Use of animal models to investigate *in vivo* biochemical functions of lycopene has allowed undertaking studies under well-defined, controlled environmental conditions where the confounding variables are minimum. Although several animal models of experimental cancer are available, very little is known about the absorption, metabolism and distribution of dietary lycopene and the possible mechanism of its effects on carcinogenesis.

Chronic dietary intake of lycopene markedly delayed the onset and reduced growth and development of spontaneous mammary tumors in a mouse strain with high incidence. This effect was associated with reduced activity of mammary gland thymidylate synthetase and lowered levels of serum free fatty acids and prolactin, a hormone known to be involved in breast cancer development that stimulates cell division. Lycopene was also shown to enhance the immune response by increasing helper T cells and normalizing intrathymic T cell differentiation caused by tumorigenesis in mice. Lycopene in small doses reduced the N-methylnitrosourea (MNU)-induced development of aberrant crypt foci (ACF) in the colon of Sprague-Dawley rats. In a dimethylbenzanthracene (DMBA)-induced mammary tumor model of rats, intraperitoneal injections of lycopene-enriched tomato oleoresin, but not of β-carotene, suppressed tumor growth as quantified by size and tumor numbers.

Diethylnitrosamine (DEN)-induced liver preneoplastic foci in rats were significantly reduced by dietary lycopene and not by any other carotenoid tested. It was hypothesized that lycopene provided protection through its modulating effect on the liver enzymes activating diethylnitrosamine, cytochrome P-450 2E1, and not through an antioxidative mechanism. Ingestion of tomato juice inhibited the development of N-butyl-N-(4-hydroxybutyl)nitrosamine (BBN)-induced development of urinary bladder transitional cell carcinomas in male Fischer 344 rats. Dietary lycopene dissolved in drinking water at a 50 ppm dose significantly decreased diethylnitrosamine (DEH)-, methylnitrosourea (MNU)- and dimethylhydrazine (DMD)-induced lung adenomas along with carcinomas in male mice.

Dietary intake of tomatoes and tomato products has been found to be associated with a lower risk of a variety of cancers in a number of epidemiological studies. In a prospective cohort study investigated the frequency of intake of different types of vegetables and cancer deaths in 1271 elderly persons from Massachusetts. High intake of tomatoes was linked to a 50% reduction in mortality from cancers at all sites. Carrots and other carotenoid-rich vegetables had no effect. High intake of tomatoes was consistently associated with reduced risk of digestive tract (especially stomach, colon and rectal) cancers in a case control study from Italy, where cases were patients with histologically confirmed cancers of oral cavity, pharynx, esophagus, stomach, colon and rectum and controls were patients with unrelated conditions.

A 2004 review that analyzed 21 observational studies (that is, not clinical trials) concluded that tomato products appear to have a weak protective effect against prostate cancer. This review did not include lycopene supplements, only tomato and tomato-based foods. Some of the individual studies, however, did consider lycopene levels in the blood. The analysis noted that the protective effect was slightly stronger for cooked tomato products and that small amount of added fat improved lycopene absorption. On the other hand, 2 studies from 2007, one of about 1,500 men and the second of more than 28,000 men, found no difference in blood lycopene levels between those in whom prostate cancer later developed and those in whom it did not. Such mixed results sometimes happen when there is no effect or only a small effect from the substance being looked at. Although there is compelling epidemiological evidence in support of the role of lycopene in cancer and heart disease prevention, it only provides suggestive evidence rather than experimental proof.

v. **Flavonoids**

1. **Epigallocatechin-3-gallate (EGCG)**

EGCG is the most abundant catechin in tea and is a potent antioxidant that may have therapeutic applications in the treatment of many disorders (e.g. cancer). It is found in green tea, but not black tea; during black tea production, the catechins are converted to theaflavins and thearubigins. Chemically it is a ester of epigallocatechin and gallic acid. An ever increasing number of preclinical investigations suggest that EGCG has the potential to confront many human diseases. Studies have shown that EGCG functions as a powerful antioxidant, preventing oxidative damage in healthy cells, an antiangiogenic and antitumor agent and as a modulator of tumor cell response to chemotherapy. Much of the cancer chemopreventive properties of green tea are mediated by EGCG that induces apoptosis and promotes cell growth arrest by altering the expression of cell cycle regulatory proteins, activating killer caspases, and suppressing oncogenic transcription factors and pluripotency maintainence factors. In vitro studies have demonstrated that EGCG blocks carcinogenesis by affecting a wide array of signal transduction pathways including JAK/STAT, MAPK, PI3K/AKT, Wnt and Notch. EGCG stimulates telomere fragmentation through inhibiting telomerase activity. Various clinical studies have revealed that treatment by EGCG inhibits tumor incidence and multiplicity in different organ sites such as liver, stomach, skin, lung, mammary gland and colon. Recent work demonstrated that EGCG reduced DNMTs, proteases, and DHFR activities, which would affect transcription of TSGs and protein synthesis. EGCG has great potential in cancer prevention because of its safety, low cost and bioavailability.

EGCG has been the subject of a number of studies investigating its potential use as a therapeutic for a broad range of disorders in addition to cancer. These include treatments for weight loss, obesity, hepatic steatosis (non alcoholic fatty liver disease), diabetes, metabolic syndrome (pathological condition related to obesity and insulin resistence) and many others. In 2005, it was reported that treatment with TEAVIGO, a green tea extract containing 94% EGCG and 0.1% caffeine, significantly reduced body weight (BW) and body fat in different strains of mice fed a high-fat diet. In addition to its weight loss effects, there are studies that have suggested that tea consumption may alleviate other metabolic abnormalities related to obesity. Several clinical investigations showed that tea treatment reduced fasting blood glucose and improved glucose tolerance in healthy and diabetic subjects. A recent clinical trial reported that when healthy subjects were given an extract of green, black, and mulberry tea concurrently with a high-starch and -lipid meal, carbohydrate absorption was significantly blunted.

There are several studies describing the beneficial effects of tea constituents in animal models of the metabolic syndrome. One study reported that oral administration of EGCG for 3 wk significantly reduced blood pressure and increased insulin sensitivity in spontaneously hypertensive rats. Green tea consumption has been shown to be inversely correlated with liver damage (a consequence of progressive hepatic steatosis) and with markers of inflammation in humans.

The effect of EGCG on improvement of glucose homeostasis is well established. Previous studies showed that green tea supplementation increased muscle glucose transporter protein expression in insulin-resistant rats (Wu et al., 2004). A study found that EGCG treatment (1.5 g/kg diet) for 7 d significantly decreased the expression of the gluconeogenic enzymes phosphoenolpyruvate carboxykinase and glucose-6-phosphatase in the livers of mice. Studies have also shown decreased expression of phosphoenolpyruvate carboxykinase and glucose-6-phosphatase by EGCG in rat hepatoma cells. These studies suggest that green tea and EGCG improve insulin sensitivity and glucose homeostasis, in part by directly increasing glucose disposal into the muscle and decreasing gluconeogenesis in the liver.

EGCG is a natural chelator and has been shown to reduce iron-accumulation in instances of neurodegenerative diseases like dementia, Alzheimer's, and Parkinson's.

2. Quercetin

Quercetin (Qu) is a well known phytochemical belonging to the flavonoid group. It is found in many fresh fruits and vegetables such as apples, onions (especially red onions), and green tea. It is also available in red grapes, citrus fruit, tomato, broccoli, leafy greens, cherries, raspberries, cranberries, and many other fruits and vegetables. Quercetin is considered an excellent free-radical scavenging antioxidant, even if such an activity strongly depends on the intracellular availability of reduced glutathione. Apart from antioxidant activity, quercetin also exerts a direct, pro-apoptotic effect in tumor cells, and can indeed block the growth of several human cancer cell lines at different phases of the cell cycle. Both these effects have been documented in a wide variety of cellular models as well as in animal models. The high toxicity exerted by quercetin on cancer cells perfectly matches with the almost total absence of any damages for normal, non-transformed cells.

Quercetin obtained from plant source is in the form of quercetin-glucose conjugates (quercetin glucosides), which are absorbed in the apical membrane of the enterocytes. Once absorbed, quercetin glucosides are hydrolyzed to generate quercetin aglycone which is further metabolized to the methylated, sulfonylated and glucuronidated forms by the enterocytic transferases. Quercetin metabolites are then transported first to the intestinal lumen, and then to the liver, where other conjugation reactions take place to form quercetin-3-glucuronide and Qu-3_-sulfate, which are the major Qu-derived circulating compounds in human plasma. It is now established that quercetin absorption in our body is more efficient in conjugated form.

Qu is considered an excellent freeradical scavenging antioxidant owing to the high number of hydroxyl groups and conjugated π orbitals by which Qu can donate electrons or hydrogen, and scavenge H_2O_2 and superoxide anion ($\bullet O_2 -$)(Heijnen et al., 2001). The reaction of Qu with $\bullet O_2$ – leads to the generation of the semiquinone radical and H_2O_2. Qu also reacts with H_2O_2 in the presence of peroxidases, and thus it decreases H_2O_2 levels and protects cells against H_2O_2 damage; nevertheless, during the same process potentially harmful reactive oxidation products are also formed. The antioxidant capability of Qu strongly depends on the intracellular availability of GSH, since, in Qu-treated cells, alterations typical of apoptosis appear when intracellular GSH is completely depleted. Indeed, in different cellular models low concentrations of Qu induce cell proliferation and increase the antioxidant capacity of the cells, whereas higher concentrations of Qu decrease antioxidant capacity and thiol content, ultimately causing cell death.

The cancer-preventive effects of quercetin have been attributed to various mechanisms, including the induction of cellcycle arrest and/or apoptosis as well as the antioxidant functions. The various means by which quercetin may act in preventing cancer are as follows:

Cell Cycle as a Possible Target

Apart from scavenging ROS, another important effect of Qu is to regulate cell cycle bymodulating severalmolecular targets, including p21, cyclin B, p27, cyclin-dependent kinases and topoisomerase II, even if the mechanisms involved have not been elucidated yet. Depending on the cell type and tumor origin, Qu is able to block the cell cycle at G2/M or at the G1/S transition.

In particular, Qu causes G2/M arrest in human esophageal squamous cell carcinoma cell line through up-regulation of p73 and p21waf1 and subsequent down-regulation of cyclin B1, both at the mRNA and protein levels. In human breast carcinoma cell lines such as SKBr3, MDA-MB-453 andMDA-MB-231 cells, low doses of Qu inhibit proliferation. Cell-cycle arrest occurs at the G1 phase through the induction of p21 and through the concomitant decrease of phosphorylation of the retinoblastoma protein (pRb). In the same cell model, Qu downregulates the cyclin B1 and cyclin-dependent kinase (CDK) 1, which are essential in the progression to the G2/M phases of the cell cycle. Similarly, in the human lung cancer cells NCI-H209, Qu glucuronides induce cell-cycle arrest at G2/M phase by increasing the expressions of proteins such as cyclin B, Cdc25c-ser-216-p and Wee1. A similar antiproliferative effect has also been observed both for highly or moderately aggressive prostate cancer cell lines, whereas no effect has been found for poorly aggressive prostate cancer cells. In HepG2 human hepatoma cells, Qu blocks cell-cycle progression at the G1 phase, and exerts this effect through the increase of p21 and p27 and p53. Similar effects on the cell cycle have also been reported in SW872 cells.

Topoisomerase II (TopoII) is another potential and delicate target of Qu. Of note, the ability of Qu to directly poison TopoII through the stabilization of double strand breaks in the TopoII-DNA cleavage complexes could account for genetic rearrangements leading primary hematopoietic progenitor cells to develop mixed-lineage leukemia.

Direct Pro-Apoptotic Effects of Qu.

Collectively, the proapoptotic effects of Qu may result from multiple pathways. First, in MDA-MB-231 cells, Qu treatment increases cytosolic Ca2+ levels and reduces the mitochondrial membrane potential (MMP), thus promoting activation of caspase-3, -8 and -9. The capability of Qu to induce apoptosis via mitochondrial pathway has been confirmed in U937 cell line. In these cells, Qu disrupts MMP, which in turn provokes the release of cytochrome c in the cytoplasm, and subsequently activates multiple caspases, such as caspase-3 and -7. Second, Qu inhibits cell growth and apoptosis by down-regulating the transcriptional activity of β-catenin/Tcf signaling, with the consequent down-regulation of cyclin D1 and surviving. The Qu-induced regulation of apoptosis through the modulation of survivin has been demonstrated to have a controversial fashion in glioma cells as well as in lung carcinoma cell lines. Thus, while in glioma cells Qu exposure results in proteasomal degradation of surviving (Siegelin & Reuss., 2009), according to another proposed model, Qu treatment raises cyclin B1 and p53 proteins that, in turn, increase survivin and p21 protein expression, thereby inhibiting apoptosis. Third, Qu likely triggers apoptosis through the generation of ROS and the subsequent activation of AMPKα1 and ASK1 which is, in turn, accompanied by p38 activation and recruitment of caspases. Fourth, the antiproliferative and pro-apoptotic effects could be related to the capability of Qu to directly bind tubulin, provoking the depolymerization of cellular microtubules. Fifth, Qu is a potent enhancer of TNF-related apoptosis-inducing ligand (TRAIL)-induced apoptosis, through the induction of the expression of death receptor (DR)-5, a phenomenon that specifically occurs in prostate cancer cells. The up-regulation of DR5, together with the down-regulation of c-FLIP (which is an inhibitor of caspase-8), are two mechanisms involved in Qu-induced recovery of TRAIL sensitivity, at least in hepatocellular carcinoma cells. It is important to note that, the enhancement of TRAIL-induced apoptosis by Qu also occurs through the inhibition of the expression of survivin in the ERK-MSK1 signal pathway.

Thus, the capability of Qu to induce apoptosis in cancer cells (via both the intrinsic and extrinsic pathways) undoubtedly renders this molecule an interesting tool in the oncology field.

Qu Influences p53 Activity.

Several studies have investigated the role of p53 in the antiproliferative and proapoptotic action of Qu on tumor cell lines. In HepG2 cells, Qu causes cell-cycle arrest and apoptosis by inducing p53 phosphorylation and by stabilizing p53 both at the mRNA and protein level. In HCT116 colon carcinoma cells, p53 contributes to Qu-mediated higher expression of NAG- 1, which in turn triggers apoptosis. It is interesting to note that the presence of p53 limits the effect of Qu, since when p53 is inhibited, cells become more sensitive to Qurelated cytotoxicity and Qu-related apoptosis. p53 elevates the p21 level, which may attenuate the proapoptotic effects of Qu in p53-wild-type tumor cells. The H1299 lung carcinoma cell line, which is a p53-null cell line, is more susceptible to Qu-induced cytotoxicity than the A549 lung carcinoma cell line, which expresses a wild-type form of p53. In A549 cells, Qu-induced cytotoxicity and apoptosis are augmented when an inhibitor of p53 or an antisense oligonucleotide targeting p53 is used.

3. Curcumin

Curcumin (diferuloylmethane), the yellow pigment in Indian saffron (Curcuma longa; also called turmeric, haldi, or haridara in the East and curry powder in the West), has been consumed by people for centuries as a dietary component and for a variety of proinflammatory ailments. Turmeric is a spice derived from the rhizomes of Curcuma longa, which is a member of the ginger family (Zingiberaceae). Rhizomes are horizontal underground stems that send out shoots as well as roots. The bright yellow color of turmeric comes mainly from fat-soluble, polyphenolic pigments known as curcuminoids. Other curcuminoids found in turmeric include demethoxycurcumin and bisdemethoxycurcumin. Curcumin was first isolated in 1815, obtained in crystalline form in 1870, and ultimately identified as 1,6-heptadiene-3,5-dione-1,7-bis(4-hydroxy-3-methoxyphenyl)-(1E,6E) or diferuloylmethane (Aggarwal et al.,2007). In 1910, the feruloylmethane skeleton of curcumin was confirmed and synthesized by Lampe. Several studies have substantiated the potential prophylactic or therapeutic value of curcumin and have unequivocally supported reports of its anti-inflammatory, antioxidant, anticarcinogenic, hepatoprotective, thrombosuppressive, cardioprotective, antiarthritic, and anti-infectious.

Curcumin's ability to influence a diverse range of molecular targets within cells has attracted the researchers over the globe towards exploring the chemopreventive and therapeutic uses of curcumin for treating several diseases and particularly cancer. Evidence suggests that curcumin suppresses all 3 stages of carcinogenesis: initiation, promotion, and progression. Several genetic targets may mediate cancer related efficacy of curcumin, but inhibition of nuclear factor kappa B (NF-κB) and subsequent downregulation of various NF-κB-related proinflammatory pathways are very likely the primary features accounting for its efficacy.

Curcumin's anti-inflammatory action

Inflammation is caused when the immune system responds to tissue damage with a complex series of actions and reactions. When the body fights infection and initiates healing, some inflammation occurs. If this inflammation becomes chronic, then the person may fall prey to a myriad of degenerative diseases like arthritis and arteriosclerosis. Curcumin works to inhibit the activity and synthesis of the enzymes implicated in inflammation, such as, cyclooxygenase-2 and 5-lipooxygenase. Its anti-inflammatory action may also be attributed to inhibition of pro-inflammatory leukotrienes, postraglandins and arachidonic acid, as well as to its neutrophil function during inflammatory states. Along with the curcuminoids, the volatile oils present in turmeric are also responsible for the anti-inflammatory activity. One of the constituents of turmeric, ar-tumerone, has been shown to arrest the growth and cytotoxic activity of human lymphocytes.

Curcumin behaves in a manner similar to aspirin, without causing vascular thrombosis. Curcumin has been compared in potency to steroidal drugs and some nonsterodial drugs as well, again without the dangerous side effects. Clinical trials show that at dosages of 400 mg per day to 1200 mg per day, curcumin is comparable to the drug phenylbutazone.

Curcumin's anti-oxidant action

Chemicals, tissue injury, infections, and auto-immune processes are all sources of free radicals which have the potential to cause damage to our body. This is where antioxidants enter the scene to provide protection from free radical-induced damage. Curcumin and other extracts of turmeric act as free radical scavengers and make for effective antioxidants. In addition, they inhibit oxidative DNA damage and relieve oxidative stress. Curcumin is a great antioxidant since it is able to regulate the formation of nitric oxide which plays a key role in inflammation and is carcinogenic. Curcumin's potency is are comparable to vitamins C and E. Curcumin was shown to be eight times more potent than vitamin E in lipid peroxidation, and three times more powerful than vitamin C in neutralizing free radicals.

Curcumin's anti-microbial properties

In India, turmeric was, and in some parts of the country still is, applied to cuts and wounds to heal them, evincing its antimicrobial properties. Laboratory studies have confirmed this traditional use of turmeric. Curcumin inhibits the growth of a variety of bacteria, parasites and pathogenic fungi. It also reduces the lesions caused by intestinal parasites, dermatophytes, and fungi. In addition to these basic functions, Curcumin also acts as a choleretic, that is, a substance that increases the volume of bile and amounts of solids secreted from the liver. More than 700 genes have been shown to be modulated by curcumin. Curcumin works well against many different kinds of cancer such as prostate cancer, colon cancer, lung cancer and breast cancer. Its anti-tumor activity appears to be due to its interactions with arachidonate metabolism and its anti-angiogenic properties.

Curcumin's Anticancer properties

Curcumin's antioxidant properties help reduce swelling and inflammation. Studies show that not only does Curcumin slow the spread of cancer (metastasis) and inhibit angiogenesis (the growth of new tumor blood vessels); it also causes cancer cells to die. Its efficacy in fighting cancer stems from the induction of detoxifying enzymes. Curcumin can suppress the initiation, promotion and spread of tumours. When angiogenesis is inhibited, the tumours are unable to nourish themselves and thus, unable to spread. Curcumin is an effective kinase-inhibitor. It keeps the "grow" signals from reaching the cancerous cell. In cell culture studies, Curcumin has been found to inhibit the activity of several matrix metalloproteinases that help cancerous cells to invade normal tissue.

Defective regulation of the cell-cycle may often result in the propogation of mutations. This aids the spread of cancer. Curcumin stops the cell-cycle and kills the cancer cells (aptosis) by its inhibitory effects on several cell-signalling pathways. There is reason to believe that Curcumin may aid chemotherapy too. In one study, the positive effects of the chemotherapy drug, paclitaxel, were enhanced and its side effects became less severe. These effects have been seen in melanoma, lymphoma and other cancers as well. Research is still in the preliminary stages and the effects of Curcumin treatment vary considerably. Results are dependent on the time of administration, the bioavailability of substance, the dose and the organ that cancer has chosen to target.

Lung cancer

Lung cancer is the leading cause of death all over the world and cigarettes are the major cause of lung cancer. Nicotine is the chemical in cigarettes that is implicated in causing cancer. Experiments on Curcumin and Nicotine showed that Curcumin halved the effects of Nicotine as a carcinogen. Research shows that Curcumin may exhibit organ-specific effects to enhance the formation of reactive oxygen species in the damaged lungs of smokers and ex-smokers. Curcumin specifically showed significant potential in the reducing the chances of lung cancer and colon cancer. Consumption of Curcumin also keeps breast cancer from reaching the lungs.

Prostate cancer

Prostate cancer, sadly, is becoming increasingly common in many countries. Curcumin appears to slow or prevent the growth of this form of cancer. In a study of prostate cancer cells, Curcumin inhibited cell growth which led the researchers to conclude that Curcumin may prove to be an important alternative to traditional prostate cancer treatment in men. It has been observed that Curcumin decelerates the rate of resistance of hormone-responsive prostate cancer cells to hormonal therapy.

Breast cancer

Curcumin has shown much potential as a treatment for breast cancer. Chinese investigations on human breast carcinoma have revealed that Curcumin exerts multiple suppressive effects on the cancer cells. Several breast tumor cell lines, including hormone-dependent, hormone-independent and drug-resistant lines, respond to the anti-proliferative effects of Curcumin. Importantly, Curcumin can interfere with commonly found pesticides, like DDT and Dioxin, which mimic estrogen. Like estrogen, estrogen-mimicking chemicals promote the growth of breast cancer. Curcumin has the power to block the cells from estrogen mimickers. In a study on human breast cancer cells, Curcumin reversed growth caused by 17b-estradiol by 98%. DDT's growth-enhancing effects on breast cancer were blocked about 75% by Curcumin. Two other estrogen mimickers, chlordane and endosulfane were tested for their ability to enhance breast cancer. Curcumin can reverse the growth caused by these chemicals by about 90%. Adding genistein to the equation causes a complete growth arrest.

Colorectal cancer

Colorectal cancer is one of the leading causes of all cancer deaths in the Western world. Naturally occurring COX-2 inhibitors such as Curcumin have been proven to be effective chemopreventive agents against colon carcinogenesis with minimal gastrointestinal toxicity. The results of phase I clinical trials in colorectal cancer patients suggest that oral supplements of Curcumin can induce biologically active levels of Curcumin in the gastrointestinal tract. Such trials provide support for further clinical evaluation in people at risk for gastrointestinal cancers. Treatment with Curcumin is easy to administer and has negligible side effects. Japanese researchers have hailed Curcumin as a wide-spectrum anticancer agent. Though a lot of the studies have been carried out on animals or in vitro, research on human subjects is underway and the results have been promising.

Antidiabetic effect of Curcumin

Curcumin is well known for its anti diabetic properties. Glucokinase enzyme plays a key role in the conversion of glucose into glycogen which is the body's primary carbohydrate store. This prevents the rise of blood sugar after a meal. After eating Curcumin, a rise in the activity of glucokinase enzyme was noted in the livers of the diabetic mice as compared to the control group which was not given any supplement. No effects on blood glucose, plasma insulin, and glucose regulating enzyme activities were reported in the non-diabetic animals. The results of the study showed that Curcumin acted as a glucose-lowering agent and antioxidant in the mice suffering from type II diabetes, while having no effect on the non-diabetic mice. Curcumin prevents galactose-induced cataract formation at very low doses. Both turmeric and curcumin decrease blood sugar level in alloxan-induced diabetes in rat. Curcumin also decreases advanced glycation end productsinduced complications in diabetes mellitus.

VI. Phenolic Acids

Phenolic acids are aromatic secondary plant metabolites, widely spread throughout the plant kingdom. The name "phenolic acids", in general, describes phenols that possess one carboxylic acid functionality. However, when describing plant metabolites, it refers to a distinct group of organic acids These naturally occurring phenolic acids contain two distinguishing constitutive carbon frameworks: the hydroxycinnamic (**Xa**) and hydroxybenzoic (**Xb**) structures. Although the basic skeleton remains the same, the numbers and positions of the hydroxyl groups on the aromatic ring create the variety. Many of the phenolic acid members have been known for their health benefits. These include gallic acid (belonging to hydroxybenzoic acid group), ellagic acid and capsaicin (phenolic amide)

Phenolic acids have been associated with color, sensory qualities, and nutritional and antioxidant properties of foods. They play a very important role in the organoleptic properties (flavor, astringency, and hardness) of foods.

Phenolics behave as antioxidants, due to the reactivity of the phenol moiety (hydroxyl substituent on the aromatic ring). Although there are several mechanisms, the predominant mode of antioxidant activity is believed to be *radical scavenging* via hydrogen atom donation. Other established antioxidant, radical quenching mechanisms are through electron donation and singlet oxygen quenching (Shahidi, 1992). Substituents on the aromatic ring affect the stabilization and therefore affect the radical-quenching ability of these phenolic acids. Different acids therefore have different antioxidant activity.

VII. Stilbenes

The most impotant stilbenes having proven chemopreventive capability is reservatol. Chemically it is called as 3,4',5-trihydroxy-*trans*stilbene and is found in red grapes (*Vitis viiefera*) in significant amounts. Numerous intracellular pathways triggered by resveratrol converge with the activation of NF-kB and AP1. More in details, resveratrol inhibited PMA-induced *COX2* expression and catalytic activity, via the cyclic AMP response element (CRE), in human mammary epithelial cells. Resveratrol also induced apoptosis and reduced the constitutive activation of NF-kB in both rat and human cell lines. The molecule was also apoptogenic in mouse JB6 epidermal cells where it caused p53 phosphorylation mediated by ERK. Resveratrol also inhibited the TNF-induced activation of MEK and JNK and abrogated TNF-induced caspase activation. Finally, resveratrol downregulated b-catenin expression in several cancer cell lines. In animal models, resveratrol has been involved in cell cycle regulation in the SKH-1 hairless mouse skin after multiple exposures to UVB (180 mJ/cm^2) radiations. The molecule was topically applied on the skin of SKH-1 hairless mice prior to UVB exposure. Topical application of resveratrol revealed that the molecule was able to downregulate UV-mediated increases in critical cell cycle regulatory proteins, such as proliferating cell nuclear antigen (PCNA), cyclin-dependent kinase (cdk)-2, -4 and -6, cyclin- D1, and cyclin-D2. Further, resveratrol was also found to cause significant decreases in UVB-mediated upregulation of MAPK. In a different study, it has been reported that resveratrol blocked UVB-mediated activation of NF-kB in dose- and time-dependent manner in the normal human epidermal keratinocytes. Resveratrol treatment of keratinocytes also inhibited UVB-mediated phosphorylation and degradation of IkBa, and activation of IKKa.

VIII.   Isoflavones

1.   Genistein

Genistein is a isoflavone found in soy. It has been identified as dietary component having an important role in reducing the incidence of breast and prostate cancers, giving a rationale for the lower incidence of these forms of cancer in Asian countries such as Japan and China that consume a traditional diet high in soy products. Genistein was first isolated in 1899 from the dyer's broom, *Genista tinctoria*; hence, the chemical name derived from the generic name. Genistein has been identified as angiogenesis formation of new blood vessels) inhibitor, and found to inhibit the uncontrolled cell growth of cancer, most likely by inhibiting the activity of substances in the body that regulate cell division and cell survival (growth factors). Various studies have found that moderate doses of genistein have inhibitory effects on cancers of the prostate, cervix, brain, breast, 2001; and colon. It has also been shown that genistein makes some cells more sensitive to radio-therapy.

Genistein's chief method of activity is as a tyrosine kinase inhibitor. Tyrosine kinases are less widespread than their ser/thr counterparts but implicated in almost all cell growth and proliferation signal cascades. Inhibition of DNA topoisomerase II also plays an important role in the cytotoxic activity of genistein. Studies on rodents have found genistein to be useful in the treatment of leukemia, and that it can be used in combination with certain other antileukemic drugs to improve their efficacy.

2.   Daidzein

Daidzein can be found in food such as soybeans and soy products like tofu and textured vegetable protein. Soy isoflavones are a group of compounds found in and isolated from the soybean. Daidzein constitutes about 37 percent of the total isoflavones found in soybean. Daidzein has both weak estrogenic and weak anti-estrogenic effects. Daizein has also antioxidant activity. The anti-estrogenic effect of daidzein may explain its anti-carcinogenic, anti-atherogenic and anti-osteoporotic activity. Epidemiological studies have long shown that people who consume a lot of soy have reduces incidences of prostate cancers. This benefit of soy could be explained by the anti-cancer and antioxidant activity of daidzein. There are also indications that daidzein may reduce the dependence on alcohol. Keung and Vallee (1998) of the Center for Biochemical and Biophysical Sciences and Medicine, Harvard Medical School, Boston, showed that an extract of Radix Puerariae suppressed the free-choice ethanol intake of ethanol-preferring hamsters. The herb Radix Puerariae contains daidzein and is used in China as a traditional Chinese medicine for alcohol addiction and intoxication. adds protective effect to the chemotherapy agent tamoxifen in animal studies of mammary cancer.

Conclusion

The population world over have the problem of facing many diseases. While some of these are beyond our control there are many which get aggravated due to the lifestyle issues. In addition to this the occurrence of cancer is increasing at an alarming rate. An estimate suggests that about 10.5 million new cases of cancer may be added to the existing ones by the year 2025 due to aging and other issues in the world. It is obvious that we need to adopt multi pronged strategies to counter the threat of these diseases. The strategy of implementation of chemoprevention by dietary phytochemicals represents an inexpensive, readily applicable, and relatively low risk approach to control and reduce cancer incidence and control many of the lifestyle diseases.

11

Pesticide Contamination in Foods

Food is essential for life. Although many people in the world do not have enough to eat, few people in the developed countries are concerned with getting enough food. For most citizens of these countries, the concern is not one of quantity but of quality. Because most citizens of these countries have enough food available to meet our needs, they can consider a variety of factors in their food selection. These include cost, preferences, ease of preparation, time for preparation, nutrient content, and appearance.

In the past, few people identified risks associated with foods as a factor in selection. However, increasing concerns of Customers about health are affecting food choices. Many people are eating less to avoid the risk of obesity, reducing sodium to lower the risk of high blood pressure, and reducing cholesterol to lower the risks of heart disease. Recently, increased attention has been focused on chemical residues in food. The presence of minute residues of pesticides in food has caused some people to ask, "Is our food supply safe?" Current evidence strongly indicates that our food is safe. Food and Drug Administration (FDA) officials recently stated that "pesticide residues occurring in foods in the U.S. pose a very minor if not negligible risk to public health." However, public perceptions of risks from pesticides differ markedly from this official viewpoint. They also differ from actual risks attributable to these products. A 1982 study compared the causes of accidental deaths, as reported to insurance companies, with the risks as perceived by college students, women voters, and business people. College students ranked pesticides as more dangerous than motorcycle riding; women voters ranked pesticides as more dangerous than hunting; and business people felt they were more dangerous than commercial aviation. The actual rankings of these in relation to all causes of accidental deaths were as follows: motorcycles (6th), hunting (14th), commercial aviation (19th), and pesticides (28th).

What Are Pesticides?

A pesticide is any product that kills or controls various types of pests. A pest is defined as a plant or animal that is harmful to man or the environment. Most of us recognize that certain insects, weeds, and rodents are pests, but the use of pesticides is not limited to the control of these pests. Other harmful pests can include birds, snails, fungi, algae, and bacteria. Inability to control pests has had a tremendous impact on world history. Millions of people died from bubonic plague (the infamous Black Death).

Because most citizen in Developed Countries like Americans have enough food available to meet their needs, they can consider a variety of factors in their food selection. These include cost, preferences, ease of preparation, time for preparation, nutrient content, and appearance. In the past, few people identified risks associated with foods as a factor in selection. However, increasing concerns of Americans informed citizens world over about health are affecting food choices. Many people are eating less to avoid the risk of obesity, reducing sodium to lower the risk of high blood pressure, and reducing cholesterol to lower the risks of heart disease.

Pesticide Residues in Foods

Most of the food produced for human consumption is grown using pesticides. Chemical control of weeds, insects, fungi, and rodents has enabled agricultural productivity and intensity to increase. However, these economic benefits are not without their risks to human and environmental health. Small amounts of some pesticides may remain as residues on fruits, vegetables, grains, and other foods. If exposures are great enough, many pesticides may cause harmful health effects, including delayed or altered development, cancer, acute and chronic injury to the nervous systems, lung damage, reproductive dysfunction, and possibly dysfunction of the endocrine (hormone) and immune systems.

Children's exposures to pesticide residues may be relatively higher than those of most adults. Pound for pound, children generally eat more than adults, and they may be exposed more heavily to certain pesticides because they consume a diet different from that of adults. For instance, children typically consume larger quantities of applesauce, milk, and orange juice per pound of body weight.

Protecting the food supply from harmful levels of pesticide residues requires the ongoing attention of government agencies, pesticide producers, and pesticide users. The U.S. Department of Agriculture (USDA) collects annual data on pesticide residues in food. Among the foods sampled by the USDA's Pesticide Data Program in recent years are several that are important parts of children's diets, including apples, apple juice, bananas, carrots, green beans, orange juice, peaches, pears, potatoes, and tomatoes. EPA evaluates the safety of all new and existing pesticides and restricts pesticide use to those applications that do not pose unacceptable human health or ecological risks.

Pesticides are not the only contaminants in food that may affect children's health adversely. Industrial contaminants (such as dioxins, PCBs, and mercury), microbial contaminants (such as *E. coli*), and natural contaminants (such as aflatoxin) also can be found in foods. The Pesticide Data Program does not analyze foods for the presence of these types of contaminants, although other government programs monitor for some of them.

The chart on the following page displays the percentage of foods with detectable pesticide residues reported by the PDP from 1994 to 1998. This measure is a surrogate for children's exposure to pesticides in foods: If the frequency of detectable levels of pesticides in foods decreases, it is likely that exposures will decrease. However, this measure does not account for many additional factors that affect the risk to children. For example, some pesticides may pose greater risks to children than others do; residues on some foods may pose greater risks than residues on other foods due to differences in amounts consumed. For some pesticides, residues at levels below detection limits may pose important risks, while for other pesticides detectable levels of residues may not pose a significant health concern. In addition, year-to-year changes in the percentage of samples with detectable pesticide residues may be affected by changes in the selection of foods that are sampled each year.

- In 1994, 62 percent of all food samples tested by the U.S. Department of Agriculture's Pesticide Data Program (PDP) had detectable levels of at least one pesticide. The proportion of samples with detections increased to 68 percent in 1996, then declined to 55 percent in 1998.

- In 1998, 29 percent of samples had detectable levels of multiple pesticides, compared with 36 percent in 1994. During the same period, the proportion of samples with detectable levels of a single pesticide remained relatively constant.

- PDP data from 1994-96 were further evaluated for the presence of pesticides in 19 foods frequently eaten by children. This analysis focused on detections of carcinogenic and neurotoxic pesticides. Twenty-five percent of the samples had detectable levels of carcinogenic pesticides, and 34 percent had detectable levels of neurotoxic pesticides (not shown).

- Each year, less than 0.2 percent of all sampled foods had residues that violated established tolerances. A tolerance is the amount of pesticide residue legally allowed to remain on a food commodity.

Pesticide Residue Monitoring and Food Safety

This fact sheet presents an overview of the federal regulations on use of pesticides, federal monitoring programs for pesticide residues in food, and outlines some issues being debated nationwide.

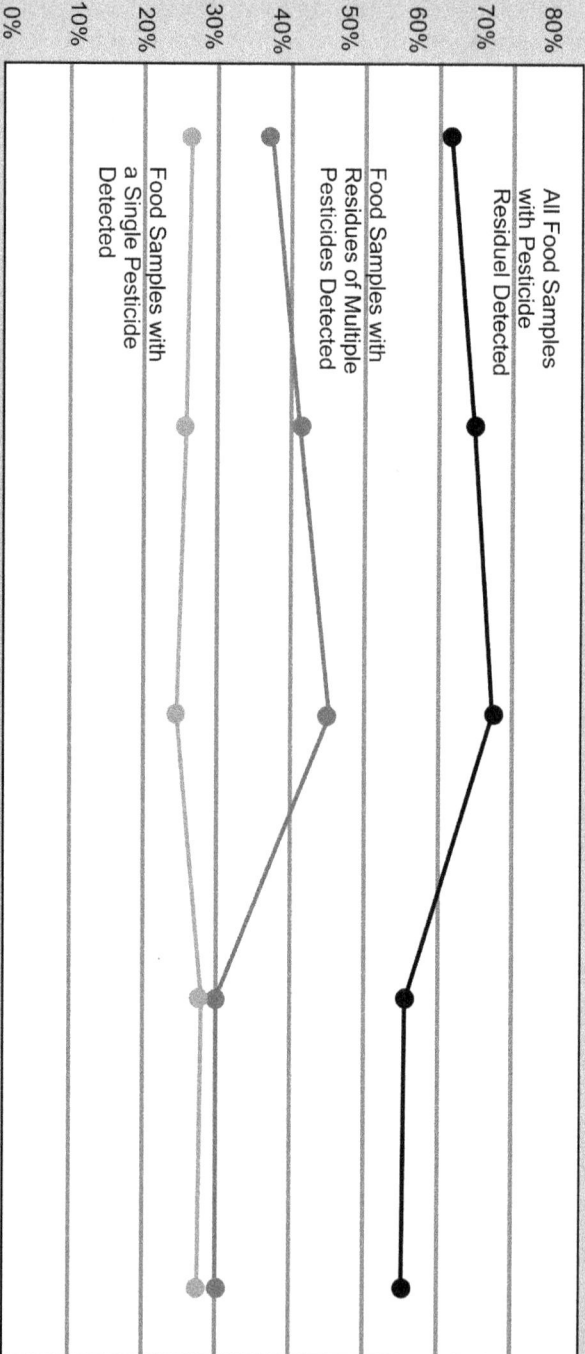

Figure 11.1

Percentage of fruits, vegetables, grains, dairy, and processed food with detectable pesticide residues.

Source: U.S. Department of Agriculture, Agricultural Marketing Service, Pesticide Data Programme Annual Summary (Calender Years 1999-1998).

Why Are Pesticides Found on Food?

Pesticides may be used in a variety of different ways during the production of food. They may be used by farmers to control the growth of weeds, or prevent crop damage by insects, rodents and molds. They may be used on food crops after harvest to prolong their storage life. Pesticides may also be used on animal farms to control insect pests. Sometimes, small amounts of pesticides used in these ways can be found in or on foods. The pesticides found in or on foods are called residues (see also BCERF Fact Sheet #24 on Consumer Concerns About Pesticides in Food). Some pesticides, even though no longer used, persist and remain in the environment. Residues of these pesticides are sometimes found on food grown on contaminated soil, or in the fish that live in contaminated waters.

Regulation of the Use of Pesticides

Before a new pesticide can be sold for use on a farm in the United States (US), it has to be registered for agricultural use by the US Environmental Protection Agency (EPA). The registration process involves a careful consideration by EPA of possible health effects from the pesticide. The manufacturer of each new pesticide is required to submit scientific data to EPA that help evaluate the risk of health effects from its use. EPA reviews the submitted data and other available studies to determine if the pesticide is likely to affect human health or the environment. All the uses that have been approved by EPA are mentioned on the pesticide label. Other uses are illegal. States also regulate the use of pesticides. The New York State Department of Environmental Conservation regulates pesticide use in New York State.

Maximum Level of a Pesticide that is Allowed on Food?

EPA sets tolerances for pesticides. A tolerance is the maximum amount of a specific pesticide or its break down products that is allowed to remain in or on foods. The tolerance is not an estimate of the residue amount that is common or typical for a food. Residue levels found in food are usually below the tolerance levels. Tolerances for a given pesticide may vary for different crops. EPA has set tolerances for about 400 different pesticides. Since a pesticide may be used on many different crops, there are about 9,700 tolerances in effect.

Safe Level of Pesticide Residue

To estimate the health risk to humans from exposure to pesticides, EPA evaluates tests done in experimental animals, and on plant, human or animal cells growing in the laboratory. EPA determines how much of the pesticide is likely to remain on foods that are grown using the recommended guidelines for pesticide use. It pays extra attention to foods that are eaten by children in large quantities, such as apple juice and milk. All this information is entered into a computer program specially developed to estimate health risks, called the Dietary Exposure Evaluation Model. EPA considers the exposure through food, drinking water, and home use of pesticides. EPA will set a tolerance level for food if the combined exposure from different sources is 100 to 1,000 times lower than the maximum level that shows no harmful effects in experimental animals. Residue levels are usually present in very small amounts that may be expressed as parts per million (ppm = 1 inch of a 16 mile-long loaf of bread) parts per billion (ppb = 1 inch of a 16,000 mile-long loaf of bread), parts per trillion (ppt = 1 inch of a 16,000,000 mile-long loaf of bread).

Levels of Pesticide Residues in Prepared Meals

FDA conducts a third kind of food monitoring called the Total Diet Studies to analyze pesticide residues that remain in a typical meal. Information on what people eat or what is a typical meal is collected by the USDAs Nationwide Food Consumption Surveys. A list of 265 food items was compiled for 1990. Some examples are: chocolate milk, boiled eggs, chicken nuggets, pork and beans, bread, banana, french fries, macaroni and cheese, ice cream, popcorn, honey, butter, lemonade, and 35 infant and childrens foods. Food monitored in the Total Diet Studies may be analyzed for nearly 200 different pesticides.

How Can Food be Analyzed for so Many Pesticide Residues?

Most food testing laboratories use methods that test for almost 200 residues at one time. These multi-residue methods make it possible to test many foods for several hundred residues at the same time.

Common Violations

More than half of the 9,843 food samples collected by FDA for monitoring in 1997 were of imported foods. Violations were detected in 85 of the 5,342 imported foods that were tested. No violative residues were found in imported milk, dairy products, eggs, seafood, bananas and apple juice. Violations were reported for 54 of 4,501 domestically produced foods that were monitored in 1997. No violative residues were found in domestic milk, dairy products, eggs, bananas, apple juice, grains and grain products, and seafood.

Is the Current Pesticide Monitoring System Ensuring a Safe Food Supply?

Consumers often voice the presence of pesticide residues in food as a concern. Important issues on food safety that concern the consumers and have become important topics of discussion is public discourse are outlined below. We have outlined below some issues on food safety that are being debated nationwide.

Should we spend more on increased monitoring of our food supply? Due to limited resources, of all the food produced or imported into the US, only 9,843 food samples were analyzed for residues by FDA in 1997. As mentioned earlier, a very small percentage of these domestic and imported food samples were found to have violative pesticide residues. Ideally, no food should have any violative residues.

What else can be done? Some people argue that a more effective way to increase food safety in the long run is to strengthen programs that guide farmers on good farm practices and proper use of pesticides, to further decrease the incidence of violative residues in food. For example, the Integrated Pest Management Program recommends a variety of strategies to reduce pesticide use for the control of pests in agriculture. Some crops are naturally more resistant to pests and lend themselves well to organic production methods without the use of any synthetic chemicals. A greater reliance on seasonal and varied local produce through local farmers markets may be another way to reduce the need for pesticides, which would be required if the food was to be shipped over great distances.

Is more information needed on health effects of pesticide residues? While the tolerances set by EPA are based on available research, there are gaps in our knowledge on the health effects of pesticides. The National Academy of Sciences published a report in 1993 recommending that more attention be paid to the estimation of risk of health effects from pesticides for infants and children. The Food Quality Protection Act passed in 1996, has special features included to assure adequate protection of children when estimates are being made for acceptable levels of a pesticide residue in food.

12

Food Additives: Traditional and Modern

Food additives are substances added to food to preserve flavor or enhance its taste and appearance. Some additives have been used for centuries; for example, preserving food by pickling (with vinegar), salting, as with bacon, preserving sweets or using sulfur dioxide as in some wines. With the advent of processed foods in the second half of the 20th century, many more additives have been introduced, of both natural and artificial origin.

To regulate these additives, and inform consumers, each additive is assigned a unique number, termed as "E numbers", which is used in Europe for all approved additives. This numbering scheme has now been adopted and extended by the Codex Alimentarius Commission to internationally identify all additives, regardless of whether they are approved for use.

E numbers are all prefixed by "E", but countries outside Europe use only the number, whether the additive is approved in Europe or not. For example, acetic acid is written as E260 on products sold in Europe, but is simply known as additive 260 in some countries. Additive 103, alkanet, is not approved for use in Europe so does not have an E number, although it is approved for use in Australia and New Zealand. Since 1987, Australia has had an approved system of labelling for additives in packaged foods. Each food additive has to be named or numbered. The numbers are the same as in Europe, but without the prefix 'E'.

The United States Food and Drug Administration lists these items as "Generally recognized as safe" or GRAS; they are listed under both their Chemical Abstract Services number and Fukda regulation under the US Code of Federal Regulations.

Categories

Food additives can be divided into several groups, although there is some overlap between them.

Acids

Food acids are added to make flavors "sharper", and also act as preservatives and antioxidants. Common food acids include vinegar, citric acid, tartaric acid, malic acid, fumaric acid, and lactic acid.

Acidity regulators

> Acidity regulators are used to change or otherwise control the acidity and alkalinity of foods.

Anticaking agents

> Anticaking agents keep powders such as milk powder from caking or sticking.

Antifoaming agents

> Antifoaming agents reduce or prevent foaming in foods.

Antioxidants

> Antioxidants such as vitamin C act as preservatives by inhibiting the effects of oxygen on food, and can be beneficial to health.

Bulking agents

> Bulking agents such as starch are additives that increase the bulk of a food without affecting its taste.

Food coloring

> Colorings are added to food to replace colors lost during preparation, or to make food look more attractive.

Color retention agents

> In contrast to colorings, color retention agents are used to preserve a food's existing color.

Emulsifiers

> Emulsifiers allow water and oils to remain mixed together in an emulsion, as in mayonnaise, ice cream, and homogenized milk.

Flavors

> Flavors are additives that give food a particular taste or smell, and may be derived from natural ingredients or created artificially.

Flavor enhancers

> Flavor enhancers enhance a food's existing flavors. They may be extracted from natural sources (through distillation, solvent extraction, maceration, among other methods) or created artificially.

Flour treatment agents

> Flour treatment agents are added to flour to improve its color or its use in baking.

Glazing agents

> Glazing agents provide a shiny appearance or protective coating to foods.

Humectants

> Humectants prevent foods from drying out.

Tracer gas

Tracer gas allows for package integrity testing to prevent foods from being exposed to atmosphere, thus guaranteeing shelf life.

Preservatives

Preservatives prevent or inhibit spoilage of food due to fungi, bacteria and other microorganisms.

Stabilizers

Stabilizers, thickeners and gelling agents, like agar or pectin (used in jam for example) give foods a firmer texture. While they are not true emulsifiers, they help to stabilize emulsions.

Sweeteners

Sweeteners are added to foods for flavoring. Sweeteners other than sugar are added to keep the food energy (calories) low, or because they have beneficial effects for diabetes mellitus, tooth decay and diarrhea.

Thickeners

Thickeners are substances which, when added to the mixture, increase its viscosity without substantially modifying its other properties.

Safety

With the increasing use of processed foods since the 19th century, there has been a great increase in the use of food additives of varying levels of safety. This has led to legislation in many countries regulating their use. For example, boric acid was widely used as a food preservative from the 1870s to the 1920s, but was banned after World War I due to its toxicity, as demonstrated in animal and human studies. During World War II, the urgent need for cheap, available food preservatives led to it being used again, but it was finally banned in the 1950s. Such cases led to a general mistrust of food additives, and an application of the precautionary principle led to the conclusion that only additives that are known to be safe should be used in foods. In the USA, this led to the adoption of the Delaney clause, an amendment to the Federal Food, Drug, and Cosmetic Act of 1938, stating that no carcinogenic substances may be used as food additives. However, after the banning of cyclamates in the USA and Britain in 1969, saccharin, the only remaining legal artificial sweetener at the time, was found to cause cancer in rats. Widespread public outcry in the USA, partly communicated to Congress by postage-paid postcards supplied in the packaging of sweetened soft drinks, led to the retention of saccharin despite its violation of the Delaney clause.

In September 2007, research financed by Britain's Food Standards Agency and published online by the British medical journal *The Lancet*, presented evidence that a mix of additives commonly found in children's foods increases the mean level of hyperactivity. The team of researchers concluded that "the finding lends strong support for the case that food additives exacerbate hyperactive behaviors (inattention, impulsivity and overactivity) at least into middle childhood." That study examined the effect of artificial colors and a sodium benzoate preservative, and found both to be problematic for some children. Further studies are needed to find out whether there are other additives that could have a similar effect, and it is unclear whether some disturbances can also occur in mood and concentration in some adults. In the February 2008 issue of its publication, *AAP Grand Rounds*, the American Academy of Pediatrics concluded that a low-additive diet is a valid intervention for children with ADHD:

"Although quite complicated, this was a carefully conducted study in which the investigators went to great lengths to eliminate bias and to rigorously measure outcomes. The results are hard to follow and somewhat inconsistent. For many of the assessments there were small but statistically significant differences of measured behaviors in children who consumed the food additives compared with those who did not. In each case increased hyperactive behaviors were associated with consuming the additives. For those comparisons in which no statistically significant differences were found, there was a trend for more hyperactive behaviors associated with the food additive drink in virtually every assessment. Thus, the overall findings of the study are clear and require that even we skeptics, who have long doubted parental claims of the effects of various foods on the behavior of their children, admit we might have been wrong."

In 2007, Food Standards Australia New Zealand published an official shoppers' guidance with which the concerns of food additives and their labeling are mediated.

There has been significant controversy associated with the risks and benefits of food additives. Some artificial food additives have been linked with cancer, digestive problems, neurological conditions, ADHD, heart disease or obesity. Natural additives may be similarly harmful or be the cause of allergic reactions in certain individuals. For example, safrole was used to flavor root beer until it was shown to be carcinogenic. Due to the application of the Delaney clause, it may not be added to foods, even though it occurs naturally in sassafras and sweet basil.

Extreme caution should be taken with sodium nitrite which is mainly used as a food coloring agent. Sodium nitrite is added to meats to produce an appealing and fresh red color to the consumer. Sodium nitrite can produce cancer causing chemicals such as nitrosamines, and numerous studies have shown a link between nitrite and cancer in humans that consume processed and cured meats.

Blue 1, Blue 2, Red 3, and Yellow 6 are among the food colourings that have been linked to various health risks in animal models. Blue 1 is used to color candy, soft drinks, and pastries and there has been some evidence that it may cause cancer in mice, but studies have not been replicated. Blue 2 can be found in pet food, soft drinks, and pastries, and has shown to cause brain tumors in mice. Red 3, mainly used in cherries for cocktails has been correlated with thyroid tumors in rats. Yellow 6, used in sausages, gelatin, and candy can lead to the attribution of gland and kidney tumors, again in animal models and contains carcinogens, but in minimal amounts. It should be noted that many animal models are poor substitutes for studying carcinogenic effects in humans because the physiology of rabbits, mice and non-human primates can be very different from humans in the relevant biochemical pathways. There has been no scientific consensus on the carcinogenic properties of these agents in humans and studies are still on-going.

Though food additives may be linked with these diseases and health risks, they also preserve nutrient value by providing vitamins, minerals, and other nutrients to foods such as flour, cereal, margarine and milk which normally would not retain such high levels. Preservatives also reduce spoilage from sources such as air, bacteria, fungi, and yeast.

In the EU it can take 10 years or more to obtain approval for a new food additive. This includes five years of safety testing, followed by two years for evaluation by the European Food Safety Authority and another three years before the additive receives an EU-wide approval for use in every country in the European Union. Apart from testing and analyzing food products during the whole production process to ensure safety and compliance with regulatory standards, to trading standards officers (in the UK) protect the public from any illegal use or potentially dangerous mis-use of food additives by performing random testing of food products.

Difference between Traditional and Modern Additives

The traditional food additives were substances like, salt, spices and herbs, smoking (yes, smoke flavor is an additive that preserves), pickling with vinegar and combinations of salt and vinegar. Believe it or not, hundreds of years ago all the way up until the 19th century, poisonous food additives were added to foods to preserve them which are ILLEGAL now. Lead, Arsenic (rat poison), and Mercuric compounds were all used to preserve foods (never mind the fact they also poisoned human beings). This may sound crazy, but if you know the history of medicine, Ludwig Von Beethoven (the German Composer) most likely died from medication his doctor gave him that was lead based. They know this by taking atomic absorption samples of Beethoven's hair in which they found huge amounts of lead in the hair. Mercuric compounds were used in medicine as the only known "cure" for the sexually transmitted disease syphillis - it was a cure alright, in which about 50% of the people who died from the treatment rather than the disease. So actually, old fashioned additives in some cases were very poisonous and toxic and part of the reason why they were used was because there were no health laws concerning whether or not they were toxic or could be used. Until the first Food and Drug Act, around the turn of the 20th century, anybody could use anything they wanted to, in any amount, in foods. This frequently leads to sickness and death. On top of that, the science of microbiology was just in its infancy and the proper canning of low acid foods had not yet been developed a result of which, people died from Botulism more frequently than you would like to know about.

With the advent of the Food and Drug law, most of these substances were banned or outlawed in food for human and animal consumption. Food additives then had to go through long, drawn out animal studies over many years to prove their efficacy, intended functionality and safety. Substances like arsenic, lead and mercury were banned. As science developed, proper heating and cooling technology was developed to retort low acid foods to prevent botulism. Yet today, as in all of history, the challenge is to preserve foods so that they are not wasted. In addition to this goal of food preservation are all of the other characteristics that we have come to enjoy in our foods, such as flavors, colors, texture modifiers, emulsifiers, acidulants, etc. Each and every one of these approved substances has been evaluated by the FDA for efficacy, intended functionality and safety. Yet the memory of the days when food additives were poisonous and could kill people, linger on. Science and medicine have progressed further, in discovering new problems, such as food allergens and sensitizers which could lead to long term allergenic reactions we know more today because of science than we have ever known before, and our food system has become much more immensely complicated and internationalized, exposing the public to a wide range of new food additives with new or improved functionalities - yet despite the fact the US has encountered a few serious food issues in the last few years, we still have the safest food system in the world. People have to realize that nothing is perfect, especially a complicated manufacturing-distributor-retailer-end user matrix. And the fact that the public demands new and exciting food trends all the time. To meet the demands, food additive companies work towards meeting those needs.

E Numbers: The Dewey Decimal System of Food Additives

Over the past century, the food industry has developed or repurposed a number of chemicals to address the issues of scaling created when producing food in large quantities. Preventing illness, maintaining freshness, controlling costs, and meeting changing consumer demands have all presented challenges. Producing larger quantities of food increases the time between harvest and consumption, increasing the chances of spoilage and the amount of time foodborne pathogens have to develop, and aggregating ingredients from a larger number of producers increases the impact that a single contaminated item can have.

Hard on the heels of World War II, when advances in food science had been applied to address these problems in the military's meal rations ("an army travels on its stomach"), the food industry found a new market in the American consumer. Convenience foods and prepared meals burst onto the scene at the same time that freezers went into mass production and television sets became the "must have" item for the American family. Instant food and instant entertainment have been married ever since.

The same family of chemicals that enabled the creation of the TV dinner (Kraft Macaroni & Cheese) also allowed for a new set of dishes to be created by haute cuisine chefs, sometimes called molecular gastronomy or modernist cuisine (we'll use the latter term). These chefs use industrial chemicals to create entirely different ways of conveying flavors and exciting the senses. When done well, the dishes are not about additives at all, but about the perceptions and emotions that all good meals strive to evoke. No one is suggesting that vegetables and whole foods should be replaced with white powders.

The demand for innovative foods at the high end of the culinary world should not be surprising. Luxury restaurants now have to compete with the enthusiastic hobbyist chef, who has been able to better approximate traditional restaurant fare as the quality of consumer gear and produce has improved. The same technological advances that have enabled the production of convenience foods have also enabled the agro-industrial food complex to deliver an ever-widening—sometimes maddeningly so—variety of food, and also to make those foods available for a longer window of time each year.

Turning to food additives for new dishes is a logical progression in the process of creating something new. Sometimes, the results are amazing; other times, they fall flat. Compare the culinary iconoclasts to the fashions that show up on the Paris runways: while it might not be "everyday" wear or cuisine, the better concepts and ideas that start out at the high end eventually make their way into the clothing shops and onto the general restaurant scene.

Many of the techniques that rely on food additives originated in Europe. Chef Ferran Adrià's restaurant elBulli, in Spain, is considered by many to be the originator of much of modern haute cuisine. Chef Heston Blumenthal's restaurant The Fat Duck, in the UK, has also established an international reputation for pushing the boundaries of food.

It's easy enough to write eggplant on the grocery list, but how does one go about writing up a grocery list for food additives? The Codex Alimentarius Commission—established by the United Nations and the World Health Organization—has created a taxonomy of food additives called "E numbers." Like the Dewey Decimal classification system, it establishes a hierarchical tree: a unique E number is assigned for each chemical compound, grouped by functional categories, with the numbering of chemicals determined by each chemical's primary usage.

Not everything has an E number; for example, neither common salt (sodium chloride) nor transglutaminase is currently included. Which additive to use for a particular effect, such as gelling, depends upon the properties of the food with which you're working and your goals. Most food additives used in modernist cuisine come from the E400–E499 range, which consists of the following:

Thickeners (e.g., cornstarch, methylcellulose, agar, carrageenan)

Provide structure to items such as gels (Jell-O), traditional French dishes (aspics and terrines), and confections (gummy candies). Food preparers also use them to prevent both water and sugar crystallization in foods such as ice creams, because thickeners inhibit the development of molecular lattices.

Emulsifiers (e.g., lecithin and glycerin)

Prevent two liquids from separating, as with oil and water in mayonnaise. The food industry uses lecithin in chocolate for similar reasons, to prevent the cocoa solids and fats from separating and to increase the viscosity of the melted chocolate during manufacturing.

Stabilizers (e.g., guar and xanthan gums)

Lend a smooth "mouth-feel" to a liquid and can also act as emulsifiers by preventing aggregates from separating. Think of how oregano stays suspended in a commercial salad dressing, instead of precipitating out and settling to the bottom.

You will also see compounds from the E300–E399 and E500–E599 ranges used, but usually as secondary additives that help the E400–E499 compounds function. A number of the E400–E499 additives require either certain pH ranges or secondary compounds to react with, such as calcium when working with sodium alginate.

Some additives work in a broad range of pHs and temperatures but have other properties that may prohibit their use, depending upon the recipe. For example, while agar is a strong gelling agent, in some gels it also exhibitssyneresis (when a gel expels a portion of its liquid—think of the liquid whey that separates out in some yogurts). Carrageenan does not undergo syneresis but cannot handle an environment as acidic as agar can. For example, if you attempt to use carrageenan to gel lime juice, which has a pH between 2.0 and 2.35, you will also need to add an acidity regulator to raise the pH.

Commercial food preparers have to balance additional variables in their recipes. In the lime gel example, if the pH is raised too much, the food becomes hospitable to bacterial activity, depending on other parameters in the food (e.g., water availability). Balancing all of this can require multiple chemicals, which is why prepared foods can have quite a number of chemicals on their ingredient labels.

E100–E199	:	Colouring agents
		(*i.e.*, food colouring, like those found in the grocery store)
E120	:	Cochineal or carminic acid ("red 4," in common use)
E200–E299	:	Preservatives
E251	:	Sodium nitrate (used in curing items like sausages)
E290	:	Carbon dioxide
E300–E399	:	Antioxidants, acidity regulators
E300	:	Ascorbic acid (vitamin C)
E322	:	Lecithin (emulsifier, typically from soy)
E330	:	Citric acid (in lemons, limes, etc.)
E327	:	Calcium lactate
E400–E499	:	Thickeners, emulsifiers, and stabilizers
E401	:	Sodium alginate

Contd (....)

Contd (....)

E406	:	Agar
E441	:	Gelatin
E461	:	Methylcellulose
E500–E599	:	Acidity regulators, anti-caking agents
E500	:	Sodium bicarbonate (baking soda)
E509	:	Calcium chloride
E524	:	Sodium hydroxide (lye)
E600–E699	:	Flavor enhancers E621: Monosodium glutamate (MSG)
E700–E799	:	Antibiotics
E900–E999	:	Miscellaneous
E941	:	Nitrogen (used in food storage)
E953	:	Isomalt (also known as Isomaltitol)
E1000–E1999	:	Additional chemicals E1510: Ethanol (alcohol)

An abbreviated table of E numbers including common food additives.

Common Uses of Additives

Impart/Maintain Desired Consistency

Alginates, Lecithin, Mono- & Diglycerides, Methyl Cellulose, Carrageenan, Glycerine, Pectin, Guar Gum, Sodium Aluminosilicate

Foods Where Likely Used

Baked Goods, Cake Mixes, Salad Dressings, Ice Cream, Process Cheese, Coconut, Table Salt, Chocolate

Impart/Maintain Desired Consistency

Alginates, Lecithin, Mono- & Diglycerides, Methyl Cellulose, Carrageenan, Glycerine, Pectin, Guar Gum, Sodium Aluminosilicate

Foods Where Likely Used

Flour, Bread, Biscuits, Breakfast Cereals, Pasta, Margarine, Milk, Iodized Salt, Gelatin Desserts

Maintain Palatability and Wholesomeness

Propionic Acid and its Salts, Ascorbic Acid, Butylated Hydroxyanisole (BHA), Butylated Hydroxytoluene (BHT), Benzoates, Sodium Nitrite, Citric Acid, Erythorbates

Foods Where Likely Used

Bread, Cheese, Crackers, Frozen and Dried Fruit, Margarine, Lard, Potato Chips, Cake Mixes, Meat

Produce Light Texture; Control Acidity/Alkalinity

Yeast, Sodium Bicarbonate, Citric Acid, Fumaric Acid, Phosphoric Acid, Lactic Acid, Tartrates

Foods Where Likely Used

Cakes, Cookies, Quick Breads, Crackers, Butter, Soft Drinks

Enhance Flavor or Impart Desired Color

Cloves, Ginger, Fructose, Aspartame, Saccharin, FD&C Red No. 40, Monosodium Glutamate, Caramel, Annatto, Limonene, Turmeric

Foods Where Likely Used

Spice Cake, Gingerbread, Soft Drinks, Yogurt, Soup, Confections, Baked Goods, Cheeses, Jams, Gum.

13

Chemical Safety of Foods

Food businesses are responsible for ensuring their food is safe, and that it complies with legislation on food additives and rules on reducing or eliminating human health risks caused by contaminants.

Chemical contaminants can come from:

- farming - *e.g.* pesticides, veterinary medicines
- packaging and other contact materials
- processing - *e.g.* acrylamides
- storage - *e.g.* naturally-occurring aflatoxins
- the environment - *e.g.* pollutants such as dioxins

Food additives must comply with specified legislation which aims to ensure that they are only used when there is a technological justification, that they do not mislead consumers, and do not have effects on consumer health.

Natural components of plants may also be toxic - such as glycoalkaloids in potatoes - while some may be harmful if not cooked properly - for example lectins in pulses. There are also some foodstuffs that can cause allergies in some people - such as peanuts.

This guide provides food businesses with information on safety rules and procedures with regard to food additives, pesticides, contact materials and processes such as high temperature cooking and irradiation.

Food Additives

Food additives are intentionally added to food for a technological purpose during its manufacture and processing. Additives may be:

- antioxidants - used in food prepared with fats or oils to protect them against deterioration caused by rancidity
- colours - used to make food look more attractive or to replace colours which have been lost during processing

- emulsifiers, stabilisers, gelling agents and thickeners - used to help mix ingredients together that would usually separate, e.g. oils and water

- flavour enhancers - used to bring out the flavour of food without adding a flavour of their own

- preservatives - used to keep food safe for longer

- sweeteners - used to replace sugar in certain foods, e.g. energy reduced products

All additives used in food must be on the EU approved list. Most additives are restricted to certain foods at maximum specified levels. EU legislation states that most additives used in foods must be labelled clearly in the list of ingredients, either by name or by an E number. If an additive has an E number, it means it has passed EU safety tests.

You must ensure that any additives you use in your food have been approved for use, and that you comply with relevant legislation about the levels of additives and the foods in which they are used.

Under the Food Labelling Regulations 1996 you must also ensure that any food you supply to caterers or consumers is clearly labelled with a list of the ingredients used, including any additives.

How to Reduce Acrylamide in Food Processing

Acrylamide is a natural by-product that forms when carbohydrate-rich foods such as potatoes and cereals - bread, biscuits and other bakery products - are fried, baked, or roasted at temperatures above 120 C.

It is not found in food that has not been heated, or that has been cooked using methods such as boiling or microwaving.

Since these foods have been cooked at high temperatures for hundreds of years, it is likely that acrylamide has been present in our food for many generations. It is thought to form from two chemicals that occur naturally in the food - an amino acid called asparagine and certain types of sugar.

Acrylamide is also found in:

- tobacco

- coffee

- raw, dried or pickled food - such as olives, prunes and dried pears

Acrylamide has been found to cause nerve damage in people who have been accidentally exposed to it whilst at work (it is used as an industrial chemical in strengthening paper and in the clarification of water). It is also considered to be a carcinogen.

There are currently no regulatory limits set for acrylamide in food. However, there is a limit for the amount of acrylamide allowed to migrate from food contact plastic into food. The specific migration limit in force means that acrylamide migrating into food from food contact plastic should not be detectable at a limit of 0.01 milligrams per kilogram of food.

The formation of acrylamide is a product of the Maillard reaction - the browning of food when cooking caused by a reaction of natural sugars. Current advice for reducing acrylamide includes:

- choosing specific varieties of raw materials - such as potatoes with a lower level of sugars

- adding asparaginase - an enzyme which reduces the production of acrylamide

- lowering the cooking temperature and reducing cooking time to reduce browning

The Confederation of the Food and Drink Industries of the EU (Confederation des industries Agro-Alimentaires de l'UE or CIAA) has produced guidance in the form of a 'toolbox' and sector specific pamphlets on how to reduce acrylamide in the processing of different types of foods - such as biscuits, bread, potato crisps and French fries.

The Acrylamide Infonet was set up following a 2002 consultation by the World Health Organization (WHO) and the Food and Agriculture Organization of the UN. It provides a single source of information on existing and ongoing research into the effects of acrylamide in food and links to external resources.

Other Contaminants in Food Derived from Food Processing

Process contaminants have the potential to increase the risk of cancer, so levels in food have to be kept as low as is reasonably practical.

The FSA is currently conducting a survey of four 'process contaminants' in food - i.e. contaminants formed during the processing of food - to gain a clearer picture of the levels of these contaminants in food normally consumed in the UK. The survey is a three-year rolling programme which started in 2007 and covers:

- acrylamide
- 3-MCPD (3-monochloropropanediol)
- 3-MCPD esters
- furan
- ethyl carbamate

The survey report is published annually. The 2007 report was published in September and the 2008 report was published in July and the report is available on the FSA website (www. food.gov.uk).

The Use of Pesticides

The use of pesticides in agriculture, horticulture, forestry and domestic gardening is regulated by the Chemical Regulation Directorate (CRD) - part of the Health and Safety Executive (HSE).

The CRD:

- regulate pesticides in accordance with national and European requirements
- actively monitor the marketing and use of pesticides and take enforcement action where necessary
- provide operational policy advice to government ministers

The CRD aims to ensure that pesticides are safe for people and the environment. They do this by regulation, encouraging best practice and researching into alternative pest control methods. The FSA works closely with CRD to make sure that consumer safety is given priority in pesticide regulation and surveillance.

Use of pesticides in the UK must be approved by government ministers and monitored through official programmes.

Pesticide Residue Levels

Rigorous safety assessments are undertaken to make sure that any pesticide residues remaining in food are not harmful to people. Residues are controlled through a system of statutory Maximum Residue Levels (MRLs).

The MRL is the maximum amount of residue likely to remain in food products when a pesticide has been used correctly. It is expressed as milligrams of residue per kilogram of food product. Before being approved for use, a pesticide must be proven to be completely safe for human consumption at its MRL - and may be safe at much higher levels.

All current EU MRLs are listed in Annex II of EC Regulation 396/2005.

In the UK, the independent Pesticide Residues Committee oversees the surveillance programme for residues in both home produced and imported food.

The purpose of this monitoring is to check that:

- no unexpected residues occur in crops
- human dietary intakes of residues in foods are within acceptable levels
- pesticide residues do not exceed the statutory MRL

The Use of Veterinary Medicines

The use of veterinary medicines in the UK is controlled and monitored by the Veterinary Medicine Directorate (VMD). The VMD is an executive agency of the Department for Environment, Food and Rural Affairs in the UK.

A high priority in the VMD's work is ensuring that veterinary medicines are used in a way that protects food safety and the environment. Their remit includes:

- regulating veterinary medicines in accordance with national and European guidelines
- putting in place and operating monitoring programmes for residues in food to ensure consumers are not exposed to unacceptable residues of veterinary medicines

- providing policy advice to government ministers
- actively monitoring the marketing and use of veterinary medicines and taking appropriate enforcement action

The VMD fulfils its remit by making scientific assessments of the safety and effectiveness of potential medicines before they are authorised, and operating systems of post-authorisation surveillance and monitoring. They work closely with the FSA to make sure that consumer safety is given priority in veterinary medicines authorisation and surveillance.

Veterinary Medicines Residue Levels

Rigorous safety assessments are undertaken to make sure that any veterinary medicines residues remaining in food are not harmful to people. For food that might contain residue of a particular medicine, an agreed Maximum Residue Level (MRL), is calculated.

The MRL is the maximum concentration of residue that is legally permitted or acceptable in or on a food. Any residues below the MRL pose no concerns for consumer health. Even when the MRL is exceeded, it is unlikely that the residues are of concern - however, an individual assessment would be made.

The VMD organises investigations on farms where residues above the MRL originated. They determine the cause and give advice to farmers.

In the UK, the independent Veterinary Residues Committee oversees the VMD's monitoring of residues in both home-produced and imported food. The purpose of this monitoring is to check that:

- the system of authorising veterinary medicines is working correctly and, when used as directed, any residues of veterinary medicines present in foods do not exceed the statutory MRLs
- residues of banned or unauthorised veterinary medicines are not present in foodstuffs

Regulations on Food Colours

Food colouring additives are used by manufacturers to change or enhance the natural colours of food. They are often used:

- to mask natural colour variations
- to replace colour lost in storage or processing
- to make the food appear more appetising
- for effect - e.g. in cake decoration

Colouring additives are used in both commercial and domestic food preparation. They can be either natural or synthetic (artificial).

The Colours in Foods Regulations 1995 define which food colour additives may be used in the UK. They list the permitted colours, set down conditions for their use and specify which colours may not be sold directly to the public.

Food Colours and Attention Deficit Hyperactivity Disorder (ADHD)

In 2008, following research that suggested a link between certain food colours andADHD in children, UK ministers and the FSA recommended that, although they remain permitted additives under EU legislation, UK manufacturers should remove six colour additives from their food by the end of 2009.

You should check whether your suppliers still use these colours, including those supplying you from abroad. The six colours are:

- sunset yellow FCF (E110)
- quinoline yellow (E104)
- carmoisine (E122)
- allura red (E129)
- tartrazine (E102)
- ponceau 4R (E124)

From 20 July 2010, most food and drink containing any of these six colours supplied to the EU market must carry additional warning information.

Many consumers now prefer to buy products with fewer artificial additives - especially in children's foods - so you may want to consider reducing your general use of colourings.

Sudan Dyes and Industrial Dyes not Permitted in Food

Certain industrial red dyes - such as Para Red and the four Sudan dyes (Sudan I, Sudan II, Sudan III and Sudan IV, otherwise know as scarlet red) - are not permitted for use in food, as they are carcinogenic. Sudan dyes are used legally in shoe and floor polish, solvents, oils, waxes and petrol.

Sudan dyes have been used illegally in spices, sauces, chutneys, vinegars and palm oil, among many other products and, in some of these cases, food products have been recalled.

The FSA provides food alerts about illegal dyes added to food to enforcement authorities who follow up with businesses that might be affected.

Other illegal dyes are:

- butter yellow
- metanil yellow
- orange G
- rhodamine B
- orange II
- toluidine red

Since 2003, all imports of dried, crushed and ground spices, curry powders, circumin and palm oil have had to be accompanied by test certificates showing that they do not contain Sudan dyes. Any consignment without relevant documentation is detained for sampling and analysis.

Random sampling must also be carried out by port and local authorities - the FSAsample over 1,000 consignments every year. Any consignment found to contain Sudan is destroyed.

From January 2010, the current rules on imported foods containing Sudan dyes will be repealed and replaced by a new system of controls and testing applicable to all imported food.

Food Contact Materials and Packaging

Food contact materials are those that are intended to, or can be reasonably expected to, come into contact with food. This can be packaging, cookware, cutlery, tableware, work surfaces or food processing machinery and equipment. Manufacturers of food packaging materials and producers and sellers of food must ensure that any food contact materials do not present a health risk for consumers.

European Regulation (EC) 1935/2004 on materials and articles intended to come into contact with food came into force on 3 December 2004. It sets out general safety requirements for materials and articles that come into contact with food - including those might come into contact with foods or transfer their constituents to food, for example printing inks and adhesive labels.

It also ensures that these materials do not change the nature, substance or quality of the food.

It includes descriptions of 'active' and 'intelligent' food packaging materials:

- active materials - release a substance into the foodstuff to extend its shelflife, or maintain or improve its condition
- intelligent materials - monitor the condition of the food or its surrounding environment inside packaging and communicate this to the consumer - e.g. a label which changes colour if it detects bacteria or gases, meaning that the food is not fresh

Future European guidelines are likely to cover:

- plastics - including packaging made from recycled plastics
- rubber
- paper and board
- glass
- metals and alloys
- wood and cork
- textiles
- waxes

The FSA is responsible for monitoring the safety of food contact materials in the UK, while the Food Contact Materials Unit carries out scientific research into detecting chemicals that have transferred to the food.

Documenting Food Packaging Materials

Food packaging materials - including those imported from outside the EU - should always have compliance documentation.

All food packaging businesses - apart from the primary materials producers - are required by law to establish and document good practices and procedures.

Understanding Irradiated Foods

Food irradiation is the processing of food by ionising radiation. The Food Irradiation (England) Regulations 2009 allow for four methods of irradiation:

- gamma rays from the radionuclide cobalt-60
- gamma rays from the radionuclide caesium-137
- X-rays generated from machine sources operated at or below an energy level of 5MeV (megaelectron volt)
- electrons generated from machine sources operated at or below an energy level of 10MeV

Irradiation is used to:

- destroy harmful bacteria - such as e-coli , salmonella, campylobacter
- delay fruit ripening
- stop potatoes and other vegetables from sprouting
- reduce spoilage of food to prolong shelf life
- rid food of organisms harmful to plants - such as fruit flies

The Food Irradiation (England) Regulations 2009 allow the irradiation of seven categories of foods:

- fruit
- vegetables
- cereals
- bulbs and tubers
- dried aromatic herbs, spices and vegetable seasonings
- fish and shellfish
- poultry

Thorough research has been carried out on food irradiation, and it has been found to be a safe and effective treatment method by the WHO, the UN Food and Agriculture Organisation and the European Community Scientific Committee for Food.

The FSA recognises irradiation as a safe processing technique and undertakes safety inspections of the food irradiation facilities in the UK, of which there is currently only one.

Effects of food additives

Food industry has continually created new chemicals to manipulate, preserve, and transform our food to feed the ever increasing population. With the use of chemicals, scientists are able to mimic natural flavors, color foods to make them look more "natural" or "fresh," preserve foods for longer and longer periods of time. There are even foods products that are made entirely from chemicals. Coffee creamers, sugar substitutes, and candies consist almost completely of artificial ingredients. Such manipulation of our food can have a profound effect on our body's unique biochemical balance. With advanced technology, our modern food industry's reliance on processing and additives continues to increase. This seemingly abundance of foodstuffs found in our supermarkets of today is deceiving our bodies by selling foods products that are chemically altered and designed to appeal to us. In this modern era foods, amongst other things (cosmetics & medications), represent a source of these toxins. Some studies have linked some food additives to hyperactivity in children. A recent British study found that children without a history of any hyperactive disorder showed varying degrees of hyperactivity after consuming fruit drinks with various levels of additives. Among those that were studied were: Sodium benzoate (E211), Tartrazine (E102), quinoline yellow (E104), Sunset yellow (E110), Carmosine (E122), Allura red (E129).

All of these additives are considered the "Dirty Dozen Food Additives" and are prohibited in countries like UK for foods marketed for children less than 36 months.

Food Safety Aspects in India

Introduction

Different Acts and orders existed in India to safeguard food safety and consumer interests. They were introduced to complement and supplement each other in achieving total food safety and quality. However due to variation in the specifications/standards in different Acts/Orders, and administration by different Departments and Ministries, there were implementation problems and a lack of importance given to safety standards over a period of time. The food industries were facing problems as different products were governed by different orders and ministries and the rules and regulations in the Country needed reorientation in its food regulation to emphasize and ensure food safety, food hygiene and food quality in an holistic manner. A new regulation was envisaged that would bring the different pieces of legislations pertaining to food safety under one roof and override the PFA, 1955 and various Quality Control Orders under Essential Commodities Act, 1955. The aim of such an endeavor was to ensure better coordination and integrate food safety controls across India to give highest level of health protection to the consumers. With this objective in vision t he Food Safety and Standards Act 2006 was introduced in India.

Food Safety and Standards Act 2006

The Food Safety and Standards Act 2006 was introduced to overcome these shortcomings and to give more importance to safety standards. This Act consolidates the laws relating to food and establishes the Food Safety and Standards Authority of India (FSSA) for laying down science-based standards for articles of food and to regulate their manufacture, storage, distribution, sale and import, to ensure availability of safe and wholesome food for human consumption.

This Act provides for the establishment of the FSSA which is an autonomous body under the Ministry of Health and Family Welfare, Government of India. FSSA's work programs ensure the provision of appropriate scientific, technical and administrative support for scientific committees and scientific panels, ensuring that the FSSA carries out its tasks in accordance with the requirements of its users, prepares statements of revenue and expenditure and executes the budget, while developing and maintaining contact with the Central Government and ensuring a regular dialogue with its relevant committees. The FSSA shall establish a Central Advisory Committee, and this committee shall advise the FSSA in drawing up proposals for the FSSA's work program, prioritization of work, identifying potential risks, pooling of knowledge and other functions specified by the regulations.

The FSSA also constitutes scientific panels and scientific committees to address various technical issues such as food additives, pesticides and antibiotics, genetically modified foods, functional foods, biological hazards, contaminants, labeling and methods of sampling. The Scientific Committee is responsible for providing scientific opinions to FSSA. Finally the FSSA is also responsible for regulating and monitoring the manufacture, processing, distribution, sale and import of food so as to ensure safe and wholesome food to consumers. The general principles to be followed by the Central Government, State Governments and FSSA while implementing the provisions of this Act shall be guided by the following seven principles:

1. The endeavour to achieve appropriate levels of protection of human life and health and protection of consumers' interests including fair practices in all kinds of food;

2. Carry out risk management based on risk assessment;

3. Adopt risk management measures necessary to ensure appropriate levels of health protection;

4. Measures adopted shall be proportionate and no more trade restrictions shall be imposed than required;

5. Measures adopted shall be revised within a reasonable period;

6. In case of suspected risks of the public consuming contaminated food, the FSSA shall take appropriate steps to inform the general public of the risk to health; and

7. If any lot of food fails to comply with food safety requirements it shall be presumed that the whole consignment fails to comply with these requirements.

Genetically modified foods, organic foods, functional foods, nutraceuticals and proprietory foods are regulated by this Act. Packaged foods, labelling requirements and advertising requirements are adequately covered along with import regulations for food articles.

There is a provision for the FSSA to establish various Scientific Panels such as:

- Food additives, flavours, processing aids, materials in contact with food;
- Pesticides and antibiotic residues;
- Genetically modified organisms and foods;
- Functional foods, nutraceuticles and foods for special dietary purposes;
- Biological hazards, other contaminants; and
- Food labelling and methods of sampling and analysis.

The Act has laid down certain broad principles for implementing the food safety, viz;

- to lay down food safety standards and to ensure fair trade practices while achieving an Appropriate Level of Protection (ALOP) of human life and health;
- for contaminants and hazards, to carry out risk analysis so as to ensure an appropriate level of protection to the consumers as well to see that such measures are least trade restrictive and are in accordance with SPS and TBT measures of WTO;
- wherever appropriate, food standards are to be specified on the basis of risk analysis;
- risk assessment is to be based on the available toxicological evaluation (e.g. JECFA) and extensive open and transparent discussion with all stakeholders, and the underlying principle is to ensure protection of consumers by preventing fraudulent, deceptive or unfair trade practices.

The Act also prescribes general provisions for articles of food:

- food additives / processing aids are to be added only in accordance with provisions / regulations under the Act;
- foods are not to contain any contaminants such as toxic metals, toxins, pesticide residues, antibiotics and veterinary drugs, in excess of limits prescribed under the regulation;
- regulations will be made for the manufacture, distribution or trade of any novel foods, GM foods, irradiated foods, organic foods, foods for special dietary uses, functional foods, nutraceuticals, health supplements, proprietary foods, etc.

The onus of safety of food production, processing, import, distribution and sale lies with the food business operator. The Commissioner of Food Safety of the state will implement rules under this Act at state level. The FSSA and the State Food Authorities will maintain a system of control, involving risk communication, food safety surveillance and other monitoring activities covering all stages of food business.

The FSSA is empowered to recognise any agency to conduct food safety audits which are a systematic and functionally independent examination of food safety measures based on food safety management systems consisting of Good Manufacturing Practices, Good Hygienic Practices, Hazard Analysis and Critical Control Points or any other such measures specified by regulation.

Food testing laboratories are required to be accredited by any accreditation agency so that the analytical results are reliable and consistent. The FSSA and State Food Safety Authorities are responsible for enforcement of this Act. Both shall monitor and verify that the relevant requirements of law are fulfilled by food business operators at all stages of food business. There is provision for food recall by the business operator if the food does not comply with the Act.

The Food Safety Authority in the State (Health Ministry) appoints a Commissioner of Food Safety, designated officers (district level) and food safety officers to implement the programmes under the provisions of this Act. The FSSIA will notify food laboratories and research institutions accredited by the National Accreditation Board for testing and calibration laboratories. It may also recognise more referral food laboratories by this Act.

This Act gives more importance for ensuring a very safe food product to consumers by providing quicker disposal of cases within the state. Punishments offered are very severe which would make the retailer/wholesaler be more cautious in their dealings. The standards for quality and safety laid down in this Act are harmonised standards and applicable throughout the country, and all other standards/specifications become null and void. This system provides for quicker corrective actions by the regulators as the problems are localised and traceable.

By 2030, people's consumption of chemicals will become negligible and will be taken over by consumption of natural, organic foods, nutraceuticals and functional foods, he said adding that the success of the pharma will be replicated by the nutra industry.

Chemical Hazards in Food

The purpose of this review is to give a broad overview of the types of chemical hazards that can occur in foodstuffs, to indicate how they arise and how they are measured and controlled. The examples given are representative of the many types of issues that the food industry has to face on a daily basis.

Origin of Chemical Hazards in Foods

It has been said that 99% of all toxins are naturally occurring, and also that all things are toxic at a sufficiently high concentration. Certainly, many food raw materials contain chemicals, which, if consumed in excess, might lead to health problems. Cooking and processing in general can remove or inactivate many chemicals (e.g. protease inhibitors, lectins) that are either directly toxic or inhibit digestion or absorption of nutrients. However, some chemicals have arisen as problems associated with food processing techniques developed in the last 100 years or so, e.g. *trans* fatty acids resulting from chemical hydrogenation of unsaturated fats, or 3-monochloropropanediol from the chemical hydrolysis of proteins. One recently publicised example of a process-derived chemical hazard in food is the formation of acrylamide in baked products. Although this has been occurring for centuries (e.g. in home baking of bread, potatoes and other starch-based foods), it was not discovered until 2002. A further area of concern is the migration of chemicals from packaging materials into foods, which has recently become a large problem for food manufacturers.

Other hazards are contaminants introduced by accident during the production of the food raw materials—sometimes these are unavoidable and sometimes they are to a greater or lesser extent caused by poor growing, postharvest or processing conditions. Mycotoxins produced by moulds on grain or nut products are one example; nitrate accumulation in leafy vegetables, and heavy metal accumulation in seafoods, are others.

Most difficult to predict or control are the chemical hazards introduced deliberately, generally as a consequence of fraudulent trading (e.g. addition of melamine to milk to boost the apparent protein content).

Chemical hazards can thus be divided into five broad categories:

- Inherent ('Natural') toxins;
- Natural and environmental contaminants;
- Process and storage-derived contaminants;
- Deliberately added contaminants; and
- Pesticides and veterinary residues.

Examples of Chemical Hazards

The examples below give a flavour of the many different chemicals that can be hazardous in food. They are chosen to give a broad picture of their nature, rather than to be exhaustive.

Natural Toxins

These chemicals occur as regular constituents of the food in question (e.g. lectins in kidney beans), or at increased levels as a response of the foodstuff to some sort of stress (e.g. glycoalkaloids in potatoes, an increased production of which can be stimulated when the tuber is exposed to light), and are inherent to the food raw material. There are also some instances of a processing regime potentially releasing a toxin from a non-toxic starting material (as occurs with cyanogenic glycosides in some canned stone fruits). The latter could be considered under the process-derived hazards category, but is essentially 'natural'. There are many types of natural toxins produced from many species of plants and the following examples serve to illustrate the importance of controlling the risk from these chemicals.

Lectins

Lectins occur in a wide variety of plants including beans of the Phaseolus genus (e.g. kidney beans and lima beans), broad beans, castor beans, soya beans, lentils, peas, field beans, peanuts, potatoes and cereals, as well as a range of non-food plants. In many cases the lectins have no or minimal toxic effect. Others are toxic to a greater or lesser extent, but in most cases normal cooking procedures eliminate this toxicity entirely, and consumption of moderate levels of most types of uncooked beans or peas will have no adverse effect. However, there are some specific exceptions, the most well known and significant of which (because of the way we consume them) is red kidney beans.

Raw kidney beans are significantly toxic due to the presence of lectins and must be cooked adequately before consumption. One form of wording suggested for the labelling of beans for sale is:

"After soaking overnight and throwing away the water, these beans should be boiled briskly for at least 10 minutes and then cooked until soft, otherwise they may cause stomach upsets. Never cook in a small casserole unless the beans have first been soaked and boiled in this way. Do not eat raw beans"

Glycoalkaloids

Potato glycoalkaloids are a good example of naturally occurring toxins that can and have caused problems when consumed in large quantities, but which we have learned to avoid without too much difficulty.

Potatoes contain two main glycoalkaloids, solanine and chaconine, with chaconine being the more toxic. Symptoms of acute poisoning can range from abdominal pain, vomiting and diarrhoea (similar to bacterial food poisoning) to confusion, fever, hallucination, paralysis, convulsions and occasionally death. There is an unofficial, but widely accepted safety limit of 200 mg glycoalkaloid/kg fresh potato. Levels of glycoalkaloids in modern varieties are usually well below this value, but they can exceed the limit under certain circumstances. The associated bitterness that accompanies these increases means that the chances of ingesting a toxic dose are small unless the bitterness has been masked with other highly flavoured ingredients.

Thus, although the chances of someone eating potatoes with high levels of glycoalkaloids are small, the possibility does exist, and hence the food industry must take precautions to eliminate the risk as far as is possible. Glycoalkaloids can only be made by the living potato tissue, and therefore will be halted by cooking and any other process that kills the tissue. However, they are heat stable and therefore preformed toxin will remain after processing. Glycoalkaloid levels in potatoes are highest in the flowers and in the sprouts on the tubers. Within the mass of the tuber itself, they are concentrated in the outer 2mm, so that unpeeled potato products are a higher risk than flesh-only products. Levels vary from one variety to another, and are generally higher in early varieties than in main crop varieties. Smaller potatoes tend to have higher levels than large potatoes, largely as a consequence of the increased surface area/volume ratio.

Increased levels arise through various stress factors, such as pest and disease damage, drought, waterlogging, and extremes of temperature. During postharvest handling, bruising, abrasion and other types of mechanical damage can all cause increases in levels, as can peeling (although the act of peeling will remove much of the glycoalkaoid content unless the peel is added back into the product). Light can also induce glycoalkaloid formation. Light also induces chlorophyll formation, causing the potatoes to turn green on the surface.

Oxalates

Oxalic acid and oxalates are widely distributed in plant foods, highest levels being found in spinach (0.3-1.2%), rhubarb (0.2-1.3%), tea (0.3-2.0%) and cocoa (0.5-0.9%). Although there is no question that the ingestion of sufficient oxalic acid as crystals or in solution can be fatal, there is considerable debate as to whether serious food poisoning from oxalate is usually due to food.

The eating of rhubarb leaves has been a well-known cause of illness for centuries. Rhubarb leaves contain high amounts of oxalate. However, the levels of oxalate in rhubarb stalks are sufficiently high that consumption of normal levels of rhubarb stalks will result in at least as much oxalate intake as from small to moderate amounts of leaves.

There is some debate as whether it is the oxalate in rhubarb leaves that is responsible for toxicity. Whatever the toxic principle, consumer perception is that rhubarb leaves are toxic, and hence consumer complaints about small fragments of leaves in canned rhubarb are well-known.

Cyanogenic glycosides

Many fruits and other plant foods contain compounds that have the potential to release cyanide. These compounds are usually glycosides, i.e. they consist of a sugar molecule linked to a cyanide group, usually indirectly through another component. The release of cyanide from these compounds occurs by enzymic hydrolysis, usually when the plant tissue is crushed or otherwise disrupted (allowing the active enzyme to reach the substrate), but it can also occur in the digestive system after the food has been eaten. Some plants are toxic because of their high levels of these compounds. Other foods are considered safe to consume, despite their having moderate levels of cyanogenic glycosides. The most well-known of these compounds is amygdalin, a cyanogenic glycoside first identified in bitter almonds, which on hydrolysis by an enzyme complex known as emulsin yields glucose, benzaldehyde and hydrogen cyanide.

Cassava or manioc is a staple food for large numbers of the world's population. It is the world's seventh largest food crop in terms of production area. The toxic potential of cassava has been known for hundreds of years, and traditional methods of food preparation from cassava have been developed to reduce cyanide content. These include leaching out the linamarin precursor, washing in running water before cooking (bruising of the cassava root during harvesting often results in considerable cyanide release), and boiling in uncovered pots so that the cyanide can evaporate. Fermentation also significantly reduces cyanogenic potential.

Trypsin inhibitors

There are substances which have the ability to inhibit the proteolytic activity of certain enzymes which are found throughout the plant kingdom. The most common of these are chemicals which inhibit the activity of the enzyme trypsin which is important for digestion of proteins in the stomach. Examples of plants containing trypsin inhibitors are Lima beans and soya beans. Most of the inhibitor molecules are proteins which are inactivated by heating, hence cooking is a key step to increasing the nutritional value of foods containing these inhibitors.

Natural and Environmental Contaminants

All plants and animals during their lifetime will accumulate various chemicals from their environment. Some of these chemicals, if they are accumulated at high enough levels, might be of toxicological significance to us when we eat the food. Specific examples that are of concern are nitrates in leafy vegetables, heavy metals in various foods, and specific toxins in shellfish. In many cases, the best way to control levels of these unwanted substances is to control the environment in which the food is produced. However, this is generally a long-term control measure and more immediate steps have to be taken to protect human health. As many of the toxins can not be 'processed out', the short term controls are usually based around the setting of maximum permitted levels, and the removal from the supply chain of food that does not meet the required standard. These contaminants are divided below into 'natural' (of biological origin) and 'environmental', but they are linked in that the food plant or animal acquires them from its surroundings during its growth.

'Natural' contaminants

Mycotoxins: Mycotoxins are a group of chemically diverse naturally occurring substances produced by a range of filamentous fungi or moulds. They have toxic effects on both humans and animals ranging from acute toxicity and death, through reduced egg and milk production, lack of weight gain, impairment or suppression of immune function to tumour formation, cancers and other chronic diseases. The mycotoxins of greatest concern are produced by mould species from three main genera–*Aspergillus*, *Penicillium* and *Fusarium*. These are mainly storage moulds affecting commodities such as nuts, dried fruits and cereals. The moulds grow and produce toxins when commodities are stored incorrectly–usually at too high moisture levels. Specific mycotoxins of greatest concern are detailed below:

- *Aflatoxins:* Aflatoxins are produced mainly by some strains of *Aspergillus flavus* and most, if not all, strains of *A. parasiticus*. There are four main aflatoxins, B1, B2, G1 and G2, plus two additional ones that are significant, M1 and M2. The aflatoxins are potent liver toxins in most animals and carcinogens in some, with aflatoxin B1 being the most toxic and carcinogenic. Mould growth and aflatoxin production are greatest in warm temperatures and high humidity, particularly in tropical and sub-tropical regions, mainly on corn (maize), peanuts, cottonseed and tree nuts.

- *Ochratoxins:* Ochratoxins are a group of related compounds produced by *Aspergillus ochraceus* and related species, as well as *Penicillium verrucosum*. The main toxin in the group is Ochratoxin A, which causes liver damage in rats, dogs and pigs. Ochratoxins are also teratogenic to mice, rats and chicken embryos, and are now thought to be carcinogenic in humans.

- *Patulin:* Patulin is produced by numerous *Penicillium* and *Aspergillus* species and by *Byssochlamys nivea*. However, the most common producer of patulin is *Penicillium expansum*, which occurs commonly in rotting apples, as a result of which patulin has frequently been found in commercial apple juice. Patulin is toxic to many biological systems, including bacteria, mammalian cell cultures, higher plants and animals. Its role in causing animal and human disease is unclear, but it is believed to be carcinogenic.

- *Cyclopiazonic acid (CPA):* Cyclopiazonic acid (CPA) is produced by several moulds which occur on agricultural products or are used in some food fermentations. It also occurs naturally in infected corn (maize) and peanuts. It affects rats, dogs, pigs and chickens, where it may cause anorexia, weight loss, diarrhoea, pyrexia, dehydration and other symptoms. Organs affected include liver, spleen, kidneys, and pancreas. It has the ability to chelate metal ions such as calcium, magnesium and iron, which may be an important mechanism of toxicity.

- *Zearalenone:* Zearalenone (also known as F-2 toxin) is produced by several *Fusarium* species. It occurs naturally in high moisture corn (maize) in late autumn and winter, mainly from the growth of *F. culmorum* in Northern Europe and *F. graminearum* in North America. Production of this and other *Fusarium* toxins is favoured by high humidity and low temperatures, conditions which often occur in temperate regions during autumn harvest. It has been found in mouldy hay, high-moisture corn (maize), corn infected before harvest and pelleted feed rations, so it is an important contaminant of animal feed. The involvement of zearalenone in human disease is unconfirmed, but it is regarded as an endocrine disruptor and hence a potential hazard.

- *Tricothecenes:* The tricothecenes are a group of over 20 chemically related toxins produced by several *Fusarium* species. These include deoxynivalenol (DON), T-2 toxin, diacetoxyscirpenal, neosolaniol, nivalenol, diacetylnivalenol, HT-2 toxin and fusarenon X. The most commonly occurring of these is deoxynivalenol or DON, which causes vomiting in animals, hence its other name of vomitoxin. It may also be a teratogen and has been found in commodities such as corn (maize) and wheat as well as some processed food products.

- *Fumonisins:* The fumonisins are a group of compounds mainly produced by *Fusarium moniliforme* and *F. proliferatum*. They have been linked to several diseases, including liver cancer and oesophagal cancer in humans.

- *Moniliformin:* Moniliformin is so called because it was first thought to be produced by *F. moniliforme* isolated from corn (maize). However, it has since been shown to be produced mainly by other species of *Fusarium*. It has been shown to be highly toxic in experimental animals, causing rapid death without severe cellular damage.

- *Other mycotoxins:* Other mycotoxins include sterigmatocystin, reported in green coffee, mouldy wheat and the rind of some hard cheese, citrinin, penicillic acid, mycophenolic acid, β-nitropropionioc acid, tremorgens (penitrem) and rubratoxin.

Shellfish toxins: There are several types of shellfish poisoning including neurotoxic (NSP), diarrhoetic (DSP), paralytic (PSP), amnesic (ASP), and ciguaterra fish poisoning (CFP). Shellfish toxins are not produced by the shellfish themselves, but are accumulated through the ingestion of planktonic dinoflagellates in the diet of the shellfish. The term shellfish generally refers to both marine crustaceans (lobsters, crab, shrimp etc), and molluscs. However, it is the bivalve molluscs – oysters, mussels, clams and scallops – which accumulate these algae by filter feeding, that are the major areas of concern. See Lawley *et al.* (2008) for a review of these different types.

Paralytic shellfish poisoning is a global problem which has increased dramatically since the 1970s. The most significant toxins in PSP are saxitoxin and its derivatives, though the exact composition differs amongst algal species and amongst regions of occurrence. Generally the population density of such algae is not sufficiently high to cause problems, but on occasion when environmental conditions (nutrients, temperature, sunlight etc) are favourable, population explosions called 'algal blooms' occur. Problems can arise if the algal bloom is of a species which produces toxins, such as the *Alexandrium* genus. Such toxins can then accumulate within the flesh of the filter-feeding bivalve at levels which cause disorder in humans after consumption. The toxins can persist within shellfish at dangerous levels for weeks or months after the algae are no longer present in the waters. Seafood containing saxitoxin looks and tastes normal, and cooking or steaming only partially destroys toxins. Therefore one of the most effective methods in preventing outbreaks of PSP is the detection of the toxins before the shellfish are harvested.

Amnesic shellfish poisoning is also caused by algae in the diet of shellfish; domoic acid is the principal toxin and is produced by various species, but the diatom *Pseudo-nitzschia* is the primary source. It can work its way up through the food chain, so illness can result from consumption of other contaminated seafood. As with PSP, decontamination of foodstuffs is not effective and detection of areas where the contamination exists is the best method of preventing problems.

Ciguatera fish poisoning is an intoxication caused by the consumption of coral reef fish which feed on certain marine plankton which contain specific toxins. It is one of the commonest marine food poisonings worldwide and a significant health problem with as many as 50,000 cases occurring each year. Toxins accumulate as they move up the food chain so that the larger carnivorous fish are more toxic. Symptoms are extremely varied and include gastrointestinal and cardiovascular problems, though most patients recover. The toxins are not easy to detect so the only effective control option is to avoid consumption of susceptible fish species.

'Environmental' contaminants

Dioxins / Polychlorinated biphenyls (PCBs): PCBs and dioxins are persistent contaminants with a wide range of chemical structures. They have been found in soil, water, sediment, plants and animal tissue in all parts of the world. Dioxins and PCBs are heterocyclic organic molecules, with PCBs being chlorinated. They have long half-lives in the environment and many have been reported to have toxicological effects in humans. PCBs and dioxins are man-made chemicals used by industry and their release to the environment is generally through by-products of fires and by some manufacturing processes. Their widespread environmental occurrence means that PCBs and dioxins are present in virtually all foods, which is the main route to human exposure. The highest concentrations are in fatty foods such as oily fish and the main sources of dioxins in the diet are meat and milk. Levels accumulate as they move through the food chain.

Control options are based on prohibiting the use of dioxins and PCBs by industry and hence their release into the environment and the EU put into force a ban on the use of most PCBs from 1978. Legislative limits have been imposed within the EU for many foods (Regulation EC 1881/2006) as have methods for sampling (EC 1883/2006). No limits exist in the USA although the FDA considers all detectable levels to be of concern.

Polycyclic aromatic hydrocarbons: Polycyclic aromatic hydrocarbons (PAHs) are a group of compounds comprising two or more fused aromatic rings. Many individual PAHs exist, the most simple of which is naphthalene. A variety of toxic properties have been related to PAH exposure, including the capacity to produce genotoxic and carcinogenic effects in mammals.

PAHs are found in petroleum and coal, and can also be formed by the incomplete combustion of these and other organic materials. These compounds have been detected in air, water, soil and foods. Foods may become contaminated through direct environmental exposure, migration from packaging material or during thermal processing of food, e.g. baking, grilling, frying and smoking.

The occurrence of PAHs in fruit, vegetables and cereals is primarily due to soil and air exposure. Although levels detected in foods of animal origin tend to be low, high levels have been recorded in smoked meats and animals farmed on contaminated land. Shellfish can accumulate PAHs from oils spilt by grounded tankers or from waste oils which have been incorrectly disposed of. PAHs can also be formed during the heating and drying processes which allow combustion products to come into contact with the food substance. Direct fire-drying and heating processes used during the production of food oils can result in high levels of PAHs.

The complexity and number of individual PAH compounds means that it is not easy to produce specific limits for regulation of levels. Benzo(a)pyrene has been used as a marker for PAH levels and limits for this have been set by the European Commission (EC 1881/2006) for a range of foods, although there is currently discussion about widening this to include other marker compounds.

Specific foods of concern are fish which are farmed in oil-contaminated waters, fats and oils including coca butter, and smoked foods. Refining processes are generally ineffective in eliminating PAHs from foods so the main control measure is to limit their production during processing and to screen out foods known to contain high levels.

Heavy metals: Heavy metals are those with a high atomic mass, including, for example, mercury, cadmium, arsenic and lead, although other metals (e.g. tin) may also be included within this category of contaminant. They are natural components which originate from the earth's crust and are found all over the world. They are toxic in low amounts and have been recognised as a health hazard for many years. There are other routes for metal contamination of products such as migration from packaging (e.g. antimony from plastic bottles, and tin in canned food).

Metals can occur in a variety of foodstuffs of plant and animal origin. Mostly, they arise indirectly in foodstuffs from the environment, e.g. they are in soil that the crop is grown in, or on the grass that a cow is eating or in the water in which a fish is living. As such, once they become incorporated into the food they cannot be removed. There is a risk to crops and animals themselves from metals in the environment (e.g. they can kill plants and reduce yields) and to humans from eating crop and livestock products. Metals which can be particularly harmful to animals and man include lead, cadmium, arsenic, mercury, copper, selenium and molybdenum. These elements can accumulate in primary products that are otherwise growing satisfactorily, but still affect animals and man.

Of particular relevance to crop products as food raw materials are lead and cadmium. Lead is a widespread environmental pollutant, deriving from such human activities as lead mining, smelting and processing, and burning of fossil fuels. The main route of crop contamination is via uptake from the soil. Soil contamination with both lead and cadmium is primarily from aerial deposition.

Maximum levels for heavy metal contaminants have been established in many countries so it is important to be aware of the legislative limits which apply if exporting. Each metal has a specific limit which is food-type-dependent and is a reflection on both the occurrence of the metal in that food and its toxicological effect. Control of raw materials is the only mechanism for ensuring that levels do not become unsafe. A particular problem has been lead and cadmium in cereals and close monitoring of levels in flour mills and maltings has been necessary to ensure that limits are not exceeded. The legislation in this area is constantly changing so food manufacturers need to keep abreast of proposed new limits and use horizon scanning methods to maintain vigilance for problems.

Nitrates: In general nitrates in agriculture are considered more of a hazard to the environment and water than in foods. However, nitrate intake from water and food has received considerable publicity because of its role in methaemoglobinaemia in infants and its reported implication in various types of cancer. Methaemoglobinaemia is caused by nitrate being reduced, under the conditions found in the infant stomach, to nitrite, which then combines with haemoglobin in the bloodstream. Methaemoglobinaemia, sometimes known as the "blue baby syndrome", can be fatal.

The possible involvement of nitrate in cancer is via its role in the generation of nitrosamines. Nitrosamines are known to be very potent carcinogens and are produced by the reaction of nitrate, when reduced to nitrite, with certain nitrogenous compounds found in proteinaceous substrates. Whilst nitrosamines can be formed in the body, the link between high nitrate exposure and the incidence of cancer is often not clear.

Nitrates in food might, therefore, have some adverse health effect, but the levels in most crops are not generally considered a food safety hazard. However, green leafy vegetables usually contain higher levels of nitrate than most other foods, and maximum levels have been set in the EU and by Codex for nitrates in spinach and fresh lettuce. There are a number of factors which affect the levels of nitrates in these crops, including nitrate availability in the soil, seasonal variations, applications of nitrate fertilisers shortly before harvest and environmental influences.

Fluoride: Fluoride can be found dissolved in waters at high levels in certain parts of the world, and in some cases is above the WHO maximum limit. There is some controversy as to whether the presence of fluoride is a benefit or a threat to human health. The benefits for protection of dental health are well known and in fact fluoride is routinely added to water and/or toothpaste in many countries. There are also reports that fluoride can be a hazard to human health with links to cancer, bone health and endocrine disruption having been cited. There is no doubt that the debate regarding fluoridation of public water supplies will continue given the emotion regarding mass medication. Information regarding the hazardous effects of long term ingestion of fluorides is required to determine whether this policy is acceptable.

Process-derived contaminants

The production of toxic chemicals in foodstuffs through processing is a recently discovered phenomenon, although historically these chemicals will have always been present. The first three examples below serve to show how unexpected contaminants may arise. In addition, the contamination of food with chemicals from packaging, pesticide and veterinary medicine applications could also loosely be described as process-derived.

Acrylamide: In 2002, Swedish scientists unexpectedly discovered acrylamide in food when they were carrying out a study into occupational acrylamide exposure. As part of the study, people who were not believed to have been exposed to acrylamide were included as controls and were also found to have significant acrylamide in their blood; further research determined that this unknown source was food. Subsequent research has now revealed that acrylamide is formed in food by traditional cooking methods such as baking, frying and roasting (i.e. high temperatures). It is formed at highest levels in starch-containing foods and varies widely among different products and between production batches of the same foods. Examples of foods most at risk are potato products such as crisps and chips, coffee, savoury snacks such as cracker type biscuits, and bread and other cereal products.

Considerable research has been carried out to understand the mechanism of acrylamide formation and a major international project took place bringing together scientists from all over the world (HEATOX). The output from this project formed the basis of industry guidelines aimed at minimising the formation of acrylamide during food processing. This guide recommends measures such as avoiding sources of asparagine (such as certain potato varieties), avoiding long cooking times and high cooking temperatures, and replacing ammonium bicarbonate as a processing aid in bread.

Although acrylamide is a known carcinogen, it is still unclear whether it has any major effect on health when consumed in food. It is certainly known that at high levels it has neurotoxic and genotoxic effects though these are unlikely at levels found in most foods. The Joint FAO/WHO Expert Committee on Food Additives (JECFA) has recommended that the food industry should use the guidelines in the CIAA 'Toolbox' to reduce acrylamide levels to as low as possible in critical food groups. Although there is not yet specific legislation, or maximum levels for acrylamide, there is a comprehensive programme on monitoring in many countries. It is possible that in future limits could be set for food manufacturers so the food industry is keen to demonstrate that it is doing all it can to reduce levels where possible through good manufacturing practice.

Chloropropanols: Chloropropanols are a group of chemical contaminants, the most notable of which is 3-monochloropropane-1,2-diol (3-MCPD). 3-MCPD can occur in foods and food ingredients at low levels as a result of processing, migration from packaging materials during storage, or domestic cooking. It has been found in a variety of foods, such as cooked/cured meats and fish, cheese, bread and toast, malt extracts and baked products, as well as in teabag paper, tissue and sausage casings. A major area of concern is its occurrence in food following the reaction between hydrochloric acid and lipids, particularly in foods processed at high temperatures such as soy sauce. In laboratory animal studies it has been shown that 3-MCPD is a carcinogen; it was originally classified as a genotoxic carcinogen, but more recent studies suggest that there is a lack of evidence of *in vivo* genotoxicity. However, the issue with 3-MCPD has meant that industry has looked to use enzymic methods of producing HVP rather than acid hydrolysis. Control of processing conditions and selection of ingredients is the main strategy being used by industry to control levels of chloropropanols. The level of 3-MCPD in the EU is prescribed by EC 1881/2006 though for other chloropropanols there are no limits and manufacturers are requested to reduce levels as far as is technically possible.

Furans: Furan is a colourless, volatile liquid used in some chemical manufacturing industries, which was occasionally found in foods. Recently, it has been discovered that furan is formed in some foods more commonly than previously thought. This discovery is probably a result of our ability to detect compounds at exceedingly low levels rather than a change in the presence of furan. It is believed that furan forms in food during traditional heat treatment techniques, such as cooking, bottling, and canning. Furan has been found in canned or bottled foods such as soups, sauces, beans, pasta meals and baby foods.

Packaging migrants: There is a risk with any packaging material that its components may be transferred in some way to the food that it is surrounding. In most cases, the level of transfer is extremely slight and the components transferred are innocuous. However, there are instances where a realistic hazard exists and must be controlled. There are no official internationally agreed guidelines, but in the EU there is a general requirement that food packaging components must not be transferred into food during its normal shelf-life to the detriment of the food (i.e. to pose a health risk, or to adversely affect the quality of the food – its flavour, texture or appearance).

Transfer of monomers and additives such as plasticisers in plastic packaging materials are the major area of concern. In the EU, there is a list of approved monomers and of additives that can be used in food contact plastic materials (this covers all contact with food, not just packaging materials) and also limits for the migration of these constituents into food. The general limit for containers and sealing devices is 60 mg per kg of food. For other contact materials it is 10 mg/dm2. To determine whether a particular plastic formulation meets these criteria, there are four model simulants that are used in laboratory trials to assess the plastic's properties. These are: distilled water; a 3% aqueous solution of acetic acid; 10% ethanol in water solution (or greater, if the alcoholic beverage in question has a higher alcohol content); and rectified olive oil. The regulations specify which simulants should be used for each category of food. In general, there are no simulants listed for dried foods, which can be considered to not take up plastics constituents from contact materials.

Tin: Tin can be considered to be a specific type of packaging-derived contaminant. Although there is no evidence that excess tin intake has any long-term health effects, some studies have shown that intake of high concentrations (above about 250 ppm) may cause short-term gastrointestinal problems. For most foods, this is of no significance, but for foods packed in cans with some unlacquered tinplate, high levels can sometimes occur. Tin dissolution in unlacquered tinplate cans is essential in that it confers electrochemical protection to the iron, which makes up the structural component of the can and so maintains the can's integrity. Without it, the can would quickly become corroded by the contents of the can; this could cause serious discoloration and off-flavours in the product and swelling of the can. Tin is also involved in maintaining product quality (it helps prevent undesirable colour changes amongst other things, by mopping up any residual oxygen left in the headspace), so there is an advantage in some products of having some exposed (i.e. unlacquered) tinplate. As tin dissolution tends to be accelerated by oxygen, for products where exposed tin is considered to be beneficial, the base, lid and ends of the can may be lacquered, with the rest being unlacquered.

Tin pick-up is normally relatively slow and does not give rise to excessive levels in the product within its shelf-life. However, certain natural variations within the product can cause problems.

Deliberately added contaminants

There is no limit to what chemical contaminants might be deliberately added to foods during manufacture in order to cause harm to the consumer. In most cases, however, the aim is not to cause harm, but to defraud for financial gain. However, potential harm can still result, as evidenced from two of the examples given below.

Illegal or unauthorised dyes: The Sudan I-IV group of chemicals are synthetic azo dyes which have been historically used in industry to colour products such as shoe polish, automotive paints and petroleum derivatives. They are not permitted food colours.

During the summer of 2003 it became apparent that chilli powder and related products in the European market, and originating from India, were contaminated with Sudan I-IV at levels between 2.8 and 3500 mg/kg. Although the Sudan dyes were deemed to be toxic, the levels at which they were found were probably not a major health concern because of the very low concentrations in which they were detected in final products. However, such dyes are not permitted for food use and were being added to the chilli powder in order to make it appear to be of better quality than it actually was. The chilli powder was incorporated into various sauces, which were themselves used as ingredients in a range of ready meals. With the significant dilution effect of this, analysing the final food for Sudan dyes became a problem, as the levels involved were now very small. A major traceability program had to be launched to identify and remove all affected products. This involved the withdrawal of over 1000 products, at a very significant cost to the food industry. However, with laboratories now routinely testing for the presence of the Sudan dyes, the contamination spread progressively to a wide range of other dyes in order to avoid detection, including Para Red, Rhodamine B, Orange II, Red G, Butter Yellow and Metanil Yellow. As well as many dyes which were not permitted for any food use, these new colours included some, such as Bixin, which were permitted in some foods, but not in the spices to which they were being added.

Melamine: Melamine is an industrial chemical found in plastics. It can be combined with formaldehyde to produce melamine resin, a very durable thermosetting plastic used in Formica, and melamine foam, a polymeric cleaning product. The end products include countertops, dry erase boards, fabrics, glues, house wares, guitar saddles, guitar nuts, and flame retardants. Melamine is one of the major components in Pigment Yellow 150, a colorant in inks and plastics. It is also used in the manufacture of plasticisers for concrete.

In 2007 it was discovered in the USA that melamine had been fraudulently added to wheat gluten and rice protein from China, which was subsequently used in pet foods. This was a widespread problem and resulted in a petfood recall initiated by manufacturers who had found that their products had been contaminated. Further vegetable protein imported from China was later implicated. It was claimed that some of the animals that had eaten the contaminated food had become ill, although melamine was not previously believed to have been significantly toxic at low doses.

Melamine has no nutritional value but because it is high in nitrogen (66% by mass), its addition to food makes it appear to have more protein than it actually does and so meet required contractual obligations. Standard tests such as the Kjeldahl and Dumas tests estimate protein levels by measuring the nitrogen content, so values obtained can be increased by adding nitrogen-rich compounds such as melamine.

By early 2006, melamine production in mainland China was reported to be in "serious surplus". In September 2008, it was discovered that melamine was present in infant milk powder produced in China. Six infants are believed to have died as a result, and over 300,000 were reported to have been made ill. Traces of melamine were subsequently found in other dairy-based products in the region. Melamine has also been detected in other products, including eggs, originating in China. Actions taken in 2008 by the Government of China have reduced the practice of adulteration, with the goal of eliminating it. Court trials began in December 2008 for six people linked to the scandal and ended in January 2009 with those convicted being sentenced to death and executed.

Melamine is described as being "Harmful if swallowed, inhaled or absorbed through the skin. Chronic exposure may cause cancer or reproductive damage. Eye, skin and respiratory irritant." However, the short-term lethal dose is on a par with common table salt with an LD50 of more than 3 grams per kilogram of bodyweight. However, it is thought that when melamine and cyanuric acid are absorbed together into the bloodstream, they concentrate and interact in the urine-filled microtubules in the kidneys, then crystallise and form large numbers of round, yellow crystals, which block and damage the renal cells that line the tubes, causing the kidneys to malfunction. Toxicology studies conducted after recalls of contaminated pet food concluded that the combination of melamine and cyanuric acid in the diet does lead to acute renal failure in cats and rats.

The European Union set a standard for acceptable human consumption of melamine at 0.5 milligrams per kg of body mass (reduced to 0.2 mg per kg in April 2010). Member States of the European Union are required under Commission Decision 2008/757/EC to ensure that all composite products containing at least 15% of milk product, originating from China, are systematically tested before import into the Community and that all such products which are shown to contain melamine in excess of 2.5 mg/kg are immediately destroyed.

More recently there has been concern about the migration of melamine from food contact materials. In addition, there have been reports of melamine residues as a result of the use of cyromazine, an insecticide derived from melamine.

Spanish toxic oil syndrome: This incident started as a deliberate act of fraudulent adulteration. A large volume of rapeseed oil had been treated with aniline to downgrade it for industrial use. Some unscrupulous traders decided to refine, decolourise and deodorise this oil, mix it with other oils, package and label it as olive oil, and then illegally introduced it on to the Spanish market. Unfortunately, the oil contained a highly toxic substance formed in a reaction between the aniline and fatty acids in the oil, resulting in the deaths of up to 600 people and over 20,000 people affected by health problems.

Pesticides and veterinary residues

Pesticides: Pesticides include chemical and biological products specifically designed to control pests, weeds and diseases, particularly in the production of food. These include insecticides, fungicides, herbicides, rodenticides and molluscicides.

Pesticides are licensed for use against specific target organisms, and their use and application are strictly regulated to control the risks to the operator involved in applying them, and the surrounding environment, and to prevent significant residues being left in or on the food. Regulations include restrictions on the target organisms the chemical may be used against, the crops on which it may be used, the concentrations that may be applied and the number of applications permitted. There are strict limits on the levels of pesticide residues allowed in food and this is closely monitored by regulatory authorities worldwide.

Pesticides can be classified by target organism, chemical structure, and physical state. They can be classed as inorganic, synthetic, or biological (biopesticides). Biopesticides include microbial pesticides and biochemical pesticides. Plant-derived pesticides include the pyrethroids, rotenoids, and nicotinoids.

Many pesticides can be grouped into chemical families. The main insecticide families include organochlorines, organophosphates and carbamates. These operate by disrupting the sodium / potassium balance of the nerve fibre, forcing the nerve to transmit continuously. Toxicities of these chemicals vary greatly, but they have been largely phased out because of their persistence and potential to bioaccumulate. The organochlorines have been largely replaced by the organophosphates and carbamates. Both of these operate through inhibiting the enzyme acetylcholinesterase, allowing acetylcholine to transfer nerve impulses indefinitely and causing a variety of symptoms such as weakness or paralysis. However, organophosphates are quite toxic to vertebrates, and they have in some cases been replaced by the less toxic carbamates. Prominent families of herbicides include phenoxy and benzoic acid herbicides (e.g. 2,4-D), triazines (e.g. atrazine), ureas (e.g. diuron), and chloroacetanilides (e.g. alachlor). Phenoxy compounds are designed as selective weedkillers to kill broadleaved weeds rather than grasses. The phenoxy and benzoic acid herbicides function in a similar way to plant growth hormones, and cause cells to grow without normal cell division, affecting the plant's nutrient transport system. Triazines interfere with photosynthesis. Many commonly used pesticides such as glyphosate are not included in these families.

In the UK, there is a national monitoring program overseen by the Pesticides Residues Committee, which measures the levels of pesticide residues in a wide range of foods, to check that they are within legal and safe limits. The limits apply both to food produced both in the UK and that imported from elsewhere. A number of different statutory bodies are involved in regulating which pesticides may be used and how. There are particularly strict limits on the levels of pesticides allowed in infant formulae and manufactured baby foods.

Veterinary residues: The use of medicines used to treat animals raised for food is regulated in a similar manner to that for pesticides used on food crops.

There are a wide variety of chemicals for different uses, including:

- antimicrobials such as sulphadiazine, enrofloxacin, ciprofloxacin, chlortetracycline, amoxicillin and oxytetracycline used to control bacterial diseases;

- pain-killers and anti-inflammatory medicines such as NSAIDs, including ibuprofen and phenylbutazone;

- dips to control external parasites, including organochlorine or organophosphorus insecticides (see above);

- wormers to control internal parasites, such as ivermectin;

- coccidiostats to control protozoal diseases, particularly in poultry, such as nicarbazin; and

- steroids such as boldenone.

How Are Maximal Limits Set?

As can be seen from the above examples, there are a variety of chemical hazards that could enter food. Some of these are unpredictable (e.g. those that are deliberately added), but most can be, and are, controlled. The main route for this is Good Manufacturing Practice and monitoring of environmental conditions and the quality of incoming ingredients and raw materials. However, part of the control at a national or international level may be in the form of the setting of maximum legal limits. What these limits are and how they are determined may vary from one part of the world to another, depending on specific circumstances, but in general three main areas are taken into consideration:

- Toxicity evidence: How toxic is the contaminant believed to be and how sound is the evidence for this belief?

- Good Manufacturing Practice: What is technologically achievable and how costly is it?

- Analytical capability: What are the limits of detection or quantification?

In all instances, safety is the primary concern, and maximum limits are usually set at about 100 times below the level at which a toxic effect is noted. However, maximum limits to control contaminant levels are only meaningful if they can be monitored by analysis (see below). In addition, even if a contaminant is only mildly toxic, it may be possible to reduce levels to well below the toxicity / 100 threshold by Good Manufacturing Practice. This approach is taken with many pesticides, where good agricultural practice (including correct application regimes and suitable intervals between application and harvesting) will result in no remaining residues. Maximum levels are therefore set at the 'limit of detection (LOD)' or 'limit of quantification (LOQ)'.

The maximum limit for a chemical will often be different for different food types – and there may well be a limited number of foods for which a maximum limit is set. It may be unnecessary to specify a maximum limit in cases where the chemical would not be expected to be found in the food. In contrast, it may very difficult to limit a chemical in some food types, and so higher limits are set, based on what is realistically achievable (bearing in mind that safety is still the over-riding factor). Nitrates provide a good example of this. In Europe, high nitrate levels are only a significant issue in leafy vegetables (spinach and lettuce), and it is these products for which limits have been set. However, levels will vary depending on growing conditions and season, and so different maxima have been set for different situations. These are typically in the range 2000-3000 ppm.

Codex Standards

The Codex Alimentarius Commission has set maximum and guideline levels for the following chemical hazards that are an inherent risk in certain foods. The figures given are typical but may vary in some cases depending on product type and whether consumed raw or further processed. In particular the levels set for foods for infants and young children are often much lower than those for the general population. The figures given are merely for illustration; for any individual contaminant in a particular foodstuff, the original text should be consulted.

Mycotoxins

Aflatoxins: 15 µg/kg in peanuts; 0.5 µg/kg M1 in milk;

Patulin: (50µg/kg in apple juice).

Heavy metals

Arsenic : typically 0.1 mg/kg;
Cadmium: typically 0.05-0.2 mg/kg;
Lead: typically 0.1-1 mg/kg;
Mercury: 0.001 mg/kg in natural mineral water; 0.1 mg/kg in food grade salt;
Methylmercury: 0.5 mg/kg in fish − 1mg/kg in predatory fish;
Tin: 150 mg/kg in canned beverages; 250 mg/kg in canned fruit and vegetables.

Radionuclides

1-10,000 Bq/kg, depending on individual radionuclide − generally 10-fold lower in infant foods.

Others

Plastic monomers: typically 60 mg/kg of food or 10 mg/dm2 of package surface;

Acrylonitrile: 0.02 mg/kg;

Vinyl chloride monomer: 0.01mg/kg.

EU Standards

As a comparison, in the EU the following have been set:

Nitrates

Typically 2000-4500 mg/kg.

Mycotoxins

Aflatoxins: typically 4-15 µg/kg in total; 0.05 µg/kg M1 in milk;

Ochratoxin A: typically 2-10 µg/kg;

Patulin: 50 µg/kg in apple juice; 25 µg/kg in solid apple products;

Deoxynivalenol: typically 500-1750µg/kg;

Zearalenone: typically 50-200 µg/kg;

Fumonisins: 200-2000 µg/kg.

Metals

Lead: 0.02-1.5 mg/kg;

Cadmium: 0.05-1 mg/kg;

Mercury: 0.5-1 mg/kg;

Tin: 100 mg/kg in canned beverages; 200 mg/kg in other canned foods'

Chloropropanols

3-MCPD: 20 µg/kg in HVP and soy sauce.

Dioxins and PCBs

Usually picogram levels per gram of fat.

Polycyclic aromatic hydrocarbons

Benzo[a]pyrene: 1-10 µg/kg.

In addition, there are limits for many components of plastic packaging materials.

Analytical Approaches

As mentioned above, robust analytical methods are essential if the occurrence of chemical hazards in food is to be monitored and controlled. The type of method used will depend primarily on the chemical concerned, as well as the levels likely to be present and the food matrix.

Analysts have at their disposal a wider range of analytical techniques than ever before, and the sophistication of many of these would have been almost unimaginable just a few decades ago. This means that the analyst can now measure lower levels of a wide range of compounds in many different sample types. But it also means that the analyst has to be careful about the approach taken. Getting the right result requires the correct approach – and this includes using the right method of analysis.

A method of analysis typically involves several stages, and can involve a combination of techniques. Following sample receipt and the associated administrative requirements, the sample may need to be pre-treated (e.g. ground or blended), before the analyte is extracted (e.g. by solvent extraction). This latter stage may involve an initial crude extraction, followed by a purification stage (e.g. on an affinity chromatography column). Only then can the analyte be measured. Following analysis, the results have to be correctly interpreted and reported. In many cases, the extraction and/or purification stages are combined with the actual analytical stages, as happens with liquid or gas chromatography techniques linked with mass spectrometry.

Given the breadth of chemical hazards that might be present in food, the variability in their nature, and the many different types of food matrices, it is impossible to describe in any detail the types of analytical techniques that could be used.

In some cases it is possible to analyse many related chemicals in one sweep - screening. This is possible for a wide range of pesticides, for example, and for some of the illegal dyes. In many other cases targeted analysis is required, i.e. a specific procedure for an individual chemical.

When looking to analyse any chemical hazard in food (or indeed any chemical), there are a few basic points to note:

- Purpose of the analysis – it is important for those commissioning the analysis to be clear about the reasons for the analysis and how the result is to be used.

- Sampling – samples should be representative of the product being analysed. Once taken, the samples should be handled, stored and prepared properly, so that they are not altered in any way that would affect the analysis.

- Method suitability – the analytical method has to be fit for purpose; even if a method has been devised for the specific hazard in question, it may have to be adapted or modified for a particular foodstuff or to take into account other chemicals present that may interfere with the analysis.

- Validation – following on from the above, the method, if it is new or modified, will have to be validated, i.e. tested to show that it works.

- Quality control and standardization – although the method itself has been shown to be fit for purpose, there needs to be evidence that it can produce consistent results over a period of time and in the hands of different analysts.

- Measurement uncertainty – no method will ever give exactly the right result all the time; in fact, in any analysis the result obtained will only ever be an approximation (adequately close, if the method is suitable) to the 'true' answer. It is important to understand where the potential sources of error might arise, and which are the most significant, when interpreting the results.

Preventing Chemical Safety Breakdowns in the Food Chain

HACCP

The most effective and efficient way of minimising the chances of chemical (and any other) safety issues arising in the food chain is through the use of HACCP (Hazard Analysis and Critical Control Points) systems. In the EU, it is a requirement throughout the industry to use HACCP-based systems to ensure food safety. In essence this means identifying which chemicals may be a problem in a particular food, and the measures to limit (or eliminate) their occurrence or remove them. It is then a case of monitoring and documenting what is being done and sampling the final product from time to time to ensure that the protocol is working.

The HACCP approach is based on seven internationally recognised simple principles:

- Conduct a hazard analysis: prepare a flow diagram of the steps in the process; identify and list the hazards associated with the process and specify how they are going to be controlled.

- Determine the critical control points (CCPs), i.e. those stages at which hazard control is essential for the production of a safe end-product.

- Establish critical limits for each hazard at each CCP, i.e. the levels for each individual hazard that must not be exceeded if a safe product is going to be achieved. This may, for example, be a requirement to boil red kidney beans vigorously for 10 minutes in order to eliminate haemagglutinin (lectin) activity.

- Set up a system to monitor control of each CCP by scheduled testing and observations, to ensure that the hazard remains within critical limits.

- Establish what corrective action needs to be taken if monitoring indicates that a particular CCP is not under control *or is moving out of control,* i.e. is going beyond critical limits – this means stopping something going wrong before it happens, if at all possible.

- Set up procedures to make sure that the overall HACCP plan is working as desired; this may include some end-product testing and a regular review of the system.

- Establish thorough documentation of the system, process and procedures, and of all measurements taken relating to the monitoring of the process.

Surveillance

General monitoring of levels of specific chemicals in foods is part of the HACCP process, but in addition to this there are general government-initiated surveillance programs for specific chemicals. These may be long-term studies to determine trends in levels of well-known hazards in the environment, such as dioxins or nitrates, or may be as a result of specific problems that arise. As an example, both the UK's Food Standards Agency (FSA) and the EU's European Food Safety Authority (EFSA) publish reports of surveillance exercises. In addition, there are also systems in place to inform the industry of specific incidents as they arise.

Traceability

Maintaining adequate traceability in the food supply chain is a prerequisite to controlling the hazards which may be present in many food ingredients. This is a mandatory requirement in many countries and should include robust supplier assurance programs as well as full records of all transactions as food is traded, processed and placed on sale. In the event of a recall due to the identification of a food hazard it will be necessary to identify through the records all possible products implicated and to remove them from sale and/or consumption.

The control of food safety hazards through "hazard analysis"

Hazard analysis is the process of identifying everything that could go wrong, in terms of food safety, and then ensures that it is prevented from happening. Your hazard analysis needs to be specific to your food business. It is not difficult or complicated. You merely trace the path of all food through the kitchen, analysing the hazards, and put in the necessary controls. It is a legal requirement. If properly done, it will have the following practical benefits:

- Reduces the likelihood of food poisoning or food complaints
- Identifies any steps where food safety could/should be improved
- Introduces the opportunity of a better way of doing things
- Provides information and instruction for all staff, so that procedures are consistent even if the manager is absent
- Improves the legal defence of "due diligence" should a complaint be made
- Demonstrates compliance with the law.

The six key elements of hazard analysis

1. Identify the various steps in the operation You may find that drawing a flow chart will help here. You need to think through the main steps in the production of food e.g. storage, preparation, cooking.

2. Hazard identification (Cross contamination, foreign bodies, etc) There are three main types of hazard; microbiological, physical and chemical.

3. Controls for microbiological hazards Hazards should be removed or reduced through appropriate controls. Whilst all controls are important, critical control points (CCPs) are controls which are essential for food safety and are the 'last chance to get it right'. CCPs will vary according to the food being prepared, but commonly encountered ones are: storage temperature which will be a CCP for cold 'high risk' foods (food which supports the growth of bacteria), e.g. fresh cream desserts and cold cooked meats.

4. Monitoring e.g visual checks on use by dates, checking for mice droppings etc. Temperature monitoring methods should be kept as simple as possible. You need at least two different thermometers: an air temperature thermometer for checking the refrigerators and freezers, and a probe thermometer for checking the temperature of food. It is critical that this equipment is thoroughly disinfected before use. Other types of thermometer include an infrared device which can be pointed directly at food to check the surface temperature without penetrating the food, and a 'between-pack' probe for frozen foods.

5. Record keeping e.g. recording the temperature on delivery of high-risk foods, cleaning schedules, cooked food temperature charts, daily cleaning

checklists and training records. Examples of a temperature monitoring log sheet and a cleaning schedule are given at the end of this booklet, and can be copied. Show staff how to complete the forms, and tell them what to do if things go wrong. Weekly verification checks should be carried out by the person in charge or other nominated person.

6. Regular review i.e. when any significant change is made to staff, menu or procedures, systems should be reassessed to ensure that the control measures are still effective.

Other controls include:

- Buying good quality products from reputable suppliers
- Ensuring that perishable products are delivered under cold/frozen conditions
- Cold storage at a maximum temperature of 8° C (better at 2-4°C)
- Thorough cooking (to a minimum temperature of 75° C at the centre)
- Hot holding at a minimum temperature of 63°C
- Preventing cross contamination of harmful bacteria from raw food to food which has been cooked or will not be cooked, e.g. cooked meats and salads
- Rapid cooking to prevent the formation of bacterial spores (some bacteria form a tough outer covering to survive adverse conditions. This is known as a spore.)
- Rapid cooling of cooked food to prevent the germination of bacterial spores and the formation of toxins
- Thaw food in refrigerator, maximum 8°C
- Proper cleaning and disinfection procedures of equipment/surfaces/ wiping cloths that may come into close contact with food
- Good personal hygiene
- Well trained staff.

14

Toxicity during Food Processing and Storage

Food processing is the transformation of raw ingredients into food, or of food into other forms. Food processing typically takes clean, harvested crops or butchered animal products and uses these to produce attractive, marketable and often long shelf-life food products. Similar processes are used to produce animal feed.

History

Food processing dates back to the prehistoric ages when crude processing incorporated slaughtering, fermenting, sun drying, preserving with salt, and various types of cooking (such as roasting, smoking, steaming, and oven baking). Salt-preservation was especially common for foods that constituted warrior and sailors' diets until the introduction of canning methods. Evidence for the existence of these methods can be found in the writings of the ancient Greek, Chaldean, Egyptian and Roman civilizations as well as archaeological evidence from Europe, North and South America and Asia. These tried and tested processing techniques remained essentially the same until the advent of the industrial revolution. Examples of ready-meals also date back to before the preindustrial revolution, and include dishes such as Cornish pasty and Haggis. Both during ancient times and today in modern society these are considered processed foods. Food processing can provide quick, nutritious meal options for busy families.

Modern food processing technology developed in the 19th and 20th centuries was developed in a large part to serve military needs. In 1809 Nicolas Appert invented a hermetic bottling technique that would preserve food for French troops which ultimately contributed to the development of tinning, and subsequently canning by Peter Durand in 1810. Although initially expensive and somewhat hazardous due to the lead used in cans, canned goods would later become a staple around the world. Pasteurization, discovered by Louis Pasteur in 1864, improved the quality of preserved foods and introduced the wine, beer, and milk preservation.

In the 20th century, World War II, the space race and the rising consumer society in developed countries (including the United States) contributed to the growth of food processing with such advances as spray drying, juice concentrates, freeze drying and the introduction of artificial sweeteners, colouring agents, and preservatives such as sodium benzoate. In the late 20th century products such as dried instant soups, reconstituted fruits and juices, and self cooking meals such as MRE food ration were developed.

In western Europe and North America, the second half of the 20th century witnessed a rise in the pursuit of convenience. Food processing companies marketed their products especially towards middle-class working wives and mothers. Frozen foods (often credited to Clarence Birdseye) found their success in sales of juice concentrates and "TV dinners". Processors utilised the perceived value of time to appeal to the postwar population, and this same appeal contributes to the success of convenience foods today.

Benefits

Benefits of food processing include toxin removal, preservation, easing marketing and distribution tasks, and increasing food consistency. In addition, it increases yearly availability of many foods, enables transportation of delicate perishable foods across long distances and makes many kinds of foods safe to eat by de-activating spoilage and pathogenic micro-organisms. Modern supermarkets would not exist without modern food processing techniques, long voyages would not be possible and military campaigns would be significantly more difficult and costly to execute.

Processed foods are usually less susceptible to early spoilage than fresh foods and are better suited for long distance transportation from the source to the consumer. When they were first introduced, some processed foods helped to alleviate food shortages and improved the overall nutrition of populations as it made many new foods available to the masses.

Processing can also reduce the incidence of food borne disease. Fresh materials, such as fresh produce and raw meats, are more likely to harbour pathogenic micro-organisms (e.g. *Salmonella*) capable of causing serious illnesses.

The extremely varied modern diet is only truly possible on a wide scale because of food processing. Transportation of more exotic foods, as well as the elimination of much hard labour gives the modern eater easy access to a wide variety of food unimaginable to their ancestors.

The act of processing can often improve the taste of food significantly.

Mass production of food is much cheaper overall than individual production of meals from raw ingredients. Therefore, a large profit potential exists for the manufacturers and suppliers of processed food products. Individuals may see a benefit in convenience, but rarely see any direct financial cost benefit in using processed food as compared to home preparation.

Processed food freed people from the large amount of time involved in preparing and cooking "natural" unprocessed foods. The increase in free time allows people much more choice in life style than previously allowed. In many families the adults are working away from home and therefore there is little time for the preparation of food based on fresh ingredients. The food industry offers products that fulfill many different needs: From peeled potatoes that only have to be boiled at home to fully prepared ready meals that can be heated up in the microwave oven within a few minutes.

Modern food processing also improves the quality of life for people with allergies, diabetics, and other people who cannot consume some common food elements. Food processing can also add extra nutrients such as vitamins.

Drawbacks

Any processing of food can affect its nutritional density, the amount of nutrients lost depending on the food and method of processing. Vitamin C, for example, is destroyed by heat and therefore canned fruits have a lower content of vitamin C than fresh ones. The USDA conducted a study in 2004, creating a nutrient retention table for several foods. A cursory glance of the table indicates that, in the majority of foods, processing reduces nutrients by a minimal amount. On average any given nutrient may be reduced by as little as 5%-20%.

Another safety concern in food processing is the use of food additives. The health risks of any additives will vary greatly from person to person; for example sugar as an additive would be detrimental to those with diabetes. In the European Union, only food additives (e.g., sweeteners, preservatives, stabilizers) that have been approved as safe for human consumption by the European Food Safety Authority (EFSA) are allowed, at specified levels, for use in food products. Approved additives receive an E number (E for Europe), which at the same time simplifies communication about food additives in the list of ingredients across the different languages of the EU.

Food processing is typically a mechanical process that utilizes large mixing, grinding, chopping and emulsifying equipment in the production process. These processes inherently introduce a number of contamination risks. As a mixing bowl or grinder is used over time the food contact parts will tend to fail and fracture. This type of failure will introduce in to the product stream small to large metal contaminates. Further processing of these metal fragments will result in downstream equipment failure and the risk of ingestion by the consumer.

Food manufacturers utilize industrial metal detectors to detect and reject automatically any metal fragment. Large food processors will utilize many metal detectors within the processing stream to both ensure reduced damage to processing machinery as well risk to the consumer. The first industrial level metal detector pioneered by Goring Kerr was introduced back in 1947 for Mars Incorporated.

Performance Parameters for Food Processing

When designing processes for the food industry the following performance parameters may be taken into account:

- Hygiene, e.g. measured by number of micro-organisms per ml of finished product

- Energy efficiency measured e.g. by "ton of steam per ton of sugar produced"

- Minimization of waste, measured e.g. by "percentage of peeling loss during the peeling of potatoes'

- Labour used, measured e.g. by "number of working hours per ton of finished product"

- Minimization of cleaning stops measured e.g. by "number of hours between cleaning stops"

De-agglomerating Batter Mixes in Food Processing

Problems often occur during preparation of batter mixes because flour and other powdered ingredients tend to form lumps or agglomerates as they are being mixed during production. A conventional mixer/agitator cannot break down these agglomerates, resulting in a lumpy batter. If lumpy batter is used to enrobe products, it causes an unsatisfactory appearance with misshapen or oversize products that do not fit properly into packaging. This can force production to a standstill. Furthermore batter mix is generally recirculated from an enrobing system back to a holding vessel; lumps then have a tendency to build up, reducing the flow of material and raising potential sanitation issues.

Using a high shear in-line mixer in place of a conventional agitator or mixer can quickly solve problems of agglomeration with dry ingredients. A single pass through a self-pumping, in-line mixer adds high shear to batter, which de-agglomerates the mix, resulting in a homogeneous, smooth batter. With a consistent, smooth batter, finished product appearance is improved; the effectiveness and hygiene of the recirculation system is increased; and a better yield of raw materials is achieved. By increasing overall product quality, the amount of raw materials needed is decreased, thereby lowering manufacturing costs.

High shear in-line mixers process food to be made faster and cheaper while increasing consistency of the finished food. Powder and liquid mixing systems are capable of rapidly incorporating large quantities of powders at high concentrations – agglomerate free and fully hydrated. Advances in technology have made processing equipment easy to clean, leading to a much safer processed food.

Trends in Modern Food Processing

Health

- Reduction of fat content in final product by using baking instead of deep-frying in the production of potato chips, another processed food.

- Maintaining the natural taste of the product by using less artificial sweetener than was used before.

Hygiene

The rigorous application of industry and government endorsed standards to minimise possible risk and hazards. The international standard adopted is HACCP.

Efficiency

- Rising energy costs lead to increasing usage of energy-saving technologies, e.g. frequency converters on electrical drives, heat insulation of factory buildings and heated vessels, energy recovery systems, keeping a single fish frozen all the way from China to Switzerland.

- Factory automation systems (often Distributed control systems) reduce personnel costs and may lead to more stable production results.

Food Processing Industries

Food processing industries and practices include the following:

- Cannery
- Fish processing
- Food packaging plant
- Industrial rendering
- Meat packing plant
- Slaughterhouse
- Sugar industry

Food Storage

Food storage is both a traditional domestic skill and is important industrially. Food is stored by almost every human society and by many animals. Storing of food has several main purposes:

- Storage of harvested and processed plant and animal food products for distribution to consumers

- Enabling a better balanced diet throughout the year

- Reducing kitchen waste by preserving unused or uneaten food for later use

- Preserving pantry food, such as spices or dry ingredients like rice and flour, for eventual use in cooking

- Preparedness for catastrophes, emergencies and periods of food scarcity or famine

- Religious reasons (Example: LDS Church leaders instruct church members to store food)

- Protection from animals or theft

Domestic Food Storage

The safe storage of food for home use should strictly adhere to guidelines set out by reliable sources, such as the United States Department of Agriculture. These guidelines have been thoroughly researched by scientists to determine the best methods for reducing the real threat of food poisoning from unsafe food storage. It is also important to maintain proper kitchen hygiene, to reduce risks of bacteria or virus growth and food poisoning. The common food poisoning illnesses include *Listeriosis, Mycotoxicosis, Salmonellosis, E. coli, Staphylococcal* food poisoning and *Botulism*. There are many other organisms that can also cause food poisoning.

There are also safety guidelines available for the correct methods of home canning of food. For example, there are specific boiling times that apply depending upon whether pressure canning or waterbath canning is being used in the process. These safety guidelines are intended to reduce the growth of mold and bacteria and the threat of potentially-fatal food poisoning.

Food Storage Safety

Freezers and Thawing Food

Freezer temperature should be maintained below 0 F. Food should never be thawed at room temperature, this increases the risk of bacterial and fungal growth and accordingly the risk of food poisoning. Once thawed, food should be used and never refrozen. Frozen food should be thawed using the following methods:

- Microwave oven
- During cooking
- In cold water (place food in watertight, plastic bag; change water every 30 minutes)
- In the refrigerator

Throw out foods that have been warmer than 40 F for more than 2 hours. If there is any doubt at all about the length of time the food has been defrosted at room temperature, it should be thrown out. Freezing does not destroy microbes present in food. Freezing at 0 F does inactivate microbes (bacteria, yeasts and molds). However, once food has been thawed, these microbes can again become active. Microbes in thawed food can multiply to levels that can lead to foodborne illness. Thawed food should be handled according to the same guidelines as perishable fresh food.

Food frozen at 0 F and below is preserved indefinitely. However, the quality of the food will deteriorate if it is frozen over a lengthy period. The United States Department of Agriculture, Food Safety and Inspection Service publishes a chart showing the suggested freezer storage time for common foods.

Refrigeration

It is important to note that safe food storage using refrigeration requires adhering to temperature guidelines:

For safety, it is important to verify the temperature of the refrigerator. Refrigerators should be set to maintain a temperature of 40 F or below. Some refrigerators have built-in thermometers to measure their internal temperature. For those refrigerators without this feature, keep an appliance thermometer in the refrigerator to monitor the temperature. This can be critical in the event of a power outage. When the power goes back on, if the refrigerator is still 40 F, the food is safe. Foods held at temperatures above 40 F for more than 2 hours should not be consumed. Appliance thermometers are specifically designed to provide accuracy at cold temperatures. Be sure refrigerator/freezer doors are closed tightly at all times. Don't open refrigerator/freezer doors more often than necessary and close them as soon as possible.

Storage times for refrigerated food

The United States Department of Agriculture, Food Safety and Inspection Service publishes recommended storage times for refrigerated food.

Storing Oils and Fats

Oils and fats can begin to go rancid quickly when not stored safely. Rancid cooking oils and fats do not often smell rancid until well after they have spoiled. Oxygen, light and heat all contribute to cooking oils becoming rancid. The higher the level of polyunsaturated fat that an oil contains, the faster it spoils. The percentage of polyunsaturated fat in some common cooking oils is: safflower (74%); sunflower (66%); corn (60%); soybean (37%); peanut (32%); canola (29%); olive (8%).

To help prevent oils from going rancid, they should be refrigerated once opened. Opened, refrigerated cooking oils should be used within a few weeks, when some types begin to go rancid. Unopened oils can have a storage life of up to one year, but some types have a shorter shelf-life even when unopened (such as sesame and flaxseed).

Dry Storage of Foods

The guidelines vary for safe storage of vegetables under dry conditions (without refrigerating or freezing). This is because different vegetables have different characteristics, for example, tomatoes contain a lot of water, while root vegetables such as carrots and potatoes contain less. These factors, and many others, affect the amount of time that a vegetable can be kept in dry storage, as well as the temperature needed to preserve its usefulness. The following guideline shows the required dry storage conditions:

- Cool and dry: onion
- Cool and moist: root vegetable, potato, cabbage
- Warm and dry: winter squash, pumpkin, sweet potatoes, dried hot peppers

Many cultures have developed innovative ways of preserving vegetables so that they can be stored for several months between harvest seasons. Techniques include pickling, home canning, food dehydration, or storage in a root cellar.

Grain

Grain, which includes dry kitchen ingredients such as flour, rice, millet, couscous, cornmeal, and so on, can be stored in rigid sealed containers to prevent moisture contamination or insect or rodent infestation. For kitchen use, glass containers are the most traditional method. During the 20th century plastic containers were introduced for kitchen use. They are now sold in a vast variety of sizes and designs.

Metal cans are used (in the United States the smallest practical grain storage uses closed-top #10 metal cans). Storage in grain sacks is ineffective; mold and pests destroy a 25 kg cloth sack of grain in a year, even if stored off the ground in a dry area. On the ground or damp concrete, grain can spoil in as little as three days, and the grain might have to be dried before it can be milled. Food stored under unsuitable conditions should not be purchased or used because of risk of spoilage. To test whether grain is still good, sprout some. If it sprouts, it is still good, but if not, it should not be eaten. It may take up to a week for grains to sprout. When in doubt about the safety of the food, throw it out as quickly as possible.

Spices and Herbs

Spices and herbs are today often sold prepackaged in a way that is convenient for pantry storage. The packaging has dual purposes of both storing and dispensing the spices or herbs. They are sold in small glass or plastic containers or resealable plastic packaging. When spices or herbs are homegrown or bought in bulk, they can be stored at home in glass or plastic containers. They can be stored for extended periods, in some cases for years. However, after 6 months to a year, spices and herbs will gradually lose their flavour as oils they contain will slowly evaporate during storage.

Spices and herbs can be preserved in vinegar for short periods of up to a month, creating a flavoured vinegar.

Alternative methods for preserving herbs include freezing in water or unsalted butter. Herbs can be chopped and added to water in an ice cube tray. After freezing, the ice cubes are emptied into a plastic freezer bag for storing in the freezer. Herbs also can be stirred into a bowl with unsalted butter, then spread on wax paper and rolled into a cylinder shape. The wax paper roll containing the butter and herbs is then stored in a freezer, and can be cut off in the desired amount for cooking. Using either of these techniques, the herbs should be used within a year.

Meat

Unpreserved meat has only a relatively short life in storage. Perishable meats should be refrigerated, frozen, dried promptly or cured. Storage of fresh meats is a complex discipline that affects the costs, storage life and eating quality of the meat, and the appropriate techniques vary with the kind of meat and the particular requirements. For example, dry ageing techniques are sometimes used to tenderize gourmet meats by hanging them in carefully controlled environments for up to 21 days, while game animals of various kinds may be hung after shooting. Details depend on personal tastes and local traditions. Modern techniques of preparing meat for storage vary with the type of meat and special requirements of tenderness, flavour, hygiene, and economy.

Semi-dried meats like salamis and country style hams are processed first with salt, smoke, sugar, acid, or other "cures" then hung in cool dry storage for extended periods, sometimes exceeding a year. Some of the materials added during the curing of meats serve to reduce the risks of food poisoning from anaerobic bacteria such as species of Clostridium that release botulinum toxin that can cause botulism. Typical ingredients of curing agents that inhibit anaerobic bacteria include nitrates and nitrates. Such salts are dangerously poisonous in their own right and must be added in carefully controlled quantities and according to proper techniques. Their proper use has however saved many lives and much food spoilage.

Like the semi-dried meats, most salted, smoked, and simply-dried meats of various kinds that once were staples in particular regions, now are largely luxury snacks or garnishes; examples include jerky, biltong, and varieties of pemmican, but ham and bacon for instance, still are staples in many communities.

Food Rotation

Food rotation is important to preserve freshness. When food is rotated, the food that has been in storage the longest is used first. As food is used, new food is added to the pantry to replace it; the essential rationale is to use the oldest food as soon as possible so that nothing is in storage too long and becomes unsafe to eat. Labelling food with paper labels on the storage container, marking the date that the container is placed in storage, can make this practise simpler. The best way to rotate food storage is to prepare meals with stored food on a daily basis.

Commercial Food Storage

Grain and beans are stored in tall grain elevators, almost always at a rail head near the point of production. The grain is shipped to a final user in hopper cars. In the former Soviet Union, where harvest was poorly controlled, grain was often irradiated at the point of production to suppress moldand insects. In the U.S., threshing and drying is performed in the field, and transport is nearly sterile and in large containers that effectively suppresses pest access, which eliminates the need for irradiation. At any given time, the U.S. usually has about two weeks worth of stored grains for the population.

Fresh fruits and vegetables are sometimes packed in plastic packages and cups for fresh premium markets, or placed in large plastic tubs for sauce and soup processors. Fruits and vegetables are usually refrigerated at the earliest possible moment, and even so have a shelf life of two weeks or less.

In the United States, livestock is usually transported live, slaughtered at a major distribution point, hung and transported for two days to a week in refrigerated rail cars, and then butchered and sold locally. Before refrigerated rail cars, meat had to be transported live, and this placed its cost so high that only farmers and the wealthy could afford it every day. In Europe much meat is transported live and slaughtered close to the point of sale. In much of Africa and Asia most meat is for local populations and is raised, slaughtered and eaten locally, which is believed to be much less stressful for the animals involved and minimizes meat storage needs. In Australia and New Zealand, where a large proportion of meat production is for export, meat is stored in very large freezer plants before being shipped overseas in freezer ships.

For emergency preparation

Guides for surviving emergency conditions in many parts of the world recommend maintaining a store of essential foods; typically water, cereals, oil, dried milk, and protein rich foods such as beans, lentils, tinned meat and fish. A basic food storage calculator can be used to help determine how much of these staple foods a person would need to store in order to sustain life for one full year. In addition to storing the basic food items many people choose to supplement their food storage with frozen or preserved garden-grown fruits and vegetables and freeze-dried or canned produce. An unvarying diet of basic staple foods prepared in the same manner can cause appetite exhaustion, leading to less caloric intake. Another benefit to having a basic supply of food storage in the home is for the cost savings. Costs of dry bulk foods (before preparation) are often considerably less than convenience and fresh foods purchased at local markets or supermarkets. There is a significant market in convenience foods for campers, such as dehydrated food products.

Secrets of the Food Processing Industry

Traditional processing has two functions: to make food more digestible and to preserve it for use during times when food isn't readily available. Nutritious, long-lasting processed foods including pemmican, hard sausage and old-fashioned meat puddings and haggis, as well as grain products, dairy products, pickles—everything from wine and spirits to lacto-fermented condiments. Farmers and artisans—bread makers, cheese makers, distillers, millers and so forth—processed the raw ingredients into delicious foods that retained their nutritional content over many months or even years, and kept the profits on the farm and in the farming communities where they belonged.

Unfortunately, in modern times, we have substituted local artisanal processing with factory and industrial processing, which actually diminishes the quality of the food, rather than making it more nutritious and digestible. Industrial processing depends upon sugar, white flour, processed and hydrogenated oils, synthetic food additives and vitamins, heat treatment and the extrusion of grains.

Breakfast Cereals

Let's look at the processing involved in the typical American breakfast of cereal, skim milk and orange juice. Cold breakfast cereals are produced by a process called extrusion. Grains are mixed with water, processed into a slurry and placed in a machine called an extruder. The grains are forced out of a tiny hole at high temperature and pressure, which shapes them into little o's or flakes or shreds. Individual grains passed through the extruder expand to produce puffed wheat, oats and rice. These products are then subjected to sprays that give a coating of oil and sugar to seal off the cereal from the ravages of milk and to give it crunch.

In his book *Fighting the Food Giants*, biochemist Paul Stitt describes the extrusion process, which treats the grains with very high heat and pressure, and notes that the processing destroys much of their nutrients. It denatures the fatty acids; it even destroys the synthetic vitamins that are added at the end of the process. The amino acid lysine, a crucial nutrient, is especially damaged by the extrusion process.

Even boxed cereals sold in health food stores are made using the extrusion process. They are made with the same kind of machines and mostly in the same factories. The only "advances" claimed in the extrusion process are those that will cut cost, regardless of how the process alters the nutrient content of the product.

With so many millions of boxes of cereal sold each year, one would expect to see published studies showing the effects of these cereals on animals and humans. But breakfast cereals are a multi-billion dollar industry that has created huge fortunes for a few people. A box of cereal containing a penny's worth of grain sells for four or five dollars in the grocery store--there is probably no other product on earth with such a large profit margin. These profits have paid for lobbying efforts and journal sponsorships that have effectively kept any research about extruded grains out of the scientific literature and convinced government officials that there is no difference between a natural grain of wheat and a grain that has been altered by the extrusion process.

The Rat Experiments

Unpublished research indicates that the extrusion process turns the proteins in grains into neurotoxins. Stitt describes an experiment, conducted in 1942 by a cereal company but locked away in the company's file cabinet, in which four sets of rats were given special diets. One group received plain whole wheat grains, water and synthetic vitamins and minerals. A second group received puffed wheat (an extruded cereal), water and the same nutrient solution. A third set was given water and white sugar. A fourth set was given nothing but water and synthetic nutrients. The rats that received the whole wheat lived over a year on this diet. The rats that got nothing but water and vitamins lived about two months. The animals on a white sugar and water diet lived about a month. The study showed that the rats given the vitamins, water and all the puffed wheat they wanted died within two weeks—even before the rats that got no food at all. These results suggest that there was something very toxic in the puffed wheat itself! Proteins are very similar to certain toxins in molecular structure, and the pressure of the puffing process may produce chemical changes that turn a nutritious grain into a poisonous substance.

Another unpublished experiment was carried out in 1960. Researchers at the University of Michigan in Ann Arbor were given eighteen laboratory rats. These were divided into three groups: one group received cornflakes and water; a second group was given the cardboard box that the cornflakes came in and water; the control group received rat chow and water. The rats in the control group remained in good health throughout the experiment. The rats eating the box became lethargic and eventually died of malnutrition. The rats receiving the cornflakes and water died before the rats that were eating the box! (The first box rat died the day the last cornflake rat died.) Furthermore, before death, the cornflakes-eating rats developed aberrant behavior, threw fits, bit each other and finally went into convulsions. Autopsy revealed dysfunction of the pancreas, liver and kidneys and degeneration of the nerves of the spine, all signs of insulin shock. The startling conclusion of this study was that there was more nourishment in the box than in the cornflakes. This experiment was designed as a joke, but the results were far from funny.

Most Americans eat boxed cereals today. Because these are fortified with synthetic nutrients, the USDA can claim that they are as healthy as the grains from which they are made. Many of these cereals contain at least 50 percent of calories as sugar. Those sold in health food stores may be made of whole grains and fewer sweeteners. However, these whole grain extruded cereals are probably more dangerous than their refined grain counterparts sold in the supermarkets, because they are higher in protein, and it is the proteins in these cereals that are rendered toxic by this type of processing.

The Extrusion Process

When we put cereals through an extruder, it alters the structure of the proteins. Zeins, which comprise the majority of proteins in corn, are located in spherical organelles called protein bodies. The scientific literature does contain one study on extruded grains, which investigated changes in protein body, shape and release of encapsulated alpha-zeins as a result of the extrusion processing. Researchers found that during extrusion, the protein bodies are completely disrupted and the alpha-zeins dispersed. The results suggest that the zeins in cornflakes are not confined to rigid protein bodies but can interact with each other and other components of the system, forming new compounds that are foreign to the human body. The extrusion process breaks down the organelles and disperses the proteins, which then become toxic. When the proteins are disrupted in this way, it can adversely affect the nervous system, as indicated by the cornflake experiment.

Old Fashioned Porridge

There is only one way to put these companies out of business, and that is not to eat their food. So, what are you going to have for breakfast instead of cheerios and corn flakes? Eggs any style are always a good choice. As for grain, old-fashioned porridges made from non-extruded grains provide excellent nourishment at an economical price. Grains such as oats should be cut or rolled and then soaked overnight in a warm, acidic medium to neutralize the many anti-nutrients naturally occurring in grains, such as irritating tannins, digestion-blocking enzyme inhibitors and mineral-blocking phytic acid. This treatment can also gently break down complex proteins in grains. You soak the grains in warm water plus one tablespoon of something acidic, like whey, yoghurt, lemon juice or vinegar. The next morning, your grain will cook in just a few minutes. It's best to eat your porridge with butter or cream, like our grandparents did. The nutrients in the dairy fats are needed in order for you to absorb the nutrients in the grains. Without the fat-soluble vitamins A, D and K_2, you cannot absorb the minerals in your food. Furthermore, the fats in butter and cream slow down the release of glucose into the bloodstream, so that your blood sugar remains stable throughout the morning.

MILK

Milk is one of nature's most perfect foods. Most of our milk comes from a sacred animal, the cow. Today, however, in the industrial system, we imprison cows indoors for their entire lives; we give them inappropriate feed such as soy, bakery waste, citrus peel cake and the swill from ethanol production, foods that cows are not designed to eat. The confinement environment and the inappropriate feed make these cows sick, so they need antibiotics and other drugs. We breed them to give huge amounts of milk, and give them hormones to increase milk production as well. These cows produce large quantities of watery milk with only half the amount of fat compared to milk produced by old-fashioned cows eating green grass. Then this milk is shipped to factories for processing.

Inside the plants, the milk is completely remade. As described by Emily Green in the *Los Angeles Times*, centrifuges separate the milk into fat, protein and various other solids and liquids. Once segregated, these are recombined at specific levels set for whole, lowfat and no-fat milks. Of the reconstituted milks, whole milk will most closely approximate original cow's milk. What is left over will go into butter, cream, cheese, dried milk, and a host of other milk products. The dairy industry promotes lowfat milk and skim milk because they can make more money on the butterfat when used in ice cream. When they remove the fat to make reduced-fat milks, they replace it with powdered milk concentrate, which is formed by high temperature spray drying.

Then the milk is sent by tanker trucks (which are not refrigerated) to bottling plants. The milk is pasteurized at 161°F for fifteen seconds by rushing it past superheated stainless steel plates. If the temperature is 230°F (over the boiling point), the milk is considered ultrapasteurized. This ultrapasteurized milk will have a distinct cooked milk taste, but it is sterile and shelf stable. It may be sold in the refrigerated section of the supermarket so the consumer will think it is fresh, but it does not need to be. The milk is also homogenized by a pressure treatment that breaks down the fat globules so the milk won't separate. Once processed, the milk will last for weeks, not just days.

Processing makes the milk difficult to digest and renders the proteins allergenic. Animals fed pasteurized milk exclusively develop nutrient deficiencies and become infertile after several generations.

Fortunately, Real Milk from pasture-fed cows, milk that is not pasteurized, processed or homogenized, is becoming more widely available. In fact, demand for Real Milk is growing rapidly.

In order to make powdered milk, fluid is forced through a tiny hole at high pressure and then blown out into the air. This causes a lot of nitrates to form, and the cholesterol in the milk becomes oxidized. Contrary to popular opinion, cholesterol is not a demon but your best friend; you don't have to worry about consuming foods containing cholesterol, except that you do not want to consume oxidized cholesterol. Evidence indicates that oxidized cholesterol can initiate the process of atherosclerosis.

Powdered milk is added to reduced-fat milks and milk products to give them body. So, when you consume reduced-fat milk or yoghurt, thinking that it will help you avoid heart disease, you are actually consuming oxidized cholesterol, which can initiate the process of heart disease.

ORANGE JUICE

Now, let's turn to the orange juice, part of our "healthy breakfast" of cereal, lowfat milk and juice. An article from *Processed and Prepared Foods*[7] describes "a new orange juice processing plant is completely automated and can process up to 1,800 tons of oranges per day to produce frozen concentrate, single strength juice, oil extracted from the peel and cattle feed." The new method of producing juice puts the whole orange in the machine. Another abstract states: "Various acid sprays for improving fruit peel quality and increasing juice yield are added to these processed oranges." These compounds are added to extract as much juice as possible, as well as the oil out of the skin. The conventional orange crop is sprayed heavily with pesticides called cholinesterase inhibitors, which are very toxic to the nervous system. When they put the whole oranges into the vats and squeeze them, all that pesticide goes into the juice. Then they add acids to get every single bit of juice out of these oranges. So commercial orange juice can be a very toxic soup. This may be one reason that consumption of fruit juice is associated with increased rates of dementia.

What about the peel used for cattle feed? The dried, left-over citrus peel from orange juice production is processed into cakes, which are still loaded with cholinesterase inhibitors. Mark Purdey, in England, has shown how this practice correlates with mad cow disease. The use of organophosphates either as a spray on the cows or as a component of their feed, causes degeneration of the brain and nervous system in the cow, and if it's doing it to the cow, there's a possibility it may be doing it to you also.

The U.S. government tries to give the impression that pasteurization of juice is necessary to ensure our safety. However, it might surprise you to learn that researchers have found fungus that is resistant to pressure and heat in processed juices. They found that seventeen percent of Nigerian packages of orange juice and twenty percent of mango and tomato juices contained these heat-resistant fungi. They also found *E. coli* in the orange juice; it was pressure resistant and had survived pasteurization. So there is plenty of danger from contamination in these pasteurized juices.

In one study, heat-treated and acid-hydrolyzed orange juice was tested for mutagenic activity. The authors found that the heating process produced intermediate products which, under test conditions, gave rise to mutagenicity and cytotoxicity. In other words, there were cancer-causing compounds in the orange juice. In another study, gel filtration and high performance liquid chromatography were used to obtain mutagenic fractions from heated orange juice.

So if you want juice with your breakfast, avoid commercial processed orange juice. Instead, squeeze yourself a couple of organic oranges or an organic grapefruit--in other words, process the juice yourself! Mix that fresh juice with sparkling water and a pinch of salt for a delicious spritzer.

NATURAL NOURISHING BROTHS

In the past, many traditional cultures made use of animal bones to make broth. They recognized the health-giving properties of bone broth as well as wonderful flavors broth gave to soups, sauces, gravies and stews. Modern science has shown us that homemade bone broths are indeed the healing wonders of the food pharmacopia; they provide minerals in abundance, strengthen bones and sinews, heal the gut and help us detoxify. The gelatin in homemade bone broth is a natural digestive aid.

INDUSTRIAL SOUPS

Most commercial soup bases and sauces contain artificial meat-like flavors that mimic those we used to get from natural, gelatin-rich broth. These kinds of short cuts mean that consumers are shortchanged. When the homemade stocks were pushed out by the cheap substitutes, an important source of minerals disappeared from the American diet. The thickening effects of gelatin could be mimicked with emulsifiers, but, of course, the health benefits were lost. Gelatin is a very healthy thing to have in your diet. It helps you digest proteins properly and is supportive of digestive health overall.

Research on gelatin and natural broths came to an end in the 1950s when food companies discovered how to induce maillard reactions--the process of creating flavor compounds by mixing reduced sugars and amino acids under increased temperatures--and produce meat-like flavors in the laboratory. In a General Foods Company report issued in 1947, chemists predicted that almost all natural flavors would soon be chemically synthesized. Following the Second World War, American food companies discovered monosodium glutamate, a food ingredient the Japanese had invented in 1908 to enhance food flavors, including meat-like flavors. Humans actually have receptors on the tongue for glutamate—it is the protein in food that the human body recognizes as meat--but the glutamate in MSG has a different configuration, which cannot be assimilated properly by the body. Any protein can be hydrolyzed (broken down into its component amino acids) to produce a base containing MSG. When the industry learned how to synthesize the flavor of meat in the laboratory, using inexpensive proteins from grains and legumes, the door was opened to a flood of new products, including boullion cubes, dehydrated soup mixes, sauce mixes, TV dinners, and condiments with a meaty taste.

The fast food industry could not exist without MSG and artificial meat flavors, which beguile the consumer into eating bland and tasteless food. The sauces in many commercially processed foods contain MSG, water, thickeners, emulsifiers and caramel coloring. Your tongue is tricked into thinking that you are consuming something nutritious, when in fact it is getting nothing at all except some very toxic substances. Even dressings, Worcestershire sauce, rice mixes, flavored tofu, and many meat products have MSG in them. Almost all canned soups and stews contain MSG, and the "hydrolyzed protein" bases often contain MSG in very large amounts.

So called homemade soups in most restaurants are usually made by mixing water with a powdered soup base made of hydrolyzed protein and artificial flavors, and then adding chopped vegetables and other ingredients. Even things like lobster bisque and fish sauces in most seafood restaurants are prepared using these powdered bases full of artificial flavors.

The industry even thinks it is too costly to just use a little onion and garlic for flavoring they use artificial garlic and onion flavors instead. It's all profit based with no thought for the health of the consumer.

Unfortunately, most of the processed vegetarian foods are loaded with these flavorings, as well. The list of ingredients in vegetarian hamburgers, hot dogs, bacon, baloney, etc., may include hydrolyzed protein and "natural" flavors, all sources of MSG. Soy foods are loaded with MSG.

Food manufacturers get around the labeling requirements by putting MSG in the spice mixes; if the mix is less than fifty percent MSG, they don't have to indicate MSG on the label. You may have noticed that the phrase "No MSG" has actually disappeared. The industry doesn't use it anymore because they found out that there was MSG in all the spice mixes; even Bragg's amino acids had to take "No MSG" off the label.

HEALTH PROBLEMS

While the industry was adding MSG to food in larger and larger amounts, in 1957 scientists found that mice became blind and obese when MSG was administered by feeding tube. In 1969, MSG-induced lesions were found in the hypothalamus region of the mouse brain. Subsequent studies pointed in the same direction. MSG is a neurotoxic substance that causes a wide range of reactions in humans, from temporary headaches to permanent brain damage. It is also associated with violent behavior. We have had a huge increase in Alzheimer's, brain cancer, seizures, multiple sclerosis and diseases of the nervous system, and one of the chief culprits is the flavorings in our food.

Ninety-five percent of processed foods contain MSG, and, in the late 1950s, it was even added to baby food. Manufacturers say they have voluntarily taken it out of the baby food, but they didn't really remove it; they just called it "hydrolyzed protein" instead.

An excellent book, *Excitotoxins*, by Russell Blaylock, describes how nerve cells either disintegrate or shrivel up in the presence of free glutamic acid if it gets past the blood-brain barrier. The glutamates in MSG are absorbed directly from the mouth to the brain. Some investigators believe that the great increase in violence in this country starting in 1960 is due to the increased use of MSG beginning in the late 1950s, particularly as it was added to baby foods.

INDUSTRIAL FATS AND OILS

The food processing empire is built on industrial fats and oils, extracted from corn, soybeans and other seeds. Crude vegetable oil which is dark, sticky and smelly is subjected to horrendous processing to produce clean-looking cooking oils, margarine, shortening and spreads. The steps involved in processing usually include degumming, bleaching, deodorizing, filtering and removing saturates to make the oils more liquid. In the process, the nutrients and antioxidants disappear--but not the pesticides. Most processors also add a hexane solvent in order to squeeze the very last drop of oil out of the seeds. Caustic refining, the most widely used process for oil refining, involves adding very alkaline, chemicals to the oil.

In order to make a solid fat out of liquid oil, manufacturers subject the oils to a process called partial hydrogenation. The oil is extracted under high temperature and pressure, and the remaining fraction of oil is removed with hexane solvents. Manufacturers then steam clean the oils, a process that removes all the vitamins and all the antioxidants—but, of course, the solvents and the pesticides remain. These oils are mixed with a nickel catalyst and then, under high temperature and pressure, they are flooded with hydrogen gas. What goes into the reactor is a liquid oil; what comes out of that reactor is a smelly mass resembling grey cottage cheese. Emulsifiers are mixed in to smooth out the lumps, and the oil is then steam cleaned once more, to get rid of the horrible smell. The next step is bleaching, to get rid of the grey color. At this point, the product can be called "pure vegetable shortening." To make margarines and spreads, artificial flavors and synthetic vitamins are added. But the government does not allow the industry to add synthetic color to margarine--they must add a natural color, such as annatto--a comforting thought. The margarine or spread is then packaged in blocks and tubs and advertised as a health food.

Saturated fat is the type of fat found in such foods as lard, butter and coconut oil. Saturated fat molecules are straight, so they pack together easily. That is why saturated fats are solid at room temperature. Unsaturated fats have a little bend at each double bond, with two hydrogen atoms sticking out on the same side. And when that molecule gets incorporated into your cells, the body wants those two hydrogen atoms to be on the same side of the carbon chain, forming an electron cloud; that is where controlled chemical interactions take place.

During the process of partial hydrogenation, one of those hydrogen atoms is moved to the other side, causing the molecule to straighten out so that it behaves chemically like a saturate—although *bio*chemically it behaves very differently. The original, unsaturated molecule is called a "cis" fatty acid, because the two hydrogens are together, and then it becomes a *trans* fatty acid, because the two hydrogens are across from each other ("*trans*" means "across"). Your body doesn't know that this new molecule is something that has never existed in nature before, and when you eat one of these *trans* fatty acids, it gets built into your cell membranes. Because of the chemical rearrangement, the reactions that should happen can't take place. Enzymes and receptors don't work anymore. The more *trans* fatty acids that you eat, the more partially hydrogenated your cells become and the more chaos that you are going to have on the cellular level.

All of the margarines, shortenings and even low-*trans*-fat spreads are made with these harmful ingredients. They're used in chips and crackers, and most restaurants use them for cooking fries. Until the early 1980s, fast food outlets and restaurants cooked the fries in tallow, which is a very safe fat, but now they use partially hydrogenated soybean oil.

In the past, when you made desserts for your kids, at least the sugar they contained came with butter, eggs, cream and nuts—all good wholesome foods. Now manufacturers can imitate the butter, eggs, cream and nuts, so all you have is sugar, industrial oils and artificial ingredients in these instant puddings, pastries and other artificial desserts.

Many diseases have been associated with the consumption of *trans* fatty acids— heart disease, cancer, and degeneration of joints and tendons. The only reason that we are eating this stuff is because we have been told that the competing saturated fats and oils—butter, lard, coconut oil, palm oil, tallow and suet—are bad for us and cause heart disease. Such assertions are nothing but industry propaganda.

THE WESTERN PRICE

Weston A. Price, DDS, discovered that as populations adopt processed foods, with each generation the facial structure becomes more and more narrow. Healthy faces should be broad. We are all designed to have perfectly straight teeth and not get cavities. When you are eating real, nutrient-dense foods, you get the complete and perfect expression of the genetic potential. We were given a perfect blueprint. Whether or not the body temple is built according to the blueprint depends, to a great extent, on our wisdom in food choices.

When primitive societies abandoned the traditional diet and began to eat processed foods, the next generation developed narrowed facial structure and many diseases. We know that if you continue this diet for three generations, reproduction ceases. This is the terrible price of the West, the Western Price. Civilization will die out unless we embrace the food ways of our ancestors. That means turning our backs on processed foods and getting back into the kitchen, to prepare real foods--containing healthy fats--for ourselves and our families.

OPTIMAL FOOD PREPARATION—MADE WITH LOVE

Food preparation is actually a sacred activity: According to esoteric lore, "If a woman could see the sparks of light going forth from her fingertips when she is cooking, and the energy that goes into the food she handles, she would realize how much of herself she imbues into the meals that she prepares for her family and friends. It is one of the most important and least understood activities of life that the feelings that go into the preparation of food affect everyone who partakes of it. This activity should be unhurried, peaceful and happy because the energy that flows into that food impacts the energy of the receiver.

"That is why the advanced spiritual teachers of the East never eat food prepared by anyone other than their own *chelas* (disciples). The person preparing the food may be the only one in the household who is spiritually advanced. An active charge of happiness, purity and peace will pour forth into the food from him, and this pours forth into the other members of the family and blesses them."

To be healthy, we need to prepare our own food, for ourselves and our families. This doesn't mean you have to spend hours in the kitchen, but you do need to spend *some* time there, preparing food with wisdom and love. If no one in the family has time to prepare food, you need to sit down and rethink how you are spending your time, because this is the only way to get nourishing foods into your children. We can return to good eating practices one mouth at a time, one meal at a time, by preparing our own food and preparing it properly.

Processed Food Pitfalls: Top 10 Toxic Food Ingredients

Most of us don't think of the food we eat as poison, but some of the ingredients commonly found in processed foods can be considered toxic. By "toxic," I mean chemicals or highly processed ingredients that aren't good for you or can cause harm to your health. I'm talking about refined grains, trans fats, high fructose corn syrup, and all the other artificial junk you can't even pronounce on the ingredient lists. Any food that has been canned, dehydrated, or had chemicals added to it is a processed food, and these foods make up about 60 percent of the average American diet. They've taken over, and we have to FIGHT BACK. Know which toxic food ingredients to avoid:

1. **Palm Oil**

    When a regular fat like corn, soybean, or palm oil is blasted with hydrogen and turned into a solid, it becomes a trans fat. These evil anti-nutrients help packaged foods stay "fresh," meaning that the food can sit on the supermarket shelf for years without ever getting stale or rotting. Eating junk food with trans fats raises your "bad" LDL cholesterol and triglycerides and lowers your "good" HDL. These fats also increase your risk of blood clots and heart attack. Avoid palm oil and other trans fats like the plague, and kiss fried foods goodbye too, since they're usually fried in one of these freakish trans-fatty oils.

2. **Shortening**

    Ditch any food that lists shortening or partially hydrogenated oil as an ingredient, since these are also evil trans fats. In addition to clogging your arteries and causing obesity, they also increase your risk of metabolic syndrome. Choose healthier monounsaturated fats, such as olive, peanut and canola oils and foods that contain unsaturated omega-3 fatty acids instead.

3. **White Flour, Rice, Pasta, and Bread**

    When a whole grain is refined, most of its nutrients are sucked out in an effort to extend its shelf life. Both the bran and germ are removed, and therefore all the fiber, vitamins, and minerals. Because these stripped down, refined grains are devoid of fiber and other nutrients, they're also easy to digest — TOO EASY. They send your blood sugar and insulin skyrocketing, which can lead to all sorts of problems. Replace processed grains with whole grains, like brown or wild rice, whole-wheat breads and pastas, barley, and oatmeal.

4. **High Fructose Corn Syrup**

    The evil king of all refined grains is high fructose corn syrup (HFCS). The amount of refined sugar we consume has declined over the past 40 years, but we're consuming almost 20 times as much HFCS. According to researchers at Tufts University, Americans consume more calories from HFCS than any other source. It's in practically everything. It increases triglycerides, boosts fat-storing hormones, and drives people to overeat and gain weight. Adopt zero-tolerance policy, and steer clear of this sweet "poison."

5. **Artificial Sweeteners**

Aspartame (NutraSweet, Equal), saccharin (Sweet'N Low, SugarTwin), and sucralose (Splenda) may be even harder on our metabolic systems than plain old sugar. These supposedly diet-friendly sweeteners may actually be doing more harm than good! Studies suggest that artificial sweeteners trick the brain into forgetting that sweetness means extra calories, making people more likely to keep eating sweet treats without abandon. Nip it in the bud. Scan ingredient labels and ban all artificial sweeteners from entering your mouth.

6. **Sodium Benzoate and Potassium Benzoate**

These preservatives are sometimes added to soda to prevent mold from growing, but benzene is a known carcinogen that is also linked with serious thyroid damage. Dangerous levels of benzene can build up when plastic bottles of soda are exposed to heat or when the preservatives are combined with ascorbic acid (vitamin C). Don't risk it.

7. **Butylated Hydroxyanisole (BHA)**

BHA is another potentially cancer-causing preservative, but it has been deemed safe by the FDA. Its job is to help prevent spoilage and food poisoning, but it's a major endocrine disruptor and can seriously mess with your hormones. BHA is in hundreds of foods. It's also found in food packaging and cosmetics. BHA has many aliases. You can look them up. Or you can follow my advice and DITCH processed foods altogether.

8. **Sodium Nitrates and Sodium Nitrites**

No that's not a typo. These two different preservatives are found in processed meats like bacon, lunch meat, and hot dogs. They're some of the worst offenders, and they're believed to cause colon cancer and metabolic syndrome, which can lead to diabetes. Protect your health by always choosing fresh, organic meats.

9. **Blue, Green, Red, and Yellow**

The artificial colors blue 1 and 2, green 3, red 3, and yellow 6 have been linked to thyroid, adrenal, bladder, kidney, and brain cancers. Always seek out foods with the fewest artificial chemicals, especially when shopping for your kids. Look for color-free medications and natural food products that don't contain artificial colors like these.

10. Monosodium Glutamate (MSG)

Monosodium glutamate is a processed "flavor enhancer." While glutamates are present in some natural foods, such as meat and cheese, the ones exploited by the processed-foods industry are separated from their host proteins through hydrolysis. The jury is still out on how harmful MSG may be, but high levels of free glutamates have been shown to seriously screw with brain chemistry. Don't fall prey to chemical flavor enhancing. Just play it safe and flavor your food naturally.

15

Marine Food Toxins

Marine toxins are chemicals and bacteria that can contaminate certain types of seafood. Eating the seafood may result in food poisoning. The seafood may look, smell, and taste normal. There are five common types of marine toxins, and they all cause different symptoms.

Food poisoning through marine toxins is rare. Every year, about 30 cases are reported to health authorities. But because milder cases are often not reported, the incidence may be greater. Marine toxin poisoning occurs most often in the summer.

How is marine toxin poisoning diagnosed and treated?

Your doctor will do a medical history and a physical exam and ask you questions about your symptoms and any fish you have recently eaten. Laboratory testing is typically not needed.

There are no specific treatments for marine toxin poisoning. Treatment generally consists of managing complications and being supportive until the illness passes. Dehydration caused by diarrhea and vomiting is the most common complication.

To prevent dehydration, take frequent sips of a rehydration drink (such as Pedialyte). Try to drink a cup of water or rehydration drink for each large, loose stool you have. Soda and fruit juices have too much sugar and not enough of the important electrolytes that are lost during diarrhea, and they should not be used to rehydrate.

Try to stay with your normal diet as much as possible. Eating your usual diet will help you to get enough nutrition. Doctors believe that eating a normal diet will also help you feel better faster. But try to avoid foods that are high in fat and sugar. Also avoid spicy foods, alcohol, and coffee for 2 days after all symptoms have disappeared.

How can marine toxin poisoning be prevented?

Always keep seafood refrigerated or on ice. If you have a weak immune system, you should consider not eating raw seafood.

To help avoid marine toxins:

- Do not eat barracuda, especially if it is from the Caribbean Sea.
- Refrigerate fresh tuna, mackerel, grouper and mahimahi. Remember that cooking does not destroy the toxins in spoiled or toxic seafood.
- Check with health officials about local advisories on algae blooms, dinoflagellate growth, or red tide.
- Do not eat fish or shellfish sold as bait. These products do not have to meet the same standards as seafood for eating.

What are the types of marine toxin poisoning?

Scombrotoxic fish poisoning:

- Is caused by bacteria. The bacteria may produce a chemical (histamine) that results in the food poisoning.
- Is usually found in finfish such as tuna, mackerel, and bonito.
- Causes symptoms within 2 minutes to 2 hours of eating the fish. The most common symptoms are rash, diarrhea, flushing, sweating, headache, and vomiting. Burning or swelling of the mouth, stomach pain, and a metallic taste may also occur. Most people have mild symptoms that are gone within a few hours. In severe cases, antihistamines or epinephrine may be needed.
- Cooking does not destroy the chemical, so buy your fish from a good source.

Ciguatera poisoning:

- Is caused by ciguatoxins, which are produced by tiny sea plants called dinoflagellates.
- Is usually found in tropical reef fish (such as barracuda) that kill other fish. But it may be found in grouper, sea bass, snapper, mullet, and other fish living in tropical waters. Common locations for these fish are the reefs surrounding Hawaii, the Virgin Islands, Puerto Rico, and Guam and other South Pacific Islands.
- Causes symptoms within a few minutes to 30 hours. Symptoms include nausea, vomiting, diarrhea, cramps, excessive sweating, headache, and muscle aches. A feeling of burning and "pins and needles" as well as weakness, itching, and dizziness can occur. You may also experience unusual taste sensations,nightmares, and hallucinations. Symptoms usually are over in 1 to 4 weeks.

- Cooking does not destroy the toxins, so buy your fish from a good source.

Paralytic shellfish poisoning:

- Is caused by a dinoflagellate, although not the same one that causes ciguatera poisoning. These dinoflagellates have a red-brown color and in large numbers can cause a red streak called "red tide" in the ocean.
- Is usually found in shellfish in colder coastal waters, such as the Pacific Northwest and New England. Shellfish that have caused the condition include mussels, cockles, clams, scallops, oysters, crabs, and lobsters.
- Usually causes symptoms within 2 hours of eating the shellfish, although symptoms may occur within 15 minutes or after as long as 10 hours. Symptoms usually begin with numbness or tingling in the face, arms, and legs, followed by headache, dizziness, nausea, and loss of coordination. Symptoms are usually mild, although severe symptoms have occurred.
- Cooking may not destroy the toxins, so buy your fish from a good source.

Neurotoxic shellfish poisoning:

- Is caused by a type of dinoflagellate.
- Is usually found in oysters, clams, and mussels from the Gulf of Mexico and the Atlantic Coast of the southern United States.
- Cause symptoms in 1 to 3 hours. They include numbness, loss of coordination, an upset stomach, and tingling in the mouth, arms, and legs. They usually last 2 to 3 days.

Amnesic shellfish poisoning:

- Is caused by toxins produced by a salt-water plant.
- Is found in shellfish such as mussels.
- Causes symptoms within 24 hours. Symptoms include an upset stomach, dizziness, headache, disorientation, and short-term memory loss. Seizures may occur in severe cases.

Food Poisoning from Marine Toxins

Seafood poisoning from marine toxins is an underrecognized hazard for travelers, particularly in the tropics and subtropics. Furthermore, the risk is increasing because of factors such as climate change, coral reef damage, and spread of toxic algal blooms.

CIGUATERA FISH POISONING

Ciguatera fish poisoning occurs after eating reef fish contaminated with toxins such as ciguatoxin or maitotoxin. These potent toxins originate from small marine organisms (dinoflagellates) that grow on and around coral reefs. Dinoflagellates are ingested by herbivorous fish. The toxins are then concentrated as they pass up the food chain to large carnivorous fish (usually >6 lb) and finally to humans. Toxins in fish are concentrated in the liver, intestinal tract, roe, and head.

Gambierdiscus toxicus, which produces ciguatoxin, tends to proliferate on dead coral reefs. The risk of ciguatera is likely to increase as more coral reefs die because of climate change, construction, and nutrient runoff.

Risk for Travelers

More than 50,000 cases of ciguatera poisoning occur globally every year. The incidence in travelers to highly endemic areas has been estimated as high as 3 per 100. Ciguatera is widespread in tropical and subtropical waters, usually between the latitudes of 35 N and 35 S; it is particularly common in the Pacific and Indian Oceans and the Caribbean Sea.

Fish that are most likely to cause ciguatera poisoning are carnivorous reef fish, including barracuda, grouper, moray eel, amberjack, sea bass, or sturgeon. Omnivorous and herbivorous fish such as parrot fish, surgeonfish, and red snapper can also be a risk.

Clinical Presentation

Typical ciguatera poisoning results in a gastrointestinal illness, followed by neurologic symptoms and, rarely, cardiovascular collapse. The first symptoms usually appear 1–3 hours after eating contaminated fish and include nausea, vomiting, diarrhea, and abdominal pain.

Neurologic symptoms appear 3–72 hours after the meal and include paresthesias, pain in the teeth or the sensation that the teeth are loose, itching, metallic taste, blurred vision, or even transient blindness. Cold allodynia (dysesthesia when touching cold water or objects) is characteristic and almost pathognomonic of ciguatera poisoning. Neurologic symptoms usually last a few days to several weeks.

Chronic neuropsychiatric symptoms resembling chronic fatigue syndrome may be disabling, last several months, and include malaise, depression, headaches, myalgias, and fatigue. Cardiac manifestations include bradycardia, other arrhythmias, and hypotension.

The overall death rate from ciguatera poisoning is approximately 0.1% but varies according to the toxin dose and availability of medical care to deal with complications. The diagnosis of ciguatera poisoning is based on the clinical signs and symptoms and a history of eating fish that are known to carry ciguatera toxin. Commercial kits are available to test for ciguatera in fish. They are sensitive but expensive. There is no test for ciguatera in humans.

Preventive Measures for Travelers

Travelers can take the following precautions to prevent ciguatera fish poisoning:

- Avoid or limit consumption of the reef fish listed above, particularly when the fish weighs 6 lb or more.

- Never eat high-risk fish such as barracuda or moray eel.
- Avoid the parts of the fish that concentrate ciguatera toxin: liver, intestines, roe, and head.

Remember that ciguatera toxins do not affect the texture, taste, or smell of fish, and they are not destroyed by gastric acid, cooking, smoking, freezing, canning, salting, or pickling. Commercial kits (if available) can be used to check if the fish is safe to eat.

Treatment

There is no specific antidote for ciguatoxin or maitotoxin. Treatment is generally symptomatic and supportive. Intravenous mannitol has been reported to reduce the severity and duration of neurologic symptoms, particularly if given within 48 hours of the appearance of symptoms.

SCOMBROID

Scombroid, one of the most common fish poisonings, occurs worldwide in both temperate and tropical waters. The illness occurs after eating improperly refrigerated or preserved fish containing high levels of histamine, and often resembles a moderate to severe allergic reaction.

Fish that cause scombroid have naturally high levels of histidine in the flesh and include tuna, mackerel, mahimahi (dolphin fish), sardine, anchovy, herring, bluefish, amberjack, and marlin. Histidine is converted to histamine by bacterial overgrowth in fish that has been improperly stored (>20 C) after capture. Histamine and other scombrotoxins are resistant to cooking, smoking, canning, or freezing.

Clinical Presentation

Symptoms of scombroid poisoning resemble an acute allergic reaction and usually appear 10–60 minutes after eating contaminated fish. They include flushing of the face and upper body (resembling sunburn), severe headache, palpitations, itching, blurred vision, abdominal cramps, and diarrhea. Untreated, symptoms usually resolve within 12 hours. Rarely, there may be respiratory compromise, malignant arrhythmias, and hypotension requiring hospitalization. Diagnosis is usually clinical. A clustering of cases helps exclude the possibility of fish allergy.

Preventive Measures for Travelers

Fish contaminated with histamine may have a peppery, sharp, salty, or bubbly taste but may also look, smell, and taste normal. The key to prevention is to make sure that the fish is promptly chilled (below 38 F) after capture. Cooking, smoking, canning, or freezing will not destroy histamine in contaminated fish.

Treatment

Scombroid poisoning usually responds well to antihistamines (H_1-receptor blockers, although H_2-receptor blockers may also be of benefit).

SHELLFISH POISONING

Several forms of shellfish poisoning may occur after ingesting filter-feeding bivalve mollusks (such as mussels, oysters, clams, scallops, and cockles) that contain potent toxins. The toxins originate in small marine organisms (dinoflagellates or diatoms) that are ingested and concentrated by shellfish.

Risk for Travelers

Contaminated shellfish may be found in temperate and tropical waters, typically during or after dinoflagellate blooms or "red tides."

Clinical Presentation

Poisoning results in gastrointestinal and neurologic illness of varying severity. Symptoms typically appear 30–60 minutes after ingesting toxic shellfish but can be delayed for several hours. Diagnosis is usually made clinically in patients who recently ate shellfish.

Paralytic Shellfish Poisoning

This is the most common and most severe form of shellfish poisoning. Symptoms usually appear 30–60 minutes after eating toxic shellfish and include numbness and tingling of the face, lips, tongue, arms, and legs. There may be headache, nausea, vomiting, and diarrhea. Severe cases are associated with ingestion of large doses of toxin and clinical features such as ataxia, dysphagia, mental status changes, flaccid paralysis, and respiratory failure. The case-fatality ratio averages 6%. The death rate may be particularly high in children.

Neurotoxic Shellfish Poisoning

Neurotoxic shellfish poisoning usually presents as gastroenteritis accompanied by minor neurologic symptoms, resembling mild ciguatera poisoning or mild paralytic shellfish poisoning. Inhalation of aerosolized toxin in the sea spray associated with a red tide may cause an acute respiratory illness, rhinorrhea, and bronchoconstriction.

Diarrheic Shellfish Poisoning

This produces chills, nausea, vomiting, abdominal cramps, and diarrhea. No deaths have been reported.

Amnesic Shellfish Poisoning

This is a rare form of shellfish poisoning that produces a gastroenteritis that may be accompanied by headache, confusion, and permanent short-term memory loss. In severe cases, seizures, paralysis, and death may occur.

Preventive Measures for Travelers

Shellfish poisoning can be prevented by avoiding potentially contaminated bivalve mollusks. This is particularly important in areas during or shortly after "red tides." Travelers to developing countries should avoid eating all shellfish because they carry a high risk of viral and bacterial infections. Marine shellfish toxins cannot be destroyed by cooking or freezing.

Treatment

Treatment is symptomatic and supportive. Severe cases of paralytic shellfish poisoning may require mechanical ventilation.

Bibliography

American Medical Association (2012). Report 2 of the Council on Science and Public Health: Labeling of Bioengineered Foods.

B.B. Aggarwal, Y.J. Surh, S. Shishodia, The molecular targets and therapeutic uses of curcumin in health and disease , Adv Exp Med Biol, 595 (2007) Springer publication.

Bull, A.T., Holt, G. and Lilly, M.D. (1982). Biotechnology : international trends and perspectives. Paris: Organisation for Economic Co-operation and Development.

Carpenter JE (2011). "Impact of GM crops on biodiversity". *GM Crops* **2** (1): 7–23.

Clive James (2009). "ISAAA Brief 41-2009: Executive Summay: Global Status of Commercialized Biotech/GM Crops The first fourteen years, 1996 to 2009".

Concon, J.M. 1988. Food Toxicology, Parts A and B. Marcel Dekker, New York.

Conner AJ, Glare TR, Nap JP (2003). "The release of genetically modified crops into the environment. Part II. Overview of ecological risk assessment". *Plant J.* **33** (1): 19–46.

CORDIS - Community Research and Development Information Service. 2005-01-06 EU project publishes conclusions and recommendations on GM foods.

D.E. Brown, N.J. Walton, (1999). *Chemicals from Plants: Perspectives on Plant Secondary Products*. World Scientific Publishing. pp. 21, 141.

Delmonte P, Rader JI (2006). "Analysis of isoflavones in foods and dietary supplements". *J AOAC Int* **89** (4): 1138–1146.

Deshpande, S.S. Food Additives. In *Handbook of Food Toxicology*; Marcel Dekker: New York, NY, USA, 2002a; pp. 219–284.

Doull, J. and Bruce, M.C. (1986). Origin and scope of toxicology. In Toxicology: The Basic Science of Poisons, 3rd ed., eds. C.D. Klaassen, M.O. Amdur, and J. Doull, pp. 3–10. Macmillan, New York.

EPA (U.S. Environmental Protection Agency). (2002). Interim Genomics Policy (June 25, 2002). Science Policy Council, U.S. Environmental Protection Agency [online]. Available: http://www.epa.gov/osa/spc/genomics. htm. Accessed on 2nd July 2013

EDF (Environmental Defense Fund). (1997). Toxic Ignorance: The Continuing Absence of Basic Health Testing for Top-Selling Chemicals in the United States. New York: Environmental Defense Fund.

Emily Marden, Risk and Regulation: U.S. Regulatory Policy on Genetically Modified Food and Agriculture, 44 B.C.L. Rev. 733 (2003).

Eric Block, (1985). "The chemistry of garlic and onions". *Scientific American* 252 : 114–9.

Greer, M.A. Goitrogenic substances in food. *Am. J. Clin. Nutr.* **1957**, *5*, 440–444.

Hutton, TC (2003) Food packaging: an introduction. CCFRA Key Topics in Food Science and Technology No. 7.

http://www.who.int/foodsafety/chem/en, Accessed on 13th July 2013

http://www.foodrisk.org/hazard/chemical/general/index.cfm, Accessed on 13th July 2013.

http://toxipedia.org/display/toxipedia/Ethical,+Legal,+and+Social+Issues+in+Toxicology. Accessed on 26th June 2013

http://www.who.int/foodsafety/chem/en, Accessed on 01 August 2013

http://www.foodrisk.org/hazard/chemical/general/index.cfm, Accessed on 01 August 2013

http://www.fda.gov/downloads/Food/FoodborneIllnessContaminants/UCM297627.pdf (Accessed

http://www.niaid.nih.gov/topics/foodallergy/clinical/Pages/default.aspx. Accessed 03 July 2013.

J. A. Milner, "A historical perspective on garlic and cancer," *Journal of Nutrition*, vol. 131, no. 3, pp. 1027S–1031S, 2001.

Jones, J (2005) Chemical analysis of foods: an introduction. CCFRA Key Topics in Food Science and Technology No. 10.

Jones, J.M.J. *Food Safety*; Eagan Press: St. Paul, MN, USA, 1995; pp. 71, 77, 84, 87.

Krishna, Vijesh V.; Qaim, Matin (2012). "Bt cotton and sustainability of pesticide reductions in India". *Agricultural Systems* **107**: 47–55.

Kukreja R and Singh BR (2009). "Botulinum Neurotoxins: Structure and Mechanism of Action". Microbial Toxins: Current Research and Future Trends. Caister Academic Press.

Lawley, R., Curtis, L. and Davis, J. (2008) The Food Safety Hazard Guidebook, RSC Publishing.

Loomis, T.A. (1978). Essentials of Toxicology. 3rd ed. Lea & Febiger, Philadelphia.

MacKenzie, Deborah (2012) Study linking GM crops and cancer questioned New Scientist.

Maga, J. A. Simple Phenol and Phenolic compounds in Food Flavor. *Crit. ReV. Food Sci. Nutr.* **1978**, *10*, 323-372.

McHugen, Alan (2000). "Chapter 1: Hors-d'oeuvres and entrees/What is genetic modification? What are GMOs?". *Pandora's Picnic Basket*. Oxford University Press.

Messina M, McCaskill-Stevens W, Lampe JW (2006). "Addressing the soy and breast cancer relationship: review, commentary, and workshop proceedings". J. Natl. Cancer Inst. **98** (18): 1275–1284.

Mishra, K Lokesh, (2012), Nutraceutical properties of vegetables in fighting human diseases: a special reference to cancer and liver diseases, Journal of Plant Science Research, 28(2), 61-64.

Mitchell, Deborah (2004). *Safe foods: the A-to-Z guide to the most wholesome foods for you and your family*. Penguin. pp. Ch. 15.

Mori, H.; Tanaka, T.; Hirono, I. Toxicants in Food: Naturally Occurring. In *Nutrition and Chemical Toxicity*; Ioannides, C., Ed.; John Wiley & Sons: West Sussex, England, UK, 1998; pp. 1–27. *Toxins* **2010**, 2 **2324.**

Muriel P, Arauz J (2010). "Coffee and liver diseases". *Fitoterapia* 81 (5): 297–305.

NRC (National Research Council). (1984). Toxicity Testing: Strategies to Determine Needs and Priorities. Washington, DC: National Academy Press.

NRC (National Research Council). (1989). Improving Risk Communication. Washington, DC: National Academy Press.

NRC (National Research Council). (2005c). Toxicogenomic Technologies and Risk Assessment of Environmental Carcinogens, A Workshop Summary. Washington, DC: The National Academies Press.

NRC (National Research Council). (2005d). Communicating Toxicogenomics Information to Nonexperts. Washington, DC: The National Academies Press.

NRC. (2004). Safety of Genetically Engineered Foods: Approaches to Assessing Unintended Health Effects. National Academies Press.

OECD (2010) Consensus Document on Molecular Characterisation of Plants Derived from Modern Biotechnology.

Ozdemir O, Mete E, Catal F, Ozol D (2009). "Food intolerances and eosinophilic esophagitis in childhood". *Dig Dis Sci* **54** (1): 8–14.

Proft T (editor) (2009). Microbial Toxins: Current Research and Future Trends. Caister Academic Press.

Rao AV, Agarwal S: Bioavailability and in vivo antioxidant properties of lycopene from tomato products and their possible role in the prevention of cancer. Nutr Cancer31: 199–203, 1998.

Roberts, HR. (1978), Principal hazards in food safety and their assessment, Fed. Proc. 37, 2575-76.

Rose, G. (1994). The Strategy of Preventive Medicine. New York: Oxford University Press.

Shibamoto, T.; Bjeldanes, L.F. Natural toxins in plant foodstuffs. In *Introduction to Food Toxicology*; Academic Press: San Diego, CA, USA, 1993; pp. 78–79, 82–84.

Singh BN, Shankar S, Srivastava RK, 2011, Green tea catechin, epigallocatechin-3-gallate (EGCG): mechanisms, perspectives and clinical applications, Biochem Pharmacol. Dec 15;82(12):1807-21.

Srivastava R, Dikshit M, Srimal RC, and Dhawan BN: Anti-thrombotic effect of curcumin. *Thromb Res* 40, 413–417, 1985.

Stewart G.C. *Staphylococcus aureus.* In: Fratamico P.M., Bhunia A.K., Smith J.L., editors. Foodborne pathogens: Microbiology and Molecular Biology. Caister Academic Press; Norfolk, UK: 2005. pp. 273–284.

Tang G, et al (2009) Golden Rice is an effective source of vitamin A. Am J Clin Nutr. 89(6) 1776-83.

Tennant. R.W. The National Center for Toxicogenomics: Using new technologies to inform mechanistic toxicology. Environ. Health Perspectives. In Press.

van Dam RM (2008). "Coffee consumption and risk of type 2 diabetes, cardiovascular diseases, and cancer". *Applied physiology, nutrition, and metabolism* 33 (6): 1269–1283.

van Eijck, Paul (2010). "The History and Future of GM Potatoes". *PotatoPro.*

Varner, J E, Bonner, J (1966). *Plant Biochemistry.* Academic Press.

Wang, C., D.J. Bowen, and S.L. Kardia. 2005. Research and practice opportunities at the intersection of health education, health behavior, and genomics. Health Educ. Behav. 32(5):686-701.

Wattenberg, L. W. (1983) Inhibition of neoplasia by minor dietary constituents. Cancer Res. 43: 2448s–2453s.

WHO. (1984).The role of food safety in health and development: A report of a Joint FAO/WHO Expert Committee on Food Safety. Technical Report Series No. 705. World Health Organization, Geneva.

Winter, CK and Gallegos, LK. (2006). University of California Agricultural and Natural Resource Service. ANR Publication 8180. Safety of Genetically Engineered Food

Wolfram S, Wang Y, Thielecke F. Anti-obesity effects of green tea: from bedside to bench. Mol Nutr Food Res. 2006;50:176–87.

Wüthrich B (1996). "[Food allergy: definition, diagnosis, epidemiology, clinical aspects]". *Schweiz Med Wochenschr* (in German) **126** (18): 770–6.

www.who.int/foodsafety/publications/biotech/20questions/ (Accessed, July 14, 2013)

www.westonaprice.org.com , Accessed on 01 August 2013.

on 09, August, 2013).

www.mycotoxins.com. (Accessed on 17, August, 2013).